P9-AQD-759

THE
LAST
FIVE
POUNDS

Other Books By Jamie Pope, M.S., R.D.

The T-Factor Fat Gram Counter, with Martin Katahn, Ph.D.
The Low Fat Supermarket Guide, with Martin Katahn, Ph.D.
The Low Fat Fast Food Guide, with Martin Katahn, Ph.D.

Available from W.W. Norton & Company, Inc.

THE LAST FIVE POUNDS

How to Lose Them and Leave Them Forever

Jamie Pope, M.S., R.D.

Foreword by Martin Katahn, Ph.D.

POCKET BOOKS

New York   London   Toronto   Sydney   Tokyo   Singapore

The author of this book is not a physician and the ideas, procedures, and suggestions in this book are not intended as a substitute for the medical advice of a trained health professional. All matters regarding your health require medical supervision. Consult your physician before adopting the suggestions in this book, as well as about any condition that may require diagnosis or medical attention. The author and publisher disclaim any liability arising directly or indirectly from the use of this book.

 POCKET BOOKS, a division of Simon & Schuster Inc.
1230 Avenue of the Americas, New York, NY 10020

Copyright © 1995 by Jamie Pope and Aimee Liu

All rights reserved, including the right to reproduce this book or portions thereof in any form whatsoever. For information address Pocket Books, 1230 Avenue of the Americas, New York, NY 10020

Library of Congress Cataloging-in-Publication Data
Pope, Jamie.
    The last five pounds: how to lose them and leave them forever/ Jamie Pope
        p.   cm.
    Includes bibliographical references and index.
    ISBN: 0-671-88453-0
    1. Reducing.   2. Low-fat diet.   I. Title.
RM222.2.P63   1995
613.2'5—dc20   94-32606
                                                       CIP

First Pocket Books hardcover printing February 1995

10 9 8 7 6 5 4 3 2 1

POCKET and colophon are registered trademarks of Simon & Schuster Inc.

Printed in the U.S.A.

To my grandparents, Gilley and Ruth Stephens,
for their unconditional love, faith, and support—

and to over half of all American women, who, like me,
struggle to make peace with the scale and themselves;
I pray this book will help.

First and foremost, I want to extend my utmost appreciation and respect to Aimee Liu for her exceptional skill, understanding, patience, and momentum during the last year as we've compiled and prepared this book for publication. Aimee pulled together (as no one else could!) my thoughts, notes, comments, and experiences with literally hundreds of highlighted scientific papers that I gathered and sent to her. She's been a friend and inspiration.

A very special thanks goes to my editor at Pocket Books, Julie Rubenstein, whose own personal weight concerns prompted the idea for this book. Her enthusiasm and support of the project and confidence in me to author such a book, made this project possible. And through the process, I believe we've both made some peace with the scale and I hope will help others do the same.

I also wish to thank my friend and colleague, Dr. Martin Katahn, who recruited me to Vanderbilt in 1986 and opened doors in writing and publishing that I never dreamed were possible. Without his guidance and belief in my abilities, I would never have had such wonderful opportunities.

Many others have made invaluable contributions, and I would like to thank:

My literary agent, Richard Pine, for connecting the idea, the people, the publishers, the contracts that make all this happen!

David Schlundt, Ph.D., for providing the foundation of research and behavioral psychology in the Weight Management Program—and for teaching me (or forcing me to learn!) computers and the behavioral aspects of weight control.

All the Weight Management Program participants, who've taught me far more about the issues of weight control than a textbook or scientific paper ever could.

My Vanderbilt Health Plus colleagues for their support, encouragement, and patience as I tried to write a book and do my job at Vanderbilt!

Kristi Elkins, for putting in many hours at home typing and editing recipes and the food guide (without complaint!).

Katie Newby, M.A., for sharing information for the exercise sections.

Special thanks to: Cea Panelle, Jean Miller, Gaynelle Doll, and Brenda Lawrence for sharing their recipes.

Sunset Grille Restaurant (Randy Rayburn and Jerry Baxter), for contributing some of its wonderful recipes.

Ted Griffith, for his encouragement and suggestions.

My mother and Jon, for being there for me and for their feedback as the book developed.

CONTENTS

II. Losing and Leaving the Last Five Pounds

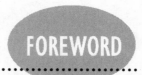

I have had the pleasure of working with Jamie Pope for the past eight years. She served as a research associate and nutrition consultant for the *T-Factor Diet* and *One Meal at a Time*, and frequently led weight management groups with me at Vanderbilt University prior to my retirement. Much of our work together has focused on the seriously overweight—people who need to lose thirty or more pounds—but it has long been clear to us both that the vast majority of people who worry about their weight have far fewer pounds to lose. When losing some weight might in reality be advantageous to their health, the target generally amounts to just five or ten pounds. Yet even this moderate goal often seems impossible to reach—or maintain. Now Jamie has written the definitive book about weight management that speaks to this majority. *The Last Five Pounds* offers a healthy, practical, and easy-to-live-with approach that ensures readers will get rid of unnecessary fat and keep it off for good.

This book covers it all: nutrition, exercise, physiology, and the emotional factors that contribute to binge eating and overeating. Jamie offers delicious recipes and menu-planning tips as well as suggestions for dining out and involving the whole family in fitness. Equally important, women will find here a deep sympathy and understanding that comes from Jamie's personal and professional experience.

While participants in Jamie's weight management groups over the years have succeeded in losing weight, they have also come away with something far more important: they like themselves better as a result of Jamie's guidance. They learn to free themselves from the obsession with weight, and they develop the skills they need to keep eating and exercising in a healthy perspective. Here, Jamie Pope extends the same invaluable guidance to you.

Take what this book says seriously. When you succeed in leaving those last five pounds behind, you just may find that your whole life becomes freer, more active, and more rewarding.

MARTIN KATAHN, PH.D.
Professor of Psychology, Emeritus
Vanderbilt University
May, 1994

THE
LAST
FIVE
POUNDS

....

Introduction: The Last Five Pounds

We've said it, we've heard it, we've thought it so many hundreds of times: *If only I could lose these last five pounds . . .* I'd look great. I'd get the job or the man (or whatever windfall seems particularly attractive and unattainable at the moment). I'd fit into the dress size I've always dreamed of wearing. I'd feel terrific, and at last I'd have control over my body.

Yet we cannot get rid of those pounds. Well, sure we can lose them. Anyone can lose five pounds, after all. But then they creep back, sometimes overnight and with two or three more pounds added on. We stand cursing the scale and feeling just this side of worthless once again.

I have stood on both sides of the scale in this perpetual battle of emotions and weight. On the one hand, I am a registered dietitian involved with Vanderbilt University's Weight Management Program. This program was started about twenty years ago by my friend, colleague, and sometime co-author Dr. Martin Katahn* and some of his health psychology students as a means of collecting information on people's experiences as they attempt weight loss and weight maintenance. Over the years, many combinations of dietary restriction and exercise have been explored. Thousands of individuals have participated in the weight management groups offered through the program. I have conducted most of these groups over the past eight years using strategies

---

*Author of the best-selling books *The T-Factor Diet, The Rotation Diet,* and *One Meal at a Time.* All of these books were based on research and strategies that came out of the Vanderbilt Weight Management Program. I was involved in follow-up research on the Rotation Diet and served as research associate and nutrition consultant on both the *T-Factor Diet* and *One Meal at a Time.*

I helped design with Dr. Katahn and health psychologist and dieting specialist Dr. David Schlundt. In this capacity and as nutrition consultant to Dr. Katahn, I have shared the frustration of thousands who had attempted—and failed at—one traditional semistarvation diet after another.

On the other side of the scale, I have to confess that I myself spent years trying to diet and exercise my way down to the magic number on the scale that would make me, somehow, as "perfect" as the models and movie stars held up by the media.

What I've learned both through my work at Vanderbilt and through my personal weight battles is that it doesn't have to be difficult or painful to lose the Last Five Pounds. In this book I will give you all the information you need to do exactly this. However, these last pounds may not be the same ones you've been chasing for years. In fact, they are not really even a measure of weight. Rather, they reflect a change of mind and lifestyle. They are the Last Five Pounds you will ever worry about.

In my work at Vanderbilt I've found, as have the vast majority of obesity specialists across the country, that the most effective and *reasonable* way to lose weight is to reduce fat intake while increasing physical activity to a moderate level. But "effective" does not mean rapid, and the amount of weight lost may not be dramatic. Rather, an effective weight loss is any weight loss that results from healthful, reasonable, and *permanent* changes in eating habits and physical activity. And an effective weight loss is sustainable.

As co-author with Dr. Katahn of several nutrition/fat gram counters, including the best-selling *T-Factor Fat Gram Counter*, I've received hundreds of letters, mainly from women, asking questions and sharing their stories. I've also worked with thousands of people—again mostly women—in weight groups under the direction of weight management expert Dr. George Blackburn and at Vanderbilt. In both cases, I've been encouraged to see that more and more women are making peace with the scale by realizing that their ideal weight is not determined by charts, envy, or wishful thinking. Instead, it is the weight they arrive at through healthy, low-fat eating and consistent physical activity. It is the natural result of a healthy lifestyle.

During my thirteen years in weight management and health promotion I have counseled individuals who are very close to their "weight goal." Many of them never even stopped to consider whether that goal was realistic, but they knew they felt fat. I have also worked with people who had hundreds of pounds to lose. At both ends of the spectrum, the solutions involve the same simple, basic changes in lifestyle. The most important point, however, and the most difficult thing for many people to accept, is that these changes must be adopted for life. Which is to say that the changes we make in the name of health and slimness must be *reasonable* and easy to maintain.

Once or twice during my own long and misdirected duel with the scale, I actually arrived at my "goal"—for a few days. But I could not and would not keep up the heroics of semistarvation and/or manic exercise I would have had to endure to stay there. This is not a moral statement implying that I lack "willpower" or determination. Rather, it is an acknowledgment that there are limits to what we can realistically expect of ourselves and to the lengths we should go in pursuing weight loss.

Over 80 percent of American women dislike their own bodies, and at least two-thirds are unhappy with their weight. Yet an overlapping 75 percent of these same women are actually within a healthy weight range! Of those currently on a diet, 20 percent of the women and 10 percent of the men are of average weight, and 9 percent of the women and 5 percent of the men are *underweight*.

So let's get real! If you are only five pounds from your target weight you deserve to be congratulated—most of the people in my weight management groups at Vanderbilt *dream* of being this close to their goal. You must already be doing something "right." Either you're emphasizing low-fat, lower-calorie foods or exercising regularly—or both. Or else you're genetically blessed! What you need is not blindly to lose more pounds in the short term but to stabilize your weight at a realistic level and prevent future gain. The even greater challenge is to put your "weight problem" into a rational perspective so it stops shadowing your life.

To this end, *The Last Five Pounds* will not give you yet another diet that feeds your preoccupation with weight. And I am not simply going to take you at your word that you need to lose five pounds. Instead, I will challenge you to establish a *realistic* weight goal—your own "personal best"—and I will help you to make the often subtle but permanent changes that will allow you to reach that goal and maintain it.

This book will teach you to:

- develop leaner, more balanced eating habits
- familiarize yourself with the fat content of foods through the revolutionary and *simple* new system of Fat-Cats (fat categories)
- cook leaner with the new low-fat foods

- live leaner with hassle-free exercise
- feel leaner by shifting focus from what you weigh to how you lead your life
- enjoy lean living as normal living.

At the same time, you will learn to *stop:*

- counting calories, pounds, and inches
- judging yourself by what you weigh
- feeling guilty about what you eat
- dwelling on your weight instead of confronting your problems
- setting impossible standards of perfection for yourself
- confusing weight loss with personal happiness
- letting the scale rule your mood and your life
- putting off the lifestyle changes that will make you leaner, fitter, healthier, and more active
- *worrying* about your weight!

Above all, I will show you ways to manage your weight and diet that will help you, not harm you, and that you can sustain for the rest of your life.

I

YOU AND YOUR WEIGHT: A RELATIONSHIP FOR LIFE

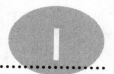

Which Five Are the Last Five Pounds?

Only five pounds. That's not much weight. Hardly enough to notice. If it weren't for the feeling you get when you step on the scale each morning, or read what your favorite fashion model weighs, or struggle to fit into last year's slacks, those five pounds wouldn't bother you at all. But they do bother you. Terribly. Persistently. So close to your goal, why can't you ever seem to get there?

There are many possible reasons, and this book will help you address them. But first you need to think carefully about why you want to lose these pounds. And which pounds are they, anyway?

The Five That You Keep Losing—and Gaining Back

At this moment, more than fifty million Americans are on a diet. Some, mostly young girls, are dieting for the first time. Others are chronic weight watchers who never quite come off their diet. But the vast majority are what researchers call yo-yo dieters.

You probably know the pattern. One day you decide you just have to lose weight. You replace a few meals with a liquid diet formula, follow the latest magazine diet plan, or cut your calories to 1,000 a day for a week. The pounds vanish relatively quickly and you feel so proud of yourself. No more diet! Sooner or later you return to your typical eating pattern and the pounds start creeping back. Before you know it you're above the weight that started you dieting in the first place. Again you lose, again you regain. With each bounce of the yo-yo the pounds seem

7

to drop off slower and come back faster. All the pounds you've lost over the years—three to fit into that cocktail dress, five before vacation, seven for a friend's wedding—and you've gained every one of them back. Will it ever end?

When you diet you are, in essence, starving your body, forcing it to pull energy from its own tissue. This is precisely what makes the pounds drop off, and if your body were programmed for thinness, all the tissue it burns would be fat. Unfortunately, that's not how crash dieting works. The human body is in fact programmed to read starvation as a threat. When the food supply is drastically reduced, it slows metabolism in order to *conserve* fat. Part of what gets burned for energy is lean body mass, namely muscle.

This starvation response was useful to early man in times of drought and famine when survival was a graver concern than obesity. Pound for pound, muscle mass burns about four to five times more calories than fat does—calories a starving body could ill afford to lose. Fat cells, on the other hand, hoard energy to see the body through long stretches of hunger. Useful for early man but not necessary today. The longer you underfeed your body and the more weight you lose, the fewer lean cells are left to burn those extra calories and the more your body slows down, trying to conserve what energy it can from the little food it's receiving. This metabolic slowdown is particularly dramatic if you diet without exercising; physical activity, by building muscle, helps offset part of the drop.

The second thing that happens when you crash diet is, quite simply, that you lose weight (a high percentage of which is water weight). This, too, causes you to burn fewer calories, because the less you weigh, the less energy your body needs to support that weight. (As a comparison, think how much less effort is required to carry an eight-pound newborn than a twenty-pound child.)

When you quit your diet, your body is left with proportionally less lean mass as well as less weight to carry and therefore continues to require fewer calories than it did to start with. If you resume eating "as usual," you will gain back on the number of calories that previously kept you stable. Even if you do not eat as many calories but return to high-fat foods (usually the very first thing people eat when they end a diet!), more of this fat intake will gravitate to your hips, thighs, and waistline. This is because, with less lean mass to burn the incoming fat from food, there are more leftovers for the body to hoard as fat deposits.

Yo-yo dieting—or weight cycling as obesity experts call it—leaves you discouraged, frustrated, and no slimmer than when you began this vicious circle. Furthermore, these repeated weight swings, even those that involve only a few pounds, put you at higher risk for heart disease and other illnesses.

The good news is that researchers have not found sufficient evidence to demonstrate that yo-yo dieting causes *permanent* adverse effects on body composition (the ratio of fat weight to lean weight). Obesity experts have found no significant differences in body fat between overweight individuals who had frequent weight swings and those whose weight had remained fairly constant. And contrary to numerous reports in the press, it now appears that your resting metabolism, distribution of body fat, and prospects for future *permanent* weight loss are unaffected by past dieting. This means that, even if you have been a yo-yo dieter for years, you needn't worry that you've ruined your metabolism, that you burn fewer calories than you did before, that you are getting progressively fatter even without gaining weight, or that you'll be stuck with your unwanted body fat forever.

Having said this, I want you to understand that it is still imperative that you get off the yo-yo. Aside from the risks to your health caused by weight cycling, the emotional and psychological impact of yo-yo dieting is just beginning to be explored. I'm sure you don't need a scientific paper to remind you how these frequent ups and downs affect your life and self-esteem. Your relationship with your body is no doubt precarious enough without the added confusion brought about by dieting. Also, while researchers have not found any metabolic reason why yo-yo dieters typically regain their weight, they have found new evidence that weight cycling may increase the preference for high-fat foods. And the stronger your "fat tooth," the more likely it is that you'll gain body fat.

But if you have succeeded in losing substantial amounts of weight over the years—even if you've regained them—then you've demonstrated that you have the power to accomplish change. What you need is not to diet "better" in the short term but to quit dieting and calorie counting and, above all, change your definition of "normal" living to mean, lean, and active living—for good.

Several years ago I had a woman in my weight program who had succeeded in losing about thirty pounds. She was delighted with her success, but one day she came in and confessed to me, "Over the weekend, I ate normal." She meant exactly that: she'd eaten a doughnut for breakfast, french fries and a hamburger and milk shake for lunch, a cream soup, cheese casserole, and apple pie for dinner. The all-American "normal" diet. Nothing unusual, and not more food than most of us eat on a given day, but well over 50 percent fat. As I'll explain in depth later in the book, dietary fat is a much more critical factor in weight control than calorie intake, and this woman was a perfect illustration. As long as she continued to think of these fatty foods as *normal* eating, she was doomed to regain all the weight she'd worked so hard to lose. In fact, she didn't change her definition of normalcy, and within two years the thirty pounds were back, plus ten more.

The good news is that the changes required to accomplish a permanent five-pound weight shift can be fairly subtle. As few as 50–100 calories or ten grams of fat a day—two pats less butter or a brisk fifteen-minute walk—can make the difference over the long run. But you have to keep it up. Reducing your calories for a few days, even a few weeks, will not give you the long-term results you desire. This new level of eating and exercise must become part of your "normal" way of life.

This does not mean you need to keep a running mental tally of every calorie and fat gram you consume, but you will need to familiarize yourself with the various food options and emphasize satisfying choices that are also lower in fat. If at the same time you reach for a higher level of physical activity in your daily life, then your body will naturally become leaner.

One word of warning: you will not see results overnight. Subtle changes in behavior inevitably translate into slow changes in body mass. Research at Vanderbilt indicates that it can take up to two years for a shift to low-fat eating (without any drop in calories) to show up as significant loss of pounds, though changes in body tone and measurements will occur much sooner. The more slowly you lose, however, the more likely you are to keep the weight off. For the sake of your health as well as to safeguard against regain, you should never lose more than two to four pounds per month, *maximum!*

If you have a history of yo-yo dieting, this "slow fix" approach may be difficult for you to accept. Minimal sacrifices and slow results are exactly the opposite of what crash diets promise. But you know from experience that the quick fix never works. If you're serious about resolving your weight dilemma once and for all, then it's time to stop pushing yourself to be heroic and start making changes you can live with.

The Five That Have Just Crept Up on You

We've all had the experience of stepping on the scale, expecting to be greeted by our usual weight, and finding the numbers off. Sometimes way off. And almost never are the numbers off the *right* way; they seem trained to err on the high side. But where do those pounds come from? Are they here to stay? Should we panic?

Physically, weight gain is simple to explain. Our bodies are like organic calculators, constantly and with relentless accuracy tracking the substances we take in, use up, and expel. Most of us gain about two pounds each day as water weight, which is gone by the following morning. On a day when we consume a great quantity of food and drink we may gain up to five pounds of temporary weight, but our bodies don't count those as real pounds. What they do count, mercilessly, are the individual grams of fat that do not evaporate overnight. We might conveniently forget the spoonful of peanut butter we ate on our morning toast or that bag of chips with lunch, but our bodies know the truth. When we consume more fat than needed, the leftovers are automatically shuttled to our bellies, hips, thighs, and backsides in the form of hard-to-lose body fat.

That's the physical reality, but in practice the reasons *why* we eat more fatty foods than our bodies need, and why our bodies need less than we eat, tend to be more complicated. Moving, falling in or out of love, having less or more free time, feeling bored, happy, or anxious can all affect our weight without our even realizing it—until the scale or the fit of our clothes alerts us to the difference. When a weight gain occurs unexpectedly it usually involves some sort of life change that, on the surface, has nothing to do with diet.

"Positive" Weight

There are plenty of positive causes of weight gain, and it would be a mistake to undercut the pleasure of these events by bemoaning the extra pounds they attract. Temporary causes of weight gain can include major celebrations such as family reunions, holiday festivities, or vacations. At these times the food supply tends to be continuous and full of high-fat delicacies, and the social setting encourages unrestricted eating. Cruises and resorts are notorious for putting on weight because rich meals and snacks are treated as central and abundant entertainment. Also, while most resort accommodations now offer everything from lap pools and racquetball courts to hourly aerobics classes, many people equate vacation relaxation with inertia, so that eating serves not only as their prime entertainment but also as their most strenuous holiday exercise. This high-fat, low-motion combination virtually guarantees weight gain.

The solution is not to become a party martyr munching morosely on carrot sticks while everyone else feasts on lobster and steak. But there is such a thing as active moderation. By taking advantage of available exercise opportunities and by maintaining balance between a few high-fat foods you really love and leaner foods, you can minimize vacation weight gain without depriving yourself.

If it's too late for preventive measures and you've already put on your holiday weight, don't panic. And most important, don't try to get rid of the gain by crash dieting. It's averages that determine your long-term body weight, not the amount you eat in a single day. Think of it as a bank loan. You've "borrowed" an extra 2,000 calories worth of fat for your vacation. The bank doesn't expect you to pay back the full 2,000 on your first day home. No, you pay back a little at a time, say 50 a day, by taking the stairs instead of the elevator at work or by eating your morning toast with jelly or jam instead of butter. In the long run, the resumption of a sensibly lean routine is the surest way to prevent celebratory weight from becoming a permanent addition.

Major changes in everyday life present a larger challenge. Marriage often results in a gain of from five to twenty pounds in early years simply because of the shift in lifestyle. More food around the house, full dinners every evening, and often a drop in activity level lead to extra pounds. Such "lifestyle gains" can best be reversed by becoming more selective about household food, more fat conscious when planning menus, and more physically active both individually and as a couple. Being happily married does not have to mean being unhappily overweight.

One of the biggest life changes that any of us will face is parenthood. For women in particular, weight gain and babies go hand in hand. Part of this is biologically imperative. For the health of her baby a pregnant woman needs to gain at least twenty-five to thirty-five pounds by the time she delivers, and some of these pounds may linger for months after the baby arrives. Having a newborn generally means less time to exercise and more time around the house with food at hand—which makes it hard to shed pregnancy fat quickly. But stringent dieting is exactly the *wrong* way to deal with unwanted pounds during pregnancy and postpartum, when the baby's health as well as the mother's full recovery depend on good nutrition. There is nothing inherent in motherhood that causes permanent weight gain, and most of these pounds will drop away naturally with resumption of a more active life. The rest can best be shed by adopting the lean eating and exercise habits I recommend throughout *The Last Five Pounds.*

Another major change that can trigger weight gain is a new job. In my weight management group at Vanderbilt I often give the example of a floor nurse who unconsciously stays thin by walking miles each day between the nurses' station and patients' rooms. She is promoted to an administrative desk job that keeps her sitting all day, and within weeks she's gained five pounds without changing any other aspect of her life. If you are making the transition from labor-intensive to brain-intensive employment you'll need to compensate by seeking out opportunities to keep your body moving both on the job and off. As long as you maintain sensible low-fat eating habits, you do not need to "go on a diet."

"Negative" Weight

The causes of sudden weight gain that I've mentioned up to this point have all been either innocuous or positive—"good news" fatteners. But often we gain because of bad news or bad feelings.

Stress and unhappiness are two of the most powerful forces that can cause us to overeat. Frustration on the job, social or professional insecurity, loneliness, boredom, and anxiety all fall within these categories. We eat to distract ourselves or smother our feelings. The trouble is, we may be so good at covering up or denying what's going on inside that we don't even realize anything is wrong until the scale sounds its warning signal.

It's important to recognize that sudden weight gain may be exactly that—a warning of other problems that have nothing to do with diet or exercise. In this case, there is little point in attacking the weight gain before addressing those other problems. Going on a starvation diet or obsessively counting calories will simply take energy and attention away from the more central tasks of identifying and changing the circumstances that prompted the weight gain in the first place. On the other hand, friends, relatives, or a professional therapist may provide critical support in dealing with the important problems. The unwanted pounds will disappear as your life shifts back into balance.

Another "negative" cause of weight gain can be illness. If you take to your bed with a bad cold you may not eat any more than ordinary, but you will be considerably less active. And while many illnesses cause such a decrease in appetite that you lose weight while sick (fever actually burns extra calories), others simply keep you low for a few days and slow for a few days longer, at the end of which your decreased activity level has allowed your weight to climb a pound or two.

Such minor temporary gains tend to vanish when life returns to an active pace, but injuries, especially chronic injuries, can have a much more profound effect on weight. Pain is a key ingredient and legacy of most injuries and is a useful signal that tells us when an activity is harming the body. Too often when we are injured, though, we interpret pain to mean that we must cease *all* activity. We take to our chair or bed as if we were sick. But out of boredom and frustration we eat more than if we were sick, and we gain weight, which makes it hurt even more when we move around on the injury. How to stop this cycle?

The crux of the problem is inactivity. While certain movements may worsen an injury, there are almost always others that not only will help keep weight down and muscle tone up but will actually aid in healing the injury. The biggest obstacle is habit. If your primary exercise for the past ten years has been jogging and you've recently sprained your ankle, you are likely to do one of two things: either stop exercising completely or go back too soon to running (without taking into account the added pounds you've gained sitting around waiting for the ankle to mend) and compound the injury. The more beneficial response would be to switch, with doctor's approval, to a low-impact exercise such as swimming, cycling, weight training, or walking.

Starting a new exercise regimen requires a change of habit that may be difficult to embrace. New equipment, new surroundings, new scheduling. It's so much easier to sit back and wait for the injury to pass and then return to business as usual. Except that some injuries can take years to heal completely; others never do, and in the meantime, your weight will continue to creep upward even if you make an effort to eat less. Lean nutrition and regular exercise are equal partners in the battle of the bulge!

Age Weight

It used to be thought that metabolism unavoidably slowed by about 10 percent for every decade of life. This theory was based on the observation that most people gain weight as they get older, particularly around middle age (hence the "middle-age spread"). But researchers now attribute most of the metabolic drop with age to a drop in physical activity and the associated drop in lean tissue. Many people, as they approach mid- to later life, become less and less active. As a result they lose calorie-burning lean mass, which in turn causes them to gain more easily even while eating the same or less.

Although it's never too late to reverse this trend, it is far better to prevent it in the first place by keeping physically active throughout life. It's a myth that older people lack the stamina or the physical ability to exercise. Not everyone is cut out for marathon running, but walking, swimming, cycling, weight training, and low-impact aerobics are just a few of the many exercise options well suited to people at all stages of life. There is no age limit to fitness, and the fitter we are at any age, the less cause we will have to worry about our weight.

The Five That Would Make You Healthy

Many of us use health to justify our perpetual concern about weight. We'll feel better if we lose a few pounds. We'll be less likely to get cancer or heart disease. We'll get fewer colds. We'll have more energy. The fitness boom, with role models such as Jane Fonda and Cher, has reinforced the notion that health is measured by how good we look in a leotard. But we are deluding ourselves.

While people who are 20 percent or more above their target weight may need to reduce for the sake of their health, being five pounds overweight in and of itself poses no medical risk. What does pose a proven health risk is strenuous dieting, especially yo-yo dieting.

Numerous long-term studies have shown that frequent dieters have a higher death rate and as much as a 50 percent higher risk of heart disease than people with stable weight who do not diet. Indeed, any large sudden weight change, either down or up (pregnancy excluded), seems to increase the risk of death due to heart disease. The message? We are better off stabilizing our weight—*stopping the gain*—and toning the pounds we have rather than continually straining to lose them over and over again.

What matters to your health is not how much you weigh but how much of your daily diet and your weight consists of fat. It also matters how that fat is distributed in your body. If most of your fat is centered around your middle, then your body type is what researchers call an "apple" type. If your largest fat deposits are located in your lower body, namely the hips, thighs, and buttocks, then your body type is considered a "pear" type. Most men are apples, most women pears.

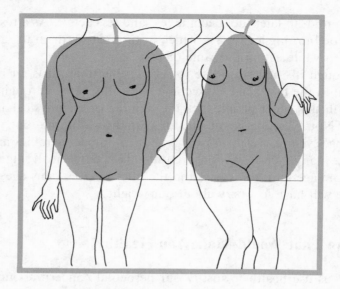

The distinction in body type is important because the fat that shapes some people like apples is chemically different from the fat that shapes others like pears. Apple fat, which collects around the middle of the body, appears to contribute to cardiovascular disease, hypertension, adult-onset diabetes, and breast cancer (especially in postmenopausal women). The fat that seems to cause the most problems seats itself deep inside the body around the major organs. Researchers think this so-called visceral fat affects the liver in a way that disrupts normal metabolism of insulin and cholesterol, thereby contributing to diabetes and heart disease.

The good news for women is that *no suspicious links* have been found between pear fat and any disease. So, while doctors believe that it is unsafe for men to gain any weight after age twenty-five (because most of the gain will show up as abdominal fat), many feel that women may safely gain up to 11 pounds as they age. The possible exception involves women at risk for diabetes because at "average" weight (with average amount of body fat) a woman's risk of developing adult-onset diabetes is 3.6 times higher than if she were lean, and the risk is highest for those who have gained significant weight during adulthood. *However*, even with these increased odds, the average-weight woman still has a minimal risk of getting diabetes—probably about the same as she would of getting struck by lightning! The critical factor is not the number of pounds on the scale but percentage of body fat.

Again, the point is to worry less about losing the pounds that are stored as apple or pear fat and work harder on redistributing them into lean mass. You can eat lots of carbohydrates and lean protein, but by reducing your fat intake you force your body to use more of its own stores of fat for energy. Happily, that apple fat around the middle will be the first to go. If, at the same time, you exercise *on a regular basis*, you will increase your lean muscle mass, causing your body to burn even more fat.

As your body mass is being redistributed you may not see a difference on the scale because muscle actually weighs three times more than fat, but your body will become more compact, stronger, fitter, and healthier. As far as the mirror and your doctor are concerned, five lean pounds "weigh less" than five pounds of fat. What the scale says is beside the point.

The Five That Would Let You Accept Yourself

Up to this point we've been looking at your extra five pounds as a physical reality, something you keep losing and gaining, or that's snuck up on you, or that may or may not threaten your health. Now it's time to consider this unwanted weight in terms of its psychological and emotional reality. *Why does it bother you so much?*

The fact is, if you think you're within five pounds of your ideal weight you are probably at or below the weight that's medically acceptable for your height and age. Yet you still feel compelled to berate yourself for not being thinner, to compare yourself constantly and automatically to people who appear leaner. You are not alone in this.

Not only has thinness become a national obsession but it seems to be fashionable—in some social circles even mandatory—to fret about weight regardless of how lean one really is. The old cliché, "You can never be too rich or too thin," is a motto that most Americans have taken to heart. In doing so, women especially have added a spin: "You can never be good enough." No wonder worrying about weight is bad for self-esteem!

Researchers who have studied the link between weight and self-esteem have found that women who have a positive sense of their own worth—who believe they are capable, popular, and bright—come in all different shapes, sizes, and weights, from fat and round to thin as a stick. The one thing they have in common is that they do not *worry* about their weight. Women who do worry, and who are dissatisfied with their overall appearance as well as specific parts of their bodies, tend to have low self-esteem. In other words, it's not what we actually weigh but rather our attitude about our bodies and weight that most directly affects our psychological health.

The first step toward balancing this attitude is to take a long, hard look at the importance our culture places on thinness. It is almost inescapable. Fashion models, popular singers, news anchors, and movie stars are generally slimmer than most of us can ever hope to be. From every magazine and newspaper and television station in the country, ads trumpet the purported benefits of miracle diet pills, plastic surgery, and wonder devices that promise to slim us in our sleep. We are conditioned by all these be-thin messages to believe that we will become more popular, more successful, more attractive, and younger in spirit as well as appearance if we just lose more weight. As if there were some magical connection between being just the next few pounds lighter and having it all.

Apart from the fact that none of these "miracle" cures has proven successful for permanent fat reduction, all losing weight will ever do for most of us is to ease the fit of our clothes. For a few that's enough, but most accept the media's messages about thinness and, deep down, are expecting much more.

To put this issue in perspective, consider that modern Western culture is virtually the only culture in history to prize thinness. Throughout Africa, South America, and Asia, a person's girth is seen as a measure of his or her prosperity, wisdom, and—yes—attractiveness. Having wealth and success means having enough to eat, so what better way to broadcast your desirability than by getting fat! Similar assumptions prevailed in this country until relatively recent decades. Even in the days of wasp waists, beautiful women were expected to be voluptuous (everyone knew and accepted that the tiny waists were the result of corsets rather than diets). And few of this century's greatest beauty queens—Marilyn Monroe, Sophia Loren, Elizabeth Taylor—come close to the standard of thinness that reigns today. Not only are these standards unrealistic for the majority of Americans, but they are, by and large, arbitrary. If the fashion gurus turned around tomorrow and instructed us that "bigger is beautiful," all our assumptions would turn inside out. And many of us would immediately quit agonizing about weight.

Unfortunately, such a societal about-face is not likely to happen. Fashion is too committed to the cult of thinness to turn it aside. So it's up to us individually. If we're finally to take control of our own weight issues we must separate the importance we personally attach to being slim from the importance slenderness has been granted by our culture. This involves asking some hard questions:

- What difference will it really make in my life if I lose five pounds?
- Can other people even tell when my weight goes up or down five pounds? (My weight management group members are astounded to learn that it takes a 5 *percent* weight change for others to notice.)
- Why do I feel proud when depriving myself of food?
- Why do I feel ashamed if I overindulge now and then?
- Why can't I feel good about myself if my weight is up?
- Why do I envy acquaintances who are thinner than I am, even when I don't respect their character?
- Why do I spend so much time worrying about my weight when I could be thinking about my work or family?
- Why does my weight overshadow other accomplishments that I deserve to feel proud of?
- Why do I let my weight keep me from doing things I really want to do?

As you answer these questions you may begin to see how irrational your attitudes about weight can be. You may also see how your feelings about your body have gotten mixed up with your feelings about your self.

In my weight management group I ask women to talk about their favorite sports. They'll tell me they love swimming or tennis or waterskiing or bowling. Then I'll ask when they last practiced those sports, and it will turn out most haven't done them in years. They feel too self-conscious to put on a bathing suit or shorts or go out where a lot of people can see them.

Then we'll talk about short-term goals. Some will say they want to confront their boss and ask for a raise, but they think they'll have more clout if they lose a few pounds. Others would like to get pregnant, but they're waiting to lose some weight first to offset what they are bound to gain during pregnancy. Still others talk about dating but say they're too embarrassed by their weight to go out with a new man.

Although most in my weight management group have more than five pounds to lose, their comments are similar to those I hear from women of all sizes who worry about their weight. What's holding these women back is not really the pounds they intend to shed but the sense of inadequacy their weight has come to represent for them. They are punishing themselves for being inferior *in their own eyes.* Ironically, by not engaging in the activities they love and by refusing to act on the desires that will make them feel successful and gratified, they end up spending more time sitting, inactive, feeling frustrated, and overeating to comfort themselves. So not only are they needlessly depriving themselves of fulfilling activities that would boost their self-worth, but the very lack of these activities perpetuates their weight problem.

Weight is not a part of our lives that we can "deal with" separately from everything else. It is in fact a reflection of everything else. When we are inactive, unhappy, spending a lot of time alone with high-fat snack foods and trying to hide from problems instead of confronting them, our weight will likely rise. When we are active, eating healthy foods, performing well, and surrounding ourselves with supportive friends and family, our weight will respond by moving downward or stabilizing. The most effective and enduring path to weight satisfaction is an active, satisfying life.

The Last Five Over That Are Really the First Five Under

There's a game many of us play with our weight that goes like this: If I just lose five pounds more than I really need to, it will give me a safety margin so I won't have to worry if I gain a little after my diet's over. This is a game that generally turns out one of two ways, both of which work against us.

The first and most common outcome, of course, is that we regain the margin of error plus a good deal more. In the bargain with our familiar unhealthy eating and exercise habits, the habits usually win. This is true whether we buy ourselves five, ten, or fifteen pounds of latitude. What we're setting ourselves up for is yo-yo dieting.

The second possible outcome is less common but more dangerous. That extra five-pound loss could be followed by yet another and another five-pound drop. The need to hang on to that "safety zone" could become so strong that it triggers habitual dieting or even a serious eating disorder such as anorexia nervosa or bulimia.

While researchers have many different opinions about the best treatment for eating and dieting disorders, they are unanimous on one point: These disorders almost always begin with a typical diet intended to lose a moderate amount of weight, and before the diet is over it turns into a compulsion and an amplified fear of fat. For anorexics, that five-pound margin of error keeps getting stretched to ten, twenty, thirty pounds, until no amount below normal really feels safe. For bulimics, the margin may remain relatively stable, but the struggle between the desire for forbidden foods and the ongoing terror of weight gain leads to a constant seesaw of bingeing and purging. Those with dieting disorders may not demonstrate such extremes of behavior, but like anorexics and bulimics, they are preoccupied with their weight, they worry about each mouthful of food, and they feel tremendous guilt about eating and shame about their bodies. Whatever diet they are currently on overshadows most other aspects of their lives.

I believe that anyone who wants to lose just a few pounds should consider carefully whether she needs to lose weight at all. I know, for instance, that many of my friends and colleagues who say they "need" to lose five pounds are actually at their ideal size or underweight. Yet they have trained themselves to believe they should be thinner.

Remember that everybody is different, and for each body there is a different ideal weight. Not even the "official" height and weight charts are an accurate gauge for everyone. There are simply too many different variables that determine individual target weight—variables such as weight history, age, bone structure, body shape, general health, lifestyle, and genetics. I'll discuss these in detail in Chapter 4, while guiding you through the process of determining the weight goal that truly is most appropriate for you, but my point here is simply that we do ourselves a great injustice by constantly trying to conform to other people's bodies. Julia Roberts is indeed a pretty woman, but she is tall and young and, by her own report, loses weight more easily than she gains it. Also her work requires her to stay exceptionally slender because the camera adds the appearance of about five pounds. So even if you're the same height as Ms. Roberts, if you also happen to be in your forties with a desk job and big bones and a long family history of abundant flesh, then her weight could be a good ten to twenty pounds too light for you.

Ultimately, your best weight will be the one you arrive at and *maintain* by incorporating low-fat eating habits and regular physical activity into your daily life. The number of pounds may well be higher than the carved-in-stone figure you've been carrying around in your head—mine certainly was!—but to reach an unrealistic goal requires drastic measures that few of us can or should submit to.

The Last Five You'll Ever Worry About

In this chapter we've looked at several of the reasons you may want to lose your five pounds. We've touched on some of the reasons why you should carefully consider whether you need to lose weight at all. But the point I've stressed most is that old-fashioned dieting—cutting calories to the bare minimum, implementing a killer exercise regimen, and agonizing, worrying, obsessing about fat—is the unhealthiest and least likely method to produce permanent weight loss.

Just consider the waste of time and energy that goes into dieting:

- The hours spent studying the scale and mirror, poring over calorie counters, daydreaming about food the counters say you can't have, calculating and recalculating how many calories you've eaten so far today
- The days spent feeling tired and weak for lack of food
- Arguments you ignite because hunger or deprivation has made you irritable
- Work that you don't get done or do poorly because you're thinking about food
- The guilt and shame and disgust you feel when your defenses are worn to the bone and you break your diet with a pint of Häagen-Dazs Rocky Road.

Now consider the benefits of being well fed and active:

- The satisfaction of never feeling hungry
- The relief of not constantly thinking about food
- The extra energy you can devote to family, friends, personal interests, and professional goals
- The confidence that your body is receiving the nutrients it needs to fight off infection and illness
- A leaner, healthier body that doesn't measure its ideal by the scale.

I'll be honest. I want you to stop needlessly depriving yourself. I want you to learn to take good care of your body instead of constantly tipping it back and forth between under- and overfeeding. I want these five pounds to be not just the last five you actually lose but the last you will ever worry about.

2

Learning to Live Low-Fat
in a High-Fat World

Chances are, if you live much like other Americans, you eat whatever is fastest or most convenient on the way to meetings or classes or child-care duties; you spend more hours in your car than you'd care to; and you often run short of time for the activities you find most rewarding. Convenience foods are a necessity, snacks a reliable way to feed your hunger or boost your spirits and energy level when you have a moment to spare. Your life is perfectly normal by modern American standards.

Unfortunately, modern American standards are guaranteed to tip your bathroom scale against you. And the sad part is, this fattening tilt has been caused by so-called "progress."

The American Diet + America's Diet Culture = Perpetual Dieting

Three or four generations back, food was treated as a life-sustaining necessity. There were few prepackaged grocery items. Ingredients were fresh and unprocessed, and most were naturally low in fat and high in fiber. It was considered normal to eat a balanced diet of fruits and vegetables, meat or poultry, dairy products, breads and cereals every day because those were the most readily available foods. High-fat packaged and fast foods such as potato chips, hot dogs, and hamburgers didn't enter the American mainstream until the 1920s and later. Once here, unfortunately, they became so popular that they dramatically altered our conception of "normal food" to mean anything high in fat that is

23

quick and convenient to eat. Not surprisingly, over the past thirty years the average adult weight for Americans has risen by more than ten pounds.

America's Fat Habit

The truth is simple: we gain unwanted pounds not because we eat too much but because we eat too much *fat* and get too little exercise. Study after study has found that the lower the percentage of fat in our diet (and the higher the percentage of carbohydrates) the lower our percentage of body fat—and "apple" or abdominal fat, in particular—will be. Why?

The short answer is that fat is designed for storage as future backup energy (which, in our society of three squares a day plus snacks, is rarely if ever needed). Only 3 percent of the total calories in a pat of butter are burned off during its passage from your mouth, through the digestive tract, to your thigh or midriff. Carbohydrates, on the other hand, are designed for immediate energy and actually resist being stored as fat. Your body must burn off 23 percent of the calories in a fat-free bagel in order to trap the remaining carbohydrate calories as fat.[1] Put another way, you get at least a 20 percent caloric discount whenever you eat carbohydrates instead of fat!

The typical American consumes about 2,000 calories per day, of which anywhere from 37 to 43 percent comes from fat. If we maintain the same, or even slightly higher, calorie intake but sharply reduce our fat intake to account for 20 percent or less of total calories, most of us will become leaner overall and healthier, in particular as our percentage of abdominal or "apple" body fat decreases. These benefits can be achieved—indeed will best be achieved—if we do *not* go on a "diet" to lower fat intake but, instead, turn our everyday eating habits around. At Laval University in Canada some 700 men and women were studied, measured, and weighed to determine the relationship between their normal fat intake, weight, and body fat. None of these people were on special eating or exercise regimens; they simply ate as they would at home. The women who normally got less than 29 percent of their total calories from fat weighed on average *ten pounds* less than the women with higher fat intake. And men who ate less fat were *twelve pounds* lighter than the male high-fat eaters.[2] So when we stare enviously at a person who seems to stay effortlessly slim, what we're often looking at is someone who routinely selects low-fat over high-fat foods as a matter of choice. That person probably also is physically active, either through intentional exercise or unplanned Lifestyle Exercise (I'll explain this term in Chapters 8 and 9, on physical activity and exercise).

But if it were really so easy to eat more and weigh less, we would all be switching our eating habits to become leaner. Clearly, we're not. So what's keeping us fat?

One of the biggest obstacles is that most of us have been programmed by our genetic makeup, taste buds, upbringing, and culture to lead high-fat lives. It's not just in our imagination that fat makes food taste good. Human beings are chemically tuned to prefer the taste of fat, because the more we like the taste, the more fat we will eat and the more body fat we will have as protection against famine and cold. We modern humans may not have to worry as our ancestors did about starvation, but that doesn't relieve us of our preference for the taste of fat. We put butter on our toast not because we need it but because we like it. That's the same reason so much fast food is fried, why the most popular cuts of meat are also high in fat, the most popular desserts high in cream or shortening. This sets up a vicious circle. Fat sells because it tastes good; the best-selling foods receive the most advertising; we tend to buy more of the foods that are widely advertised; we all end up eating more fat. And we are what we eat!

Another factor that contributes to our preference for fat is conditioning. We were raised on fat. Hot dogs, hamburgers, peanut butter sandwiches. These kid foods, all more than 40 percent fat, set the standard by which we continue eating as adults. These kid foods are also largely responsible for the fat cells we acquired as children, which we continue to "host" to this day. While these fat cells may expand or shrink as weight is gained or lost, they do not go away. Fat cells are with us for life.

Researchers have dubbed this phenomenon the Fat Ratchet. If we consume more fat than our existing cells can accommodate, we may gain new fat cells as adults, but no matter how little we eat we can never completely eliminate a fat cell. Thus, if we keep eating more fat than we need, we will continually "ratchet" our body fat upward. The treatment of choice against the Fat Ratchet is prevention. Guide a child to prefer lean foods, and that child will have fewer fat cells to worry about as an adult. Stop weight gain in adulthood, and your existing fat sites will begin to shrink instead of spawning new fat cells.

The Exercise Connection

The other proven effective weapon against the Fat Ratchet is physical activity. As I'll explain in detail later, when you exercise regularly your body burns more calories both during and between workouts—and anywhere from 30 to 60 percent of these calories will come from fat. The more active you are in your daily life, the more fat you will burn, and if you eat less fat than you burn off, then the remainder will come from body fat.

In our country as recently as two or three generations ago, physical exercise was built into daily life by necessity. There were fewer cars, fewer washing machines, fewer automatic gadgets and labor-saving devices. Before inventors began coming up with machines to exterminate physical movement, Americans actually benefited from all those extra steps and strokes and reaches they had to perform to get the job of living done.

But just as America's current taste habits steer us away from lean eating, our convenience-based lifestyle discourages even moderate physical activity. We drive instead of walking. We let machines do our housework. More and more of us spend our days sitting at desk jobs, and when we come home we continue sitting and stare at the television. From cave people to pioneers, most of our ancestors had trouble finding time to sit down, whereas most of us have to strain to find an occasion to get up!

Now that technocrats have saved us from all the labor we used to accept as a matter of course, they have taken to inventing new machines to make us sweat during recreation. America is the first and still one of the few places on earth where people rely on mechanical devices to get them to use their bodies. But still, we have now been so thoroughly conditioned to avoid physical effort that most of us—women especially —would rather diet than step on a treadmill or exercise bike. And that's how we spend much of our lives: dieting and gaining—and dieting and regaining.

According to the Department of Health and Human Services, women who do not exercise regularly are seven times more likely to gain *twenty-eight pounds or more!* over the next ten years than are women who exercise for an hour at least three times per week.[3] And a survey of more than 18,000 Americans found that people who regularly walk, jog, cycle, or do aerobics weigh less than people who do not exercise, *regardless of calorie intake*, height, race, smoking status, or education.[4]

While dieting alone may burn lean muscle tissue, exercise will both preserve and build new lean muscle mass, which in turn will burn more calories, making it harder for you to regain the lost fat! And you may be surprised and encouraged to learn that lengthy low- to moderate-intensity workouts can take off fat more effectively as high-powered sprints. Exercise that goes slowly and for a long time also helps to change the distribution of fat, significantly reducing the percentage of abdominal fat and thereby lowering the risk of heart disease and other associated health problems.

Fat's Best Friend

Of all the machines ever invented, the one that has contributed most to our national weight problem is television. Quite simply, TV is fat's best friend. Nearly 20 percent of people who watch more than three hours of television a week are overweight, compared to just 4.5 percent of those who watch less than an hour. Among adolescents in one study, the prevalence of obesity increased by 2 percent for every additional hour of television watched per day.[5] And according to the A. C. Nielsen company, the average American teenager today watches up to forty hours of television per week, compared with just eighteen hours in 1968. At this rate, each new generation will be about 6 percent fatter than the last. So far, this "growth rate" seems to be holding true.

But television is an inanimate object. Why should it be more fattening than, say, reading? For one thing, television nourishes passivity in the form of a virtual trance. You don't need to hold a book or a pen or even lift your head up. You hardly have to move your eyes. TV encourages your metabolism to drop to its minimum resting rate, lower even than when you are sleeping (most of us get pretty active in our sleep!), and the lower your metabolic rate, the fewer calories burned and the less body fat is disturbed.

Another of television's fattening tendencies is to bombard you with ads for high-fat foods. The obvious objective of these ads is to persuade you to buy those potato chips, frozen pizzas, snack cakes, and pies, but in the meantime they also tempt you to rush right into the kitchen *now* and grab something—anything—to munch on before the program resumes. This you frequently, obediently, do before settling back to sit motionless for another twenty minutes.

Unfortunately, when the Fat Ratchet is combined with our inactive lifestyle and our cultural love affair with fatty foods, the result does not bode well for dramatic weight loss or even for weight maintenance. On the one hand, our childhood habits would seem to have doomed us to a certain minimum body fat level. On the other, our way of life seems destined to push us to our maximum body fat level.

America's Diet Culture

At the same time, there is that other force at large, a force that constantly pushes us to want exactly what the Fat Ratchet and our cultural habits deny us. Ironically, it comes at us most aggressively via the same television that is so good at unconsciously fattening us up. That force, of course, is the media with its battalions of wafer-thin celebrities, as well as "ordinary people" who insist that we, too, can lose fifty pounds if we'd just try the liquid diet that worked so well for them. The weight loss industry, expected to exceed $50 billion in 1995, encourages us to believe that we can buy thinness without making substantial lifestyle changes.

Along with our eating and exercise habits, the expectations we place on ourselves have changed radically over recent decades. Everything happens so fast today that we feel compelled to look for instant solutions, instant results, even for the most difficult, persistent problems —even when the results we desire are completely unrealistic.

Why We Can't Have Our Cake and Lose It, Too

Here are a few of the commonly accepted attitudes and beliefs that make it so difficult to maintain a healthy weight *and* healthy eating habits.

Morality myths about weight make us long to lose.
• You can never be too rich or too thin.
• You have to be thin to be truly successful.
• Being thin makes you a better person.
• Thin people get to eat satisfying food.
• Thin people don't have to work at it.
• Not being thin is "bad."

Programmed messages about food set us up for failure.
• Food is for comfort and escape.
• Food is a reward and means of celebration.
• You can't have fun without food.
• Fatty food tastes better than lean food.
• Food is more fun than exercise!
• Food helps numb bad feelings, such as shame.

It would seem obvious that we can't keep the fat, eat the fat, and lose the fat all at the same time. Yet the conflicting cultural messages are so powerful and so persistent that that's precisely what many of us spend our lives trying to do. We literally want to have our cake and lose it, too. The resulting internal "fat wars" lead to a variety of unhealthy behaviors that are all too common among Americans, especially women.

I have found that these behaviors tend to follow certain patterns, which are important to recognize because each one requires a different weight management approach. As you read the following case studies you probably will recognize people you know—including yourself. Pay special attention to the individualized goals at the end of each case.

Who "Needs" to Lose: Four Weight-Behavior Profiles

The following profiles are composites of people I have worked with at Vanderbilt and known in my personal life. Taken together, they reflect the most common problems faced by people who worry about their weight.

HANNAH: THE COMPULSIVE DIETER

Hannah is typical of a majority of women in America. She became dissatisfied with her body during her teens and began dieting in an attempt to "fix" it. She has tried the Scarsdale, Beverly Hills, and Atkins diets, Weight Watchers, Jenny Craig, and Slimfast. She's used diet pills and diet bars and diet formulas. She's spent several fortunes on packaged diet foods and programs. She may even have gone through desperate periods when she purged with laxatives and vomiting. But try as she does to control herself and the cravings that seem to overwhelm her when she's dieting, she can't help occasionally bingeing. Well, more than occasionally . . .

Over the years Hannah's weight has fluctuated up and down, with a general upward trend. At age forty, she weighs 135 pounds, which she considers at least five pounds too heavy for her five-foot-five frame. She exercises in fits and starts, throwing herself into daily aerobics classes for a couple of weeks, then injuring herself or burning out and doing nothing for a month. She's daydreamed about plastic surgery and liposuction, but the combination of cost and cowardice has kept her from these drastic options. So, while she suffers constant guilt about practically everything she eats, she keeps searching for the perfect diet that will keep her effortlessly and forever thin.

Control is a critical issue for the compulsive dieter. Hannah perceives control to be a good thing, even if she is trying to restrict herself to an unnatural degree. Thus, she limits her eating so that she consumes less than her body needs to stay healthy and active. She strives to be thinner than her genetic makeup or lifestyle would naturally lead her to be. And she imposes such strict rules on her life that she has no reasonable margin for self-indulgence or impulsive behavior. The problem with Hannah's emotional setup is that by being so rigid she actually pushes herself to violate her own rules—by bingeing.

It may sound paradoxical, but psychologists over and over have found it to be true: the more severe the controls imposed on us, the more likely we are to violate them. When we go on an 800-calorie diet, permit ourselves no dessert, no snacks, no sugar, no salt, no fat, and on and on, then we are virtually doomed to react the same way as a teenager whose parents tell him he can have no phone calls, no contact with the opposite sex, and must spend all his free time either studying or cleaning his room. If the rules are unreasonable, the logical response will be to rebel. And the stricter the rules, the more extreme the rebellion will be. Which is why compulsive dieters like Hannah also tend to be compulsive bingers. If dieting is an unnatural version of undereating, bingeing is an equally unnatural version of overeating; the two behaviors are mirror images of each other.

Goals That Will Free Hannah from Her Compulsion and Keep Her Lean
(And the chapters in *The Last Five Pounds* that will guide her to these goals!)

- Learn how to eat, not how to diet. (Chapter 5)
- Determine if weight loss is really desirable or reasonable. (Chapter 4)
- Learn to lose gradually and *sensibly*. (Chapter 6)
- Cultivate other sources of personal satisfaction. (Chapter 2)
- Exercise regularly and moderately. (Chapters 8 and 9)

NELLIE: THE EMOTIONAL EATER

Nellie loves food. She was chubby as a child. Her family life centered around the kitchen, and her parents used to give her treats to cheer her up whenever she was feeling low. She never became really fat, and she's never seriously dieted—she likes eating too much to starve herself—

but at 125 pounds and five feet three inches tall, she does wish she could look like the models in those fashion magazines.

Nellie's weight, like Hannah's, goes up and down, but her highs and lows generally correspond to her life. When things are going well at work and at home, she eats sensible meals, works hard, exercises a few times a week, and her weight dips. But when she's overworked or nervous or upset she turns to food for comfort. She'll eat a couple of doughnuts in the car on the way home from work, then break open a can of peanuts, work her way through a half-pound of cheese instead of dinner, and finish up with cookies and milk. By the end of the week Nellie will be several pounds heavier.

Even on the best of days, though, Nellie still has a weakness for food. Bakeries, street vendors, and ice cream trucks are her downfall. The sight or smell of food make her hungry even if she's just come from a meal, and she doesn't try all that hard to restrain herself. When she thinks about it, it's a wonder she's not two hundred pounds, but still, it would be nice to lose just five.

While control is Hannah's bugaboo, temptation is Nellie's. Hannah tries too hard to control herself, but Nellie doesn't really try at all. The solution for an emotional eater like Nellie is not to impose a lot of rigid rules. Certainly, there is no advantage to turning her into a Hannah or encouraging her to become obsessed with diet. Nellie doesn't binge per se, but she does use food for more than nutrition. The solution for Nellie is to develop interests and coping skills that will balance her tendency to rely on eating for comfort and distraction.

She needs to use nonfood treats to lift her spirits, at least some of the time. Instead of driving home with a bag of doughnuts, she might go home with a friend and spend the evening watching an old movie. Instead of snacking she might go to a museum or out for a long walk. And instead of leaving herself open to the threat of boredom or anxiety, she might develop a new hobby or craft that would occupy those restless moments and divert her from impulse eating. She might buy a dog!

Note that I did not say Nellie should resist the pleasure she gets from eating. Food is a fundamental source of human pleasure, and that pleasure should not be diminished. But someone with a true love of food can easily turn that passion toward healthy low-fat eating, just as some of the world's great chefs—Julia Child and Craig Claiborne to name just two—have done in recent years. The secret for Nellie is to master the fine art of substitution (which will be discussed in Chapters 6 and 7, on low-fat cooking), replacing her high-fat favorites with low-fat equivalents. She also needs to restock her kitchen so that the foods on hand for cooking and for snacking are as lean and healthy as possible.

Finally, Nellie needs to increase her level of physical activity, making it part of her everyday routine, whether things are going well at work or not. Exercise can be especially beneficial when things are *not* going well because it helps to relieve stress and offers a mental time-out. (So, for that matter, will Nellie's new dog, and Nellie will be forced to get more exercise by taking the dog out for regular walks.) Exercise will take up time when Nellie might otherwise be snacking and step up her metabolism to make her feel more energetic as well as become leaner.

Goals That Will Help Nellie Cope with Stress Without Gaining Fat

- Practice "environmental control" by stocking low-fat foods. (Chapters 5 and 6)
- Cultivate nonfood interests, distractions, and sources of comfort and relaxation. (Chapter 2)
- Learn to use the new low-fat food products in cooking. (Chapters 6 and 7)
- Use exercise to buffer stress. (Chapters 8 and 9)

CARL: THE OVEREATER

Carl eats like a "typical American," which is to say he gives little thought to how, when, where, or what he eats. He doesn't care a great deal about food but was raised on hamburgers, hot dogs, and potato chips, with an occasional steak and milk shake thrown in for special occasions. That pretty much describes how he still eats today. The guys at his local McDonald's know him by name, and the barbecue works all summer.

Carl's wife gets annoyed with him for mindlessly snacking. He rarely goes in search of food, but if there's a cake on the counter he'll saw off a wedge. If she's making biscuits he'll grab one on his way through the kitchen. If the kids have left a sandwich he'll inhale it in passing. And when they're at a party Carl will spend the whole time by the food table, eating steadily without paying the slightest attention to what goes into his mouth. Moreover, after polishing off a basket of chips, a tub of dip, countless chunks of cheese, and several trays of hors d'oeuvres, he'll turn to his wife and ask what she's got planned for dinner.

Carl has gained ten pounds in the eight years since he got married, and he points the finger of blame at his wife's cooking. He'd love to get back down to his college "fighting weight," but in his mind, that would require a divorce.

The only contribution Carl's marriage has made to his weight gain is to put more food in his path. It's not his wife's fault that he consumes whatever is in front of him. Or that he was raised to favor high-fat meat and fast foods. Or that his hands and mouth seem to function without any connection to his brain. Carl does not eat compulsively or emotionally; his problem is that he eats unconsciously, and consumes huge quantities of calories and fat without even realizing he's eaten. Until that link between his brain and his mouth is restored, he hasn't a prayer of stopping his gain, much less actually losing weight.

If Carl is serious about taking charge of his weight, then, his first step must be to notice what he's eating and when. "Because it's there" is not a defensible reason for bolting down half a cheesecake. Cleaning up after the kids is not justification for consuming a second or third sandwich at lunch. And the hand does not have an inalienable right to bring food to the mouth unless commanded specifically to do so by the brain. Which gives the brain ultimate responsibility for every bite the mouth sends to the stomach. And that's Carl's brain, not his wife's.

Carl's challenge is not to diet or deprive himself. It is simply to eat when he's hungry, preferably at regular intervals throughout the day. And to recognize when he's full, even if he's standing in front of a plate of brownies. He may choose to take a brownie anyway, but that's different from *automatically* reaching for one, then another, then another.

Choice is the key word here. Once Carl realizes that he doesn't have to eat everything he sees, he is ready for the next startling revelation: that he is not locked into eating the same foods he was trained to eat as a child. He can choose from a host of foods that are lower in fat and richer in basic nutrition, such as grains, vegetables, and fruits—foods that will help bring his weight down.

Finally, Carl can choose to move away from food when he's not hungry, and keep moving, substituting exercise for the aimless, habitual eating that has filled his spare moments up to now. Washing the car, riding the exercise bike, and walking around the block may require as little mental effort as munching a bag of corn chips, but they're a lot less fattening!

Goals That Will Increase Carl's Eating Awareness

- Monitor eating patterns and food choices until eating becomes a conscious process. (Chapter 5)
- Learn Fat Categories—Fat-Cats—of foods (i.e., what's Low, Regular, and Full Fat)—not necessarily specific numbers of fat grams. (Chapter 6)
- Use low-fat alternatives. (Chapter 7)
- Use exercise instead of eating as a diversion. (Chapters 8 and 9)

SUSAN: THE NONEXERCISER

Susan could be Carl's wife. She eats a varied, reasonably low-fat diet and makes an effort to keep healthy food in the house, but she has two kids and a full-time job, and nutrition often takes a backseat to convenience. She rarely preplans meals or snacks and often picks up take-out food for the family on her way home from work. She also cooks a lot of frozen dinners.

Still, Susan manages to keep her weight more or less under control. It's her shape that really bothers her. All flab. Hips, thighs, stomach, dangling arm flesh, the works. There's not a spare minute in her weekday for exercise, and though she tries to be a weekend athlete, she's so out of shape that most of her marathon workouts last only fifteen or twenty minutes before she's winded or has pulled a muscle and put herself out of commission. As Susan sees them, her choices are to quit her job, give away her kids, or simply put up with the flab and bulges. But her body really disgusts her.

Susan's is a common plight, but it's not quite as dire as she perceives it. Her biggest advantage is that she's not locked into an emotional battle with food. She understands that her problem is lack of exercise more than diet.

Susan's mistake is to think of exercise as a chore to be added on top of all her other duties. The marathon is a race few of us are capable of running. We don't have the time or the stamina or the will. Besides, we don't need to run marathons to stay in shape. We don't need to run at all. For busy women like Susan, the key to fitness is to *enhance* the activities of daily life so they require a little more physical exertion on a consistent basis. She might walk instead of taking the bus to work, or if she drives, park at the far end of the parking lot. Take the stairs instead of the elevator. Walk the long way around to the copy machine. Stand and pace while talking on the phone. Stretch every half hour or so. Go to a nearby park and speed-walk on her lunch break instead of sitting in the coffeeshop. At home, Susan's body and spirits, as well as her relationship with her kids, would benefit from a game of catch or a family swim at the local Y in place of the family's usual habit of collapsing on the couch in front of prime-time TV. Fitness is easiest to achieve if it is integrated into daily life rather than being pushed into a separate slot.

Increasing her level of ordinary activity will help Susan reshape her body, but some simple adjustments to her food choices can also help this process along. She doesn't have to settle for high-fat foods in the name of convenience. For openers, some of the healthiest and leanest foods— raw fruits and vegetables—require minimal preparation. And now more than ever, it is possible to find low-fat replacements for most high-fat foods in supermarkets and on fast-food menus. From Lean Cuisine to Burger King's broiled chicken sandwiches, the alternatives are there. By substituting these leaner choices for her standard convenience fare, Susan can cut her fat intake—and the amount of fat she'll need to reduce through exercise.

Goals That Will Help Susan Shape Up Her Lifestyle

- Make fitness a family affair. (Chapter 10)
- Incorporate exercise into the daily routine. (Chapter 8)
- Substitute lean for high-fat convenience foods. (Chapter 6)
- Focus on fitness, not weight. (Chapter 9)
- Learn the simple "tricks" of eating and living that promote lifelong leanness. (Chapter 12)

Weight and Stress

Nutritious food is one of the most effective antidotes to stress. Others are regular rest and recreation, and ongoing human contact, support, and intimacy. These natural stress reducers are as essential for humans as shelter and warmth. But our society does not respect these necessities. The pace of modern life offers too little time for regular, nourishing meals. The load of work we are expected to accomplish offers too few opportunities for rest and exercise and fun. The result is greater and greater stress, to which many of us respond by overindulging in high-fat foods. Or by throwing ourselves into a new cycle of dieting and overeating. Or by binge eating. This is why so many of us gain weight under pressure.

Stress is an inevitable part of modern life. None of us can eliminate it entirely, but we can develop *constructive* strategies for coping with it. In doing so, we may also gain an advantage in the body fat battle.

Yale researchers have found that women in particular who do not cope well with stress tend to have fatter bellies—more apple fat—than less stressed women. There may be a physiological explanation, since the higher stressed women also produce more of the hormone cortisol, and researchers suspect a link between this hormone and production of body fat. But it doesn't take an Ivy League scientist to prove that many of us eat more when we are feeling anxious or frustrated—particularly if we see no more effective way to combat these feelings. In my weight management groups at Vanderbilt, I have noticed over and over that the women who are least successful in reducing and especially in *maintaining* a lower weight also tend to be the least willing to confront problems and make changes in other areas of their lives.

Too many of us conduct our lives according to what we feel we should do rather than what we want to do. And when we try to make a dramatic change, such as losing weight, we do it by heaping more should-dos on our already overloaded plates instead of focusing on the things we want to do that might lead us to the same goal. We tell ourselves we have to go on a liquid fast, for example, instead of making more time to play ball in the park with our kids. The liquid fast, which is self-punishing and highly stressful, may pull our weight down in the short term, but we're virtually doomed to gain it back. The calories we burn off at the park, on the other hand, will be a pleasure to lose *and* will bring the family closer together. And the exercise, unlike the diet, will reduce stress and alleviate tension.

As for immediate, highly specific tactics to reduce the impulse to eat in response to stress, the key is to develop an array of constructive nonfood responses to both negative and positive emotions. The best antistress response I've found is exercise. A good workout relieves tension, alleviates mild depression, and directly counteracts that stressed-out belly fat! Other proven, nonfattening stress-reduction methods include prayer, yoga, meditation, biofeedback, deep-muscle relaxation, and massage. You can also read, take a hot bath, go for a stroll, paint, write, talk to old friends, do crossword puzzles, or simply lie outside and watch the clouds—these are all more satisfying and more constructive responses to stress than eating is. And they serve equally well as rewards for hard work or as outlets for anger or frustration.

Generally what you want when you overeat, particularly when you binge, is escape. But exercising, doing something creative, connecting with other people, and seriously relaxing can serve as escapist activities, too, and they tend to leave you in a much better frame of mind than will overeating. It's all about replacing that list of punitive "should-dos" with positive "want-to-dos." Which, of course, translates into a new view of yourself, not as someone who deserves to be controlled, pushed, and possibly punished, but as someone who deserves to be encouraged, treated well, and rewarded often.

Smoking and Weight

One route commonly used to allay stress that I do *not* recommend is smoking. Cigarette consumption has decreased dramatically thanks to new awareness of the health risks related to tobacco use, but there are still some 48 million smokers in this country, and the habit is rapidly *gaining* ground among teenage girls and women under the age of twenty-five. Given the strong proven link between cigarettes and heart disease, cancer, and emphysema, it's hard to justify continued smoking and even harder to justify taking up the habit. Why, then, are so many young women choosing to take that first puff? For some the push comes from increased stress or peer pressure, but many are also motivated by the desire to lose weight.

There is a widespread misconception that smoking helps with weight control. In part this notion has arisen because so many people who quit smoking subsequently gain weight. In part it has come from scientific studies that reflect only half of the relationship between smoking and body fat. Here is the truth about that relationship, at least as much as we know right now.

There is evidence that smoking may boost the metabolism by about 6 percent, or some five calories per hour.[1] However, this effect on metabolism lasts no more than 30 minutes after the cigarette is finished.[2] So a chain smoker, while increasing her risk of death through cancer tenfold and reducing her life expectancy by eight years or more, might conceivably burn an extra hundred calories a day. For some weight-obsessed women, cancer and hastened death may seem a slight price to pay for that caloric advantage. But wait. This "advantage" is not all it appears.

Several recent studies, including one of over 5,000 young adults[3] and another that compared smoking and nonsmoking twins[4], have shown that, while smokers tend to have smaller bodies overall, they are no leaner than nonsmokers and consistently have *more* of the worst kind of fat—"apple fat." It appears, in other words, that smoking somehow affects the distribution of fat, increasing the amount in the middle of the body, where it's least attractive and most likely to contribute to future heart disease or diabetes. Furthermore, recent studies examining the diets of smokers and nonsmokers found that smokers in general, especially women smokers, consume more calories, fat, saturated fat, cholesterol, caffeine, and alcohol, and less fiber than people who do not smoke.[5] Thus, smoking is not the dieting boon that many young women believe, and it may lead to even more health problems than are now recognized.

Why do many smokers gain pounds when they quit cigarettes? The basic reason is that people tend to eat more to subvert the oral craving for a cigarette. Gum, candy, snacks, and sodas are the ex-smoker's staples. Also, because smokers tend to use cigarettes to relieve stress, they must find alternative emotional outlets, and one of the most common is eating. Finally, if no adjustment is made either to eat less or exercise more, those "free" calories that used to go up in smoke will now turn to body fat. It's not hard to see why the average postsmoking weight gain is twelve pounds. *However*, the health risks caused by smoking are equivalent to the health risks of carrying seventy to eighty pounds of excess body fat. And ex-smokers' proportion of abdominal fat is almost as low as in people who've never smoked.

I've had several individuals join my weight management group as a way of preventing weight gain while they quit smoking. In the group they learned to follow the same guidelines for eating and activity that are described in this book and, while they did not lose at quite the same rate as other group members, not one of them gained. Moreover, the strategies they learned through the group actually made it easier for them to kick the cigarette habit for good. That's because the reduction in fat intake and increase in physical activity made them feel more energetic, less stressed, and more confident that they could succeed in making the healthful changes they desired a permanent part of their lives.

If you currently smoke, I urge you, for your health's sake, to quit. Your doctor can recommend the smoking-cessation plan that will work best for you. And the exercise and eating recommendations in this book can help you eliminate cigarettes from your life without paying in unwanted weight gain.

The Mind-Life-Body Connection

There is a direct connection between your mind and your life and your body. Your health as a whole person depends on this being a healthy connection.

Many people overeat—or become obsessed with weight and dieting —as an unconscious way of filling a larger social, emotional, or spiritual void in their life. Lacking a balanced perspective on life or on themselves, they can become consumed with a relatively minor goal such as losing five pounds even when they are among the 75 percent of Americans who are already at their healthy weight. Lacking a strong sense of their own human value, they may think it perfectly acceptable to attack these few pounds by abusing their bodies and minds. But self-abuse in the name of weight loss is *not* acceptable! Not for fifty pounds, and certainly not for five.

No matter how badly you want to lose weight, if you succeed at the expense of your physical or emotional well-being, or of your family or your job, you will not be pleased with the results. Moreover, you will probably gain back the weight. On the other hand, if you focus on improving your overall health and outlook across your professional and personal lives, then your weight will find its own realistic level—and any fine-tuning can be accomplished with subtle changes in eating and exercise.

Being part of a supportive community, whether that community consists of a biological family, a network of friends, neighbors, or a more formalized support group, is absolutely vital. One of the most powerful attractions of weight control programs is that they provide a group setting where people can discuss their problems openly and without fear of criticism, where they believe they can find solutions to at least some of the issues surrounding their weight. These programs offer a sense of community, which is sometimes a more critical factor in the resulting weight control than any specially packaged meals, weigh-ins, or professional instruction. It's only fair to ask, though, if people might be better served by addressing their emotional and spiritual needs directly.

For myself, I've found spiritual foundation and expression in my Christian faith, but spiritual expression does not necessarily mean going to church or temple. It can be found in music, art, writing, reading, nature, just to name a few examples, as well as open and generous human contact.

The feelings of accomplishment you gain from performing tasks in which you have a strong emotional investment, whether this involves raising a child, getting a degree, earning a promotion, or planting a garden, will contribute directly to your sense of well-being. The more you do to raise your estimation of your own worth and the more you do to demonstrate your value both to yourself and to the world at large, the more satisfied you will be with yourself as a whole, and the less the numbers on the scale will matter. Believe in yourself! This is the first and most important step not only in achieving your ideal weight but in bringing your life as a whole into a healthy balance.

Putting Your Weight into Perspective: A Human-Needs Pyramid

Human companionship and intimacy
Balanced, nutritional eating
Regular physical activity
Meaningful interests
Shelter and clothing
Relaxation
Sleep

3

Women and Weight

If you have bought this book in the hope of losing weight, chances are you're a woman. As a woman, you have a very special relationship with your body, whatever the scale may say. I cannot give you the information you need to get rid of your unwanted pounds without first exploring this relationship in some detail. Only by understanding what has created your feelings about weight will you acquire the power to change them, and if you're like most women, the only way you'll finally put an end to this struggle is to redefine dramatically your attitude toward your body, the scale, and yourself.

Thinner Is Better—or Is It?

Far more frequently and insistently than men, we women are told by our culture that being thin will make us attractive, sexy, successful, and happy. Dieting, calorie counting, nibbling "daintily" at food, and pretending not to be hungry are all accepted as typical feminine behavior. Only among women is a slender body viewed as a mark of power and control—and a healthy appetite grounds for shame.

What is it about fat that can make otherwise bright and accomplished people feel discouraged, insecure, and unhappy? It's not the fat that does it. It's our culture. What's more important, it's our own mind-set, which buys into this culture.

Because of this mind-set:

- We berate ourselves for not being able to bring our weight down even as we establish careers, raise families, build friendships, and construct otherwise rich and fulfilling lives.
- We wake up smiling, step on the bathroom scale, and immediately fall into a pit of gloom where we stay for the rest of the day.
- We blame our weight whenever things go wrong in our lives: "If only I were ten pounds lighter, he wouldn't have broken up with me!"
- We condemn ourselves when we overeat, as if we've committed a sin: "I could just shoot myself, I was so bad last night, I ate three helpings of cake."
- We hide our weight, as we hide the true shape of our bodies, feeling embarrassment about both: "I'd rather die than wear a bikini in public."

We use weight, in other words, as a moral hammer that pounds down other, more troublesome aspects of life. When we're feeling upset about a relationship we eat too much, and then we feel so guilty about eating too much that we worry about that instead of the relationship problem. Or we feel frustrated at having been passed over for a promotion, so we gain four pounds, and then the shame of gaining weight persuades us we didn't really deserve the promotion anyway.

Men don't beat themselves up emotionally over *their* unwanted pounds. Only women do. Why?

Women's Distorted Body Image

When you look in the mirror, what do you see? Does it change depending on whether you're clothed or naked, wearing a bathing suit or a business suit, getting ready to go out to lunch with a friend or to address a group of business colleagues? Do you see yourself as lean and mean one morning, and the next as flabby and downright grotesque? If you were a man, such variability would make you abnormal, but as a woman you have practically been programmed to have a distorted body image.

Body image begins to form in infancy and is largely a reflection of how we are received by our parents, our peers, and society. Children learn at an early age to categorize themselves as skinny or stocky, gangly or chubby. Often that body image becomes an integral part of their identity. When the body changes during puberty, it can cause a severe shock to that sense of identity.

Many women's weird relationship with their own bodies dates directly to the adolescent eruption of fat deposits around the hips and breasts. A girl's body fat *normally* increases by 50 percent between the ages of nine and sixteen. And with that first unexpected development comes the realization that normal girls are not like fashion models. The shock of it!

A healthy reaction might be to yawn: "So what? It's reality." Instead, most teenage girls try to take on nature. Dieting, excessive exercising, compulsive overeating, anorexia, and bulimia are all patterns that typically start during adolescence. According to some estimates, 70 percent of American girls begin dieting between the ages of fourteen and twenty-one, and that includes underweight, normal-weight, and over-weight girls alike. At one suburban high school in New York, two-thirds of the female students thought they were too heavy—though only 13 percent of the girls were in fact overweight.[1] By contrast, less than 15 percent of teenage boys diet or worry about their weight.[2]

Translation: Our society has created a model of feminity that requires us to fret about our figures and pick at our food, or better yet, go hungry, *regardless of what we actually weigh.*

When taken to heart, this pattern can have a catastrophic effect on women's mental and emotional as well as physical health. If we feel ashamed of our bodies, we are not going to feel particularly good about ourselves. Nor are we going to treat our bodies with care and respect. Proof: a survey of more than 300 college women found that one-fifth had used diet pills, and 13 percent had used vomiting, laxatives, or diuretics as purgatives for weight control. Sixty percent were currently on a diet, and in the prior seven months nearly 30 percent had crash dieted or fasted.[3]

Crash dieting means eating less than 1,000 calories a day, and fasting means eating none (or, if juice fasting, only the calories contained in a few glasses of juice). To put this in perspective, as Naomi Wolf did so well in her book *The Beauty Myth*, in India, the very poorest women eat 1,400 calories a day. In Jewish concentration camps during World War II it was determined that 900 calories was the minimum required to sustain human functioning. Given female America's widespread use of poten-tially life-threatening measures to lose weight, perhaps it should come as no surprise that more women are afraid of becoming fat than fear death, but in their quest to avoid fat they could well be hastening their own demise.

Women agonize over that image in the mirror, actively looking for bad news and disregarding the good, almost as if *afraid* to see the best in themselves. In spite of the fact that three-quarters of American women are within their recommended weight range and do not need to lose weight at all, less than one-fifth of grown women ever achieve their "desired" weight! This, by the way, is rarely the healthy weight most men desire in women. Regardless of how their boyfriends and husbands may ogle voluptuous "pinup" models, women persist in believing that men are most attracted to superthin bodies—and then strive to become thinner than that!

Signals of a Distorted Body Image

- It doesn't matter how much you weigh, you still think you're too big or parts of your body are too large.
- Other people don't seem to see your body the way you do.
- You never believe people really mean it when they compliment you.
- You feel fatter on days when you're upset, and thinner on good days.
- You feel as if your body changes dramatically from one day to the next.

Why Do We Do This to Ourselves?

Body image has more to do with what's going on in the mind than in the mirror, and, like those other products of the mind—thoughts and feelings—it changes from one situation to the next. We may feel pretty good about ourselves while getting dressed in the privacy of home, but that feeling of satisfaction dissolves when we're trying on bathing suits in front of a store mirror or when we're walking past an exceptionally slender and attractive woman. We tend to dislike our bodies right after eating, even if the meal was not fattening. And we feel fatter before and during menstruation, or when we're in a bad mood or under stress. Most of us dislike our bodies the most when we feel we are losing control, even if what we want to control has nothing to do with our appearance.

Women's common pattern is to become self-critical when we're feeling threatened or anxious. Unlike men, who most often respond to the same feelings by lashing outward, we turn this negative power against ourselves. We use eating and weight to punish ourselves and to avoid confronting more serious problems. It's a form of narcissism, really: the more energy we concentrate on our bodies, even if it's negative energy, the less attention we pay to the outside world, and the less vulnerable we feel to potential risks, hurts, and disappointments.

I see this pattern frequently among my weight management group members. Miriam, for example, had a number of personal problems in addition to being overweight. She had a troubled relationship with her teenage son and was overwhelmed by financial difficulties. She talked about seeking professional counseling with her son. She talked about taking the courses she needed to complete her college degree, which would pave the way to a promotion and pay raise. But ultimately she did neither. Her problems continued to fester. And her weight continued to climb.

On the other hand, women who successfully cope with the problems of living also tend to have an easier time managing their weight. Ellen's story contrasts sharply with Miriam's. Ellen had gained a significant amount of weight over a period of two years before joining the group. When she examined the possible reasons for this gain, she found that her children had left home for college during this same period, and she had been promoted at work under a new, often difficult supervisor. These life changes had altered her eating habits and led to more anxiety-induced eating. Once she saw this connection, Ellen took action. She downscaled her weekly shopping list and adjusted her cooking methods to reflect the fact that she and her husband were now cooking—and eating—for two instead of four. And she took the initiative to have a formal discussion with her boss about reasonable work hours and demands. The result? Ellen felt more in control of her life. The anxiety that had triggered her overeating diminished. At her last follow-up group meeting she was almost back to her original weight.

What this means is that we women have got to learn to cope with the problems of living—to face the inevitable conflicts in life instead of ducking or denying them. We must develop positive ways to soothe ourselves when we are feeling down, to steady ourselves when nervous, and to reward ourselves (regularly!) for jobs well done. We have to stop picking ourselves apart and dwelling on our shortcomings, and instead build on our strengths and accept ourselves as complete individuals— regardless of the messages we pick up from those around us. Only then can we finally free ourselves from the constant, senseless obsession with weight.

The Physiological Truth

Women's cultural obsession with thinness flies directly in the face of our physiology. Being female means being fat. Not obese. Not overweight. But comfortably padded. We are constructed for the purpose of reproducing the human species, after all, not to pose in swimsuit editions of *Sports Illustrated!* The mechanism of human reproduction requires us to carry extra reserves of fat to ensure the nourishment of future babies. Given this biological reality, the connection between superthinness and femininity is absolutely perverse! Real women are not all muscle and bone but are rounded, curving, and supple. This is not a moral statement. It is nature. We resist it at our own peril.

At birth, before they've even tasted their first doughnut or french fry, girl babies have 10 to 15 percent more body fat than boys. This discrepancy increases at puberty, when the ratio of muscle to fat increases in boys and falls in girls. By age twenty, the average woman has about 29 percent body fat, by middle age 38 percent. These figures remain fairly constant, despite variations in cultural eating or dieting patterns, throughout the world.

More than 20 percent of the fat deposits in men but only 8 percent in women are located in and around the abdomen. So, while men gain readily in the belly, women gain most easily in their hips and thighs; while men *lose* fat readily from their hips and thighs, women drop it most easily from the midriff. There does appear to be some connection in women between having too much—or too little—overall body fat and certain health complications such as osteoarthritis, osteoporosis, and menstrual irregularities. In the end, however, women come out ahead, because the smaller percentage of abdominal fat gives them a much lower risk than men for certain killer diseases.

Still, women fret over their fat. And no fat is cursed more than the "cottage cheese" most of us wear around our thighs and backsides. The location, size, and number of fat deposits in these regions, combined with the relative thinness of women's skin, create this dimpled composition, which we call cellulite. In fact, cellulite is just plain fat, but because the deposits in the hips and thighs are close to the skin (fat in the midsection is stored deeper in the body) and because these storage ports are both large and numerous, the actual consistency of the fat tends to mottle the surface of the skin. There is some evidence that the structure of fat cells in these areas causes the skin to retain water, giving it a slightly swollen appearance. But no amount of rubbing, buffing, or pounding will change the texture of cellulite. Toning the muscles in the buttocks and thighs can help, but unless you also lose fat you will simply end up with firmer limbs underneath the cellulite. The only effective way to combat this "cottage cheese" appearance is to reduce the total amount of fat in your body.

Genetics, Hormones, and Fat

How does the female body know it's supposed to be fatter than a man's? We still haven't identified all the contributing mechanisms, but the two most powerful influences appear to be genetics and hormones. The same genetic map that determines our sex also determines to a substantial degree how much fat our grown bodies will carry. In fact, if we consider all the factors that can affect our weight, genetics controls at least one-quarter of them. Thus, even if a woman with a family history of obesity eats minimal fat in her diet, works out vigorously for an hour each day, and leads an otherwise active life, she might never become as lean as another woman whose whole family for generations have been reed thin. It's not unfair, it's not immoral, it's biology.

There seems to be a direct link between female hormones, body fat, and body weight. As the hormone levels shift throughout the menstrual cycle, many women experience related changes that affect appetite and weight:

• Basal body temperature changes significantly in response to different hormone levels. Fever of any kind burns more calories, so when a woman's body temperature climbs after ovulation, so does her caloric consumption. And so does her appetite, which may more than compensate for any benefits of the thermostat.
• Water weight shifts with hormonal swings. Most women gain one to two pounds through fluid retention in the days leading up to each period.
• Hormones sometimes trigger cravings at specific times of the month. Many women who have PMS crave chocolate. Others crave carbohydrates.

Hormones appear also to affect the distribution of body fat. Specifically, they instruct the fat sites in the hip and thigh area to hoard a certain minimum amount of fat. Needless to say, the hormonally prescribed minimum is considerably more fat than most of us desire. By the time we get within five pounds of our target, our hormones have most likely already kicked into their shutdown mode, and it will take extreme measures to reduce our thighs and hips much further. It's called being female, and most of us are better off accepting the curvature of our bodies than fighting nature.

One of the first casualties when a woman drops significantly below her natural level of body fat is her fertility. That's because crucial sex hormones are stored in fat. When a woman's body fat drops below 20 percent, her risk of infertility and menstrual irregularities directly increases, while her sexual appetite and ability to be sexually aroused dramatically decrease. Women undergoing treatment for fertility are routinely warned not to lose too much weight, and if they're underweight, they're often told to gain.

Pregnant Fat

The body requires extra fat during pregnancy. Of the twenty-five-pound weight gain that is recommended as an absolute *minimum* for a healthy pregnancy, up to ten pounds consist of new fat deposits around the internal organs, abdomen, back, and upper thighs. This fat ensures the fetus's nutrition through the end of pregnancy and, after birth, safeguards the mother's ability to breast-feed. This extra fat is vital for the health of the baby. Underweight women are twice as likely as plumper mothers to have low birthweight babies. And low birthweight babies are much more susceptible to illness and developmental problems than chubbier infants.

While hormones trigger the increase in fat during pregnancy, after birth they prompt the fat deposits to shrink. Just how fast fat decreases varies from woman to woman, but some new mothers lose as much as twenty pounds in the first two weeks after birth. This loss includes amniotic fluid, water from swelling, and blood, as well as fat.

Further fat is lost during breast-feeding. Nursing requires an extra 500 to 1,000 calories a day on top of the mother's own caloric needs. The chemistry of fat in her hips and thighs reverses after birth so that fat can readily deliver some of the necessary calories. In addition, breast-feeding triggers the contraction of the uterus back to its normal size, thus helping to tone the abdominal muscles. Contrary to what used to be popular opinion, breast-feeding actually helps the new mother lose weight and regain her figure. According to one study, by six months after birth, nursing mothers weighed on average six pounds less than bottle-feeding mothers, and a year after birth the difference was seven pounds. Furthermore, the breast-feeding mothers still were considerably leaner and lighter two years after giving birth.[4]

This is all normal and natural, and has little to do with the mother's diet or exercise. If a woman has one or two children, the cycle of pregnant fat leaves little lasting impact on her shape or weight. In fact, women who have one or two children statistically have less fat overall and less abdominal fat than women who have never given birth. Unfortunately, women who have more than two children do tend to retain some of that fat. A survey of nearly 41,000 women found that those who had three or more children tended to have more overall body fat and porportionally more abdominal fat than women with fewer children.[5]

Good News About Menopause

It's a common assumption that we gain weight as we age, and that it becomes more difficult to trim down as we get older. While it's statistically true that most Americans expand with age, women tend to gain the most during the childbearing years.[6] Weight gain then tapers off. Once the reproductive years are over, and the female body no longer hoards that extra "fertility padding" around the hips, thighs, and breasts, it may actually be easier for women to lose weight because the body no longer *resists* fat loss. Studies of women in weight loss programs have found that younger women lose less fat and more lean body mass than women who have gone through menopause, and the older women tend to lose fat from all over the body, while younger women lose mainly from the abdomen.[7] In my own weight management groups at Vanderbilt, I've noticed that as older women slim down they typically lose from the hips and thighs and from the upper body, producing a significant change in overall body shape. Younger women, on the other hand, tend to lose from the waist but otherwise retain their basic body shape—perhaps smaller but still proportionally the same.

Unfortunately, if women put on weight after menopause, they will tend to gain around the waist, and with this gain will come the same increased health risks associated with abdominal fat in men. The best way to prevent this shift, of course, is not to gain the weight.

Exercise seems to be the most powerful weapon against unwanted fat after menopause, just as it is earlier in life. One study found that elderly women who do not exercise weigh on average more than twenty-four pounds more than women the same height who work out regularly![8] Low-fat eating, too, can help prevent the shift of fat from hips to belly. Taking supplementary estrogen can reverse the hormonal patterning and with it the tendency to store fat around the middle. Women who have taken estrogen typically weigh less and have less abdominal fat than women who have never taken it. However, synthetic hormones must be taken under a doctor's supervision and may not be medically advisable for all women. Exercise and lean eating, on the other hand, are recommended for just about everyone!

The Urge to Binge

If we believe what the TV ads tell us, we are supposed to eat loads of high-fat foods and yet look as fit and lean as Jane Fonda. The commercials never acknowledge that the female body was designed to be fatter than the male's. And they never suggest we put our health ahead of either our appetites or our pursuit of thinness. Is it any wonder that many of us treat our health as the least important of these three driving forces? If we can lose weight by abusing our bodies, so be it. If we can lose weight *and* feed our appetite for fat, that's an even greater incentive to abuse our health. So we learn to purge, or alternate between liquid fasts and Big Mac attacks, or take laxatives, or become addicted to exercise, or smoke. The more we push to control our weight, the more out of control our lives become. And the more likely we are to develop an eating disorder.

The most common eating disorder, and a behavior that is shared by bulimics and many anorexics, is binge eating. Diagnosed as Binge Eating Disorder (BED), this involves eating large quantities of food in a short period of time with a feeling of loss of control. BED is estimated to affect approximately one-third of overweight individuals, especially women, and millions more "normal-weight" women who appear on the surface to have balanced eating patterns. In my weight management groups at Vanderbilt alone, between one-third and one-half of the women are binge eaters. More than half of teenage girls binge periodically.[9] And the problem seems to be occurring more and more frequently among women who have no history of emotional distress or visible weight problem.

I have found that among women who complain of just five or ten unwanted pounds, binge eating is often the primary cause of that extra weight. You probably know the drill:

You've been "good" all day, maybe even all week. You've eaten light and lean. You haven't had time to exercise but that hardly seems to matter since you'd dropped three pounds as of this morning. You were confident you'd be able to keep up the good work—confident, that is, until you came home to an empty house and an evening with zero plans. Now you have a craving for ice cream that just won't quit. Satisfying it will mean a trip to the store, during which you'll probably end up buying not just the ice cream but some of that prefab cookie dough or maybe a pound cake. After which, you'll devour every single crumb and spoonful. You'll hate yourself for it, but you know how this will end up. It always does. . . .

STOP! Enough guilt, shame, and fatalism. The monster that makes you binge is not weakness, nor is it your destiny. According to the research that is just beginning to emerge regarding dietary cravings, there may actually be a link to certain hormones and brain chemicals that are released in response to inadequate nutrition, stress, and conditioning. By learning what causes your craving for "forbidden" foods you will discover the keys to managing the monster.

Dietary Restriction

Restricting your food intake and especially your caloric intake makes you a prime candidate for binge eating. Restriction may simply mean skipping breakfast, or it may mean intentionally omitting certain foods or entire groups of foods. Or it may mean crash dieting and fasting. Here are a few of the ways this can lead to bingeing.

To break a fast. When you have gone without eating for a number of hours, as when you wake up in the morning, high levels of a brain chemical called neuropeptide Y and low levels of the hormone serotonin trigger a preference for carbohydrates. This is why toast, cereal, waffles, pancakes, and fruit are breakfast favorites. Bread for breakfast, of course, does not qualify as a binge, but the same brain chemicals will kick in if you've been dieting or fasting or simply forgetting to eat. The longer you go without feeding yourself, the stronger your craving for carbs will become and the stronger your feelings of deprivation, which can lead to a binge. *Do not skip meals, especially not breakfast.*

To hoard energy. The brain chemical galanin triggers a desire for fatty foods and works with other hormones to convert dietary fat into body fat. Levels of galanin rise throughout the day and, ironically, seem to jump even higher after fatty foods are eaten. In women, galanin levels also rise after ovulation each month, in conjunction with estrogen. But galanin levels really soar during "quick weight-loss" diets when the body is not receiving adequate calories through carbohydrates and is forced to burn its own fat; that's when the craving for high-fat foods is strongest. Coupled with the simultaneous diet-induced craving for carbs caused by the imbalance in neuropeptide Y and serotonin, the rise of galanin heightens the psychological sense of deprivation and makes bingeing almost irresistible.

To maintain reproductive function. Women's bodies, in particular, produce cravings in the face of starvation—even semistarvation—in order to maintain the levels of body fat required for reproduction. High estrogen levels may contribute to the craving for high-density calories and may produce less severe cravings even when the body is well fed. What are the most likely targets of a starving woman's cravings? Yes, those high-fat *and* sugary favorites such as doughnuts, ice cream, iced cakes, brownies, pie. . . . This explains the frequent binges of adolescent girls, whose bodies are fighting to pack on fat even as the girls unsuccessfully attempt to diet against it. And it may be part of the reason why women in general are more prone to bingeing than men are.

High Stress

When your body is stressed, the adrenal glands release stress hormones such as corticosterone and norepinephrine, which spur a rise in galanin and neuropeptide Y. The resulting "stress craving" for high-fat, high-carb foods help explain why boredom, anxiety, frustration, and unhappiness so often trigger binges.

Conditioning and Habit

In addition to all the chemistry that contributes to binges, of course, everyone is susceptible to emotional and behavioral cues. Here are just a few examples of how this works:

• If your mother used cookies and milk to comfort you throughout your childhood, you may still turn to these foods for solace—but without the maternal nurturing that used to go with them, you may find that you eat vastly more cookies as an adult.

• If you were an overweight teenager, you might have trained yourself to eat very little at meals and around other people, but whenever you were alone you gorged. Having established this pattern of behavior, you may feel tempted to binge whenever you're alone.

• If you and your ex-husband ate a large meal every night, you may continue to eat a large quantity of food each evening even after breaking up. The difference is that you don't bother to cook a healthy meal for yourself; you just binge to fill the mealtime.

Managing the Binge Monster

If you are an occasional binge eater, you will go a long way toward managing your cravings by following the nutritional and exercise routines I have recommended throughout this book. A low-fat, high-carbohydrate, high-activity, eat-when-you're-hungry lifestyle will minimize your urge to binge, if not eliminate it altogether. Here's why:

1. Delivering a steady supply of complex carbohydrates to your bloodstream via healthy snacks and regular meals will keep the levels of neuropeptide Y and serotonin within a normal range, thus preventing cravings for more carbs than you really need.

2. Raising carbohydrate intake while lowering fat intake to about 20 percent of total calories helps to keep galanin levels down, thus minimizing the craving for fat.

3. Permitting yourself occasional indulgences in modest portions helps to curb your cravings. The craving control works best when you substitute low-fat versions of high-fat favorites—chocolate frozen yogurt, say, instead of chocolate ice cream. Remember, you are most likely to binge on a food if you feel deprived of it.

4. Physical activity helps to reduce stress and maintain a proper balance of brain chemicals, thus minimizing the urge to binge on high-fat foods.

5. Permitting yourself satisfying foods whenever you're hungry removes the emotional anguish and sense of desperation from the process of eating. When you feel good *and* you genuinely enjoy the food that makes you feel good, you are less prone to binge. And more likely to stay fit and lean.

When Dieting and Bingeing Become a Disease

People who have a genuinely positive body image and a healthy relationship with food tend to eat because they're hungry, because food tastes good, because eating makes them physically feel better than going hungry does. They view eating as a *good thing*. But women for whom binge eating has become a disease tend to view eating as something forbidden, and binge eating as the ultimate wrong.

Chronic binge eaters—who may binge eat several times each day—do not generally binge when hungry; they do not savor the food they consume when bingeing; and rather than feeling better after bingeing, they feel physically and emotionally terrible. Disgust, guilt, depression, panic, and despair are just a few of the emotions that typically follow a binge, whether or not that binge is followed by bulimic purging. Bingeing unleashes a desperate feeling of being out of control, frenzied, and helpless to stop. It can also:

- impair performance in work or social life
- lead to obsession with weight and body shape
- create general psychological distress
- increase dieting
- contribute to depression, alcohol or drug abuse, and emotional problems.

Many doctors now believe that the mere act of dieting, which for most women means starving themselves below the minimum human caloric requirement, can trigger binge eating and other eating disorders. The reasons a woman starts dieting, of course, may have more to do with stresses and strains in personal relationships, work, family life, and surrounding community and cultural concerns than it does with her actual weight. But once eating and dieting get out of control, another layer of problems is added, and these require specialized treatment or counseling in and of themselves. It is easier to prevent an eating disorder than it is to stop it after the cycle has begun.

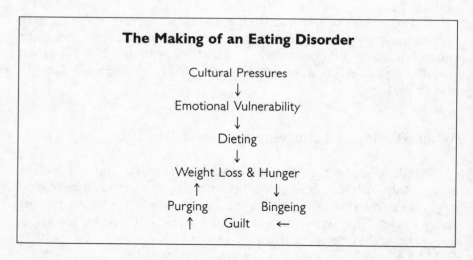

The best way to prevent extreme dieting is to follow the low-fat eating and exercise guidelines described in *The Last Five Pounds*. But if you suspect that it's too late for preventive strategies because you or a loved one already have an established eating or dieting disorder, *please* get help. Start by reaching out to your family physician, health care provider, family members, or friends you can trust. If you need further information or assistance in locating counseling or treatment facilities, contact:

National Association of Anorexia Nervosa
and Associated Disorders
PO Box 7
Highland Park, IL 60035
(708) 831-3438

Food and Weight: Keep Them in Perspective

Do	*Don't*
• Give attention and energy to meaningful life goals.	• Don't weight yourself!
• Eat healthy meals, get regular exercise, and appreciate your body.	• Don't count calories.
• Take pride in your appearance, whatever your weight.	• Don't allow food, weight, and body image to consume your thoughts.
• Give priority to your health, personal values, and integrity.	• Don't try to force your body to conform to someone else's standards.
• Be a friend to yourself rather than criticize or judge yourself.	• Don't diet! It can actually lead to weight *gain*.
• Build on your strengths instead of your frailties.	• Don't expect a thin body to provide inner beauty.
• Accept the weight you achieve by eating balanced meals and exercising regularly.	• Don't focus on your mistakes and failures, but have the courage to learn from them.
• Focus on yourself as a whole human being instead of dwelling on your parts.	• Don't berate your natural weight.
	• Don't forget that your most valuable qualities have nothing to do with the size or shape of your body.

It Doesn't Have to Be This Way

Many of us are so conditioned by our immediate friends and culture, or by the version of our society portrayed through the media, that we assume *everyone* wants to be hyperthin and lean and fit. Nothing could be further from the truth. Thinness is not generally considered a hallmark of beauty in the African-American or Hispanic culture. And among lower income groups and upper age groups weight is given much less importance than it is among younger middle- and upper-income women.

The fashion industry is largely responsible for distorting white culture's view of the ideal woman's body. You might say it has played a hoax on women's self-image. HOAX. These letters spell out the four basic female body types. At one end are the H women, straight up and down and usually narrowly built. At the other are the X, or hourglass, figures. Most fashions are designed for these two body types, with the emphasis on the slender H.

But the vast majority of women fall in between, with rounded O or bottom-heavy A shapes. And there's little they can do to change this. Body type is, for the most part, genetically determined. We can gain or lose weight, become larger or smaller overall, but unless we take this size change to extremes, our basic shape will remain the same.

Regardless, the fashion industry has singled out body types that are least representative of the female species and has used them for decades as the basis for clothing design. Not only do we beat ourselves up for not looking like models who, for the most part, are underfed adolescents, but we then have to suffer the further indignity of squeezing ourselves into garments designed for somebody else's body. How often do you find a dress that looks as good on you as it did in the newspaper or catalog? No wonder we have a collective inferiority complex!

It Hasn't Always Been This Way

Fashion standards have changed radically throughout history. Here, to give you some perspective, is an overview of body types considered "ideal" in different eras.

- Mid-1800s: Small, curvaceous, and corseted. Scarlett O'Hara in *Gone With the Wind* stood 5'4" and 110 pounds with a 32-22-33 figure trussed into a whalebone girdle.
- 1880s: The curves intensified with the concept of "wasp waists," and so did the use of corsets. The hourglass now measured 38-18-38.
- 1890s: Gibson Girls and Lillian Russell made heft desirable. Lillian Russell stood six feet tall and weighed in at 200 pounds!

- 1900: Full-bodied comfort was the name of the game. The Flora Dora girls in Ziegfield's Follies, selected on the basis of their looks, averaged 130 pounds at 5'4".
- 1920s: With women's growing emancipation, increased enrollment in college and the professions, fashions deemphasized curves and introduced women to the adolescent, flat-chested look of the flappers.
- 1930s: The professional woman became the arbiter of style, with models appearing glamorous, voluptuous, and competent.
- 1940s: With men off to war and women shifting into the workplace, the feminine image became synonymous with strength, ability, and courage.
- 1950s: As soon as the men returned and women were directed back toward the home, the female figure again was given more attention than female brainpower or competence. Blond bombshells such as Marilyn Monroe, Jayne Mansfield, and Kim Novak were the new ideals. The measurements to have were 36-26-36. Miss America stood 5'8" and weighed 132 pounds.
- 1960s: Another surge of women into colleges and professions once reserved for men, and in response a drastic downscaling of the models representing feminine beauty. Twiggy, 92 pounds at 5'6", set fashion's standards. At the end of the decade diet-related articles in women's magazines shot up 70 percent.
- 1970s: California girls reign as America's ideal women. Models such as Cheryl Tiegs, Farrah Fawcett, and Christie Brinkley may not be as skinny as Twiggy, but they're no Lillian Russell!
- 1980s: Jane Fonda, Cher, Raquel Welch and other workout stars launch beauty's fitness wave. Now women must be not only thin but muscular, sculpted, buff! The simultaneous rise of the Yuppie status model requires that true superwomen must, in addition to being lean and sculpted, be professionally independent, perfectly groomed and coiffed, and designer dressed.
- 1990s: Cindy Crawford, with big hair, big lips, and a very big presence, sets one feminine standard for the decade. The nouveau Twiggy "waif look," which Mademoiselle magazine describes as "thin, pale, and slightly bruised," sets quite another. Which will win out? Neither, if American women learn to stand up and set their own healthy and realistic beauty standards!

The solution, of course, is to stop trying to dress—and reshape yourself—according to the dictates of the fashion world, and to start choosing your wardrobe to help you look and feel your best.

Here are a few suggestions:

• Create a personal style of your own by collecting garments you know flatter you. When they wear out, replace them with similar designs instead of attempting trendy fashions.

• Find the hem length that feels comfortable and stay there, regardless of what's "in" this season.

• Wear clothes that allow you a full range of motion without binding or pinching but at the same time reveal your figure's strong points.

• Don't force yourself into a size 8 when you need a 10; nobody can see the size tag, and the smaller size will actually make you look bigger if it doesn't fit properly.

• On the other hand, don't hide under oversized clothes; that only perpetuates a sense of shame and embarrassment about your body.

• Accept the fact that fashion models belong to a different species, and stop using them as a yardstick for your own appearance.

• Accept the fact that fashions and "ideal" body types have changed dramatically through history and will continue to change. Whatever the ideal, relatively few of us will measure up to it; we must strive for our bodies' Personal Best condition instead of trying to reshape them according to cultural ideals.

The Times—Are They Changing?

I am happy to close this chapter with some evidence that the message of sanity may finally be getting through to American women. The good news comes from, of all sources, that unlikely champion of women's self-improvement, *Glamour* magazine. Seems like every issue of *Glamour* I've ever read offers a new diet or weight loss section as a prescription for thinness. But recently *Glamour* has stopped emphasizing weight loss and has embraced health as the goal young women should aim for. According to the magazine's own survey of 17,000 women under the age of thirty-five, this new emphasis reflects a trend in *Glamour* readers:

• Today almost half of the readers report that their weight is just right, compared to only 15 percent in a poll conducted in 1983. The average weight in this survey was 135 pounds for an average height of 5'5".

• If given their choice of several life goals 43 percent of today's women would choose to be loved by a man, 20 percent would choose to be rich, and only 19 percent would choose to be ten pounds thinner. A decade ago, losing weight ranked number one.

• Only one-third of today's readers said they'd recently been on a low-calorie diet to lose weight, 78 percent said they exercised, and 64 percent cut fat rather than calories when they did want to reduce. A decade ago, crash dieting and calorie counting were the most popular methods of weight control, and only 57 percent of women exercised.[10]

Unfortunately, the *Glamour* survey also suggested that more than half of young American women still harbor "food secrets," such as a passion for chocolate, private binges on sweets, and eating disorders. And 16 percent of underweight women still think they weigh too much. So there's plenty of work to do, but with more women learning that a low-fat, high-activity lifestyle can provide a *sane* way to trim down without sacrificing health or energy, we may be seeing the beginning of a new and positive era in women's weight consciousness. An era when we can enjoy feeling strong and lean and healthy and let the last five pounds take care of themselves.

LOSING AND LEAVING
THE LAST FIVE POUNDS

4

The Ideal You

When I was in high school most of my friends weighed between 105 and 118 pounds and stood under 5′6″. Although I was five inches taller than that, I was ashamed to be 140 pounds. I began to skip lunch, eat half servings at dinner, and avoid all sweets. Hunger was the hallmark of my first diet. Helped along by a bout of flu, semistarvation brought my weight down to 124. Was I proud. My clothes hung on me; I could pull the waist of my school uniform out like a magazine before-and-after picture. My family told me I was too thin, and a boyfriend said my arms looked like twigs, but it was all music to my ears. The dieting might have spiraled into full-blown anorexia if I didn't enjoy eating so much—and if I hadn't joined the school track team.

I imagined that running must burn countless calories, and therefore stopped dieting! I rejoined my friends at lunch, took normal helpings at dinner, and indulged in ice cream on a regular basis. By summer my weight was back up to 140. Fortunately, I'd stopped agonizing about it.

But life events inched my weight upward over the next few years. My parents' divorce and a steady boyfriend added five pounds, going off to college another ten. After Christmas of my freshman year I brought a scale (a gift from my family) into my dorm room and became obsessed with counting calories, weighing myself several times a day. I fasted periodically and decided to major in nutrition—surely, if I became a dietitian I'd get rid of those extra pounds! But, for the moment, nothing seemed to slim me down.

Twenty years old and feeling fat, I joined a local health spa. The "counselor" calculated that I should weigh 100 pounds for the first five feet of my height, and three pounds for every inch above. That made my target weight 133. And gave me twenty pounds to lose! Dressed in oversize clothes to hide my "fat body," I worked every machine in the gym, including the rollers that "vibrate the fat away." I went on the then-popular low-carbohydrate diet and broke 150, then 145, and finally, after breaking up with a boyfriend, hit 137. Two months, a trip to Florida, and a new boyfriend later, I was back at 150 pounds.

Academic demands gave me an excuse to eat on the run and skip exercise, and my weight edged up to 157 in graduate school. One day in Exercise Physiology class we were told to divide, for fitness testing, into weight groups: those who weighed less than 150 went to one end of the football field, those 150 and above went to the opposite end. I just couldn't bear to be in the Big Group, so I lied and was sure they would not conduct a mass weigh-in right there. Realistically, I did need to lose five pounds, but I found that by lengthening my morning jogs to a total of 15 miles per week, the pounds vanished without dietary sacrifice.

After graduate school I moved to Boston where I knew no one and started a new job as a dietitian specialist. As a Southerner wintering north of the Mason-Dixon line, I felt stranded. I turned to food for company and entertainment, and my weight reached an all-time high of 167 pounds. But gradually, I made friends; spring's warm weather urged me back into running; the extra pounds retreated without "dieting." Within a year, my weight leveled off again at 152.

Four years later I returned to Nashville, a new job, and old friends. I was recovering from a relationship breakup and running more than usual; my weight dipped to 145. But marriage and stability pulled my life back to normal and my weight back up. That's right: 152 pounds.

You see my point. When I'm active and choose low-fat foods 80 percent of the time, the weight of my 5'11" body naturally settles between 148 and 152 pounds, with a body fat level of about 21 percent. Whenever it's dropped below this I've either been aggressively dieting or exercising or else my life has been out of whack. To maintain a lower weight would require heroic measures and more stress and anxiety than I am willing to trade for unnatural thinness. So at long last I've stopped tormenting myself with calculations of how much I'd have to lose to look like someone skinnier. And I've accepted a natural weight range that is healthy and reasonable—and therefore ideal for me.

Now it's time to take a closer look at your weight, your body, and your lifestyle, and determine what's realistically ideal for you.

Reality Check: Bring Your Goal Within Reach

One reason people so often fail on weight loss programs is that they set a goal unreasonably low for their bodies and for their way of life. The frustration of not meeting this goal can cause a rebound effect, sometimes leading them to a net weight *gain*.

Is your goal too low? To answer this, you need to understand that your weight is influenced by a variety of factors, many of which are beyond your control. It's important to take them all into account when evaluating your individual "ideal."

Think of the people you most admire. Visualize their eyes, their noses, the color and cut of their hair, the way they dress and talk. Chances are, each person's characteristics are different. Moreover, you expect and admire the differences. Why, then, when it comes to weight, should everyone strive for the lowest common denominator? In reality, weight is as individual and variable a characteristic as skin or hair color. Ultimately, the weight that's right for you must be both attainable and maintainable, and must be a weight at which you can be happy and healthy and productive.

To determine where, precisely, this ideal goal lies, we'll start with some general, objective measures and then narrow down your target to fit your individual needs and lifestyle.

Basic Body Mass

Equal rights notwithstanding, men's and women's bodies are not alike. Women are *supposed* to carry more fat than men; men are supposed to carry more muscle and therefore weigh more than women of the same height. Of course, there's wide variation in muscularity in both sexes, but nevertheless this presumed gender difference is the reason weight tables reflect higher acceptable weight ranges for men than for women. Traditionally, most physicians have used the old Metropolitan Life Insurance tables to determine whether patients are within a healthy weight range, but in recent years those tables have been in dispute. For a quick and *very general preliminary measure,* I prefer to use recommendations I learned years ago through the American Dietetic Association. I feel these targets are realistic for most people, and they do not require the use of a table.

For women, then, assume an acceptable midpoint weight of 100 pounds for the first five feet of height, plus five pounds per inch of additional height. The acceptable range is from 10 percent below to 10 percent above this midpoint, depending on your body frame, bone structure, and weight distribution (more on these variables in a moment).

I am 5′ 11″ tall, so I'd calculate:

$$\begin{array}{rl} 100 & \textit{(pounds for the first 5 feet)} \\ +\ \ 55 & \textit{(5 pounds} \times \textit{11 inches)} \\ \hline 155 & \textit{pounds (my recommended midpoint)} \end{array}$$
plus or minus 10%

• *140 to 170 pounds (my "acceptable" weight window—and also, almost exactly, the range of my actual weight fluctuations over the years)*

For men, the first five feet of height are worth 105 pounds. Then six pounds are added for each additional inch to arrive at the midpoint. The acceptable range is from 10 percent below that midpoint to 10 percent above.

Now, a thirty-pound range is too general to use as a weight goal and does not reflect your body composition, weight distribution, or frame. It can serve *only* as a baseline.

An alternative, slightly more specific way to assess your overall weight is by using the body mass index. BMI is a widely accepted measure often used by health professionals.

To calculate your body mass follow the steps below. It will be easier if you use a calculator.

1. Convert your weight to kilograms by dividing your pound weight (without clothes) by 2.2.
My 152 pounds divided by 2.2 equals **69.**
2. Convert your height to meters by dividing your total inches (without shoes) by 39.4. Take the dividend and square it.
My 71 inches divided by 39.4 equals **1.8,** *and 1.8* × *1.8 equals* **3.24.**
3. Divide your kilogram weight by your metric height squared to find your body mass.

My weight in kilograms, **69,** *divided by my height squared,* **3.24,** *results in a body mass of* **21.29.**

For women, a body mass of 21 to 23 is considered desirable. Lower body mass is considered underweight. A body mass of 27.5 or above is considered overweight. Health risk associated with excess weight increases as BMI climbs over 30, rising sharply above 35. But if you feel you only have five pounds to lose, I expect that your BMI is probably in the low to mid twenties, so the health risk is not a consideration for you.

For men, a body mass of 22 to 24 is considered desirable. Above 28.5 is overweight. Again, health risk increases proportionally above this level of BMI.

Body mass index is more precise than the calculated weight-for-height method, but both measures fail to distinguish between lean and fat body mass. So if you're a serious athlete or body builder, or if you have very large bones, you may have a relatively high body mass and still be exceptionally lean. As we work through the rest of this chapter you will factor in your specific characteristics to arrive at a much narrower weight window that is your personal ideal. I believe this individualized approach is the wave of the future in weight management, and will ultimately replace weight tables and standardized calculations as the preferred method of determining "ideal" weight.

Bone Structure

The size of your skeletal frame and the heaviness of your bones can make a big difference to your weight. A person with small bones might weigh twenty pounds less than someone with heavy bones and yet be fatter! That's why the standard height and weight charts presented three categories for small, medium, and large frames, with different recommended weight ranges for each.

But how do you know which frame category is yours? A variety of measures and standardized dimensions are used to assess frame size, but I've found that the simplest way to gauge bone structure is by the size of a person's wrist. To check your own bone structure take one hand and wrap it around the opposite wrist. Try to touch the thumb to the middle finger of the wrapping hand.

- If your thumb and middle finger overlap easily, you likely have a *small frame.*
- If the thumb and finger just meet, you have a *medium frame.*
- If the thumb and middle finger don't meet, you have a *large frame.*

Each step up in frame size is "worth" about six to ten pounds. Referring to your body mass computations, this means that, if you have small bones, your "ideal weight" will probably be located within the first third of the thirty-pound target weight range for your height. If you have a medium frame, you can aim for the middle third, and a large frame will push you toward the top third of the recommended weight range. But even after taking bone structure into account, you may still want to carry a higher than recommended weight if you are extremely fit and muscular.

Body Fat Percentage

The critical issue, when it comes to your health, fitness, and good looks, is not how much you weigh but how much of your total body mass consists of fat. As you can see from the reference box below, there's a great deal of "mass" in your body that you would not and should not want to lose. In fact, the only tissue that it's safe or desirable to lose is fat, and not even all of that! For this reason, it's essential to know approximately how much of your body mass is fat before you can decide how much to reduce.

The Lean and the Fat of It

Your Lean Body Mass
- Bones, cartilage, and teeth
- Water
- Muscle
- Blood
- Protein
- Carbohydrate/glycogen

Essential Fat
- Bone marrow fat
- Protective fat around heart and lungs
- Nerve sheath
- Reproductive fat
- High-density lipoprotein cholesterol (about 30 percent of blood cholesterol)

Nonessential Storage Fat
- Subcutaneous (just under the skin)
- Intramuscular (between muscles)
- Intraorganic (around internal organs)

Unfortunately, there is no quick, easy, and precise way to measure body composition. There are special calipers that measure the thickness of skin folds to determine fat percentage, but these measurements must be taken by a doctor or clinician with special training. Even then, accuracy varies with the instrument and the individual taking the measurement. Fat readings using calipers must be taken from at least seven different sites on the body and require tremendous precision. You should *not* try to use calipers to measure your own body fat because there is no way to ensure the accuracy of your results.

Other elaborate and expensive methods of measuring body fat include the use of infrared light rays, bioelectrical impedence, molecular "labeling" of potassium in the body, and underwater weighing. If you use one of these methods you can expect to pay anywhere from $10 to well over $100 per reading. And with all of this science, researchers still haven't found a fail-safe way to determine exactly what percentage of your body is fat. What to do?

I recommend using the Body Fat Chart on page 70 as a means of gauging your *approximate* body fat percentage. I can't guarantee that your reading will be precise to the percentage point, but it will be close enough to tell you whether you're near your ideal. Remember that if your body fat registers *anywhere* in the low to mid 20 percentile range, you should consider yourself acceptably lean.

Body Fat Chart

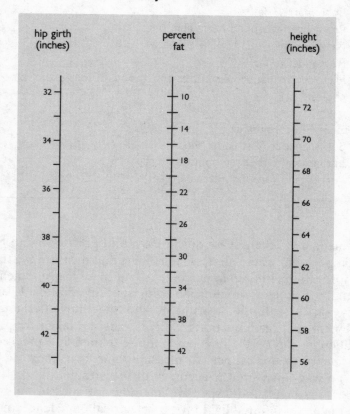

Adapted from *Sensible Fitness, 2nd edition* (p. 31) by J.H. Wilmore, Ph.D. Champaign, IL: Human Kinetics Publishers. Copyright © 1986 by Jack H. Wilmore. Reprinted by permission.

Here's how to use the Body Fat Chart:

1. Mark your height in the right-hand column.
2. Measure the circumference of your hips at the widest point, and mark this measurement in the left-hand column.
3. Use a ruler to draw a line connecting the two marks. The point where the line crosses the middle column is your estimated body fat percentage.

If I am 71″ tall and my hips measure 38″ this chart tells me that my body fat percentage is between 22 and 23 percent. More elaborate, "precise" methods have given me readings of anywhere from 18 to 23 percent, so I feel the chart is plenty accurate enough.

How about translating this body fat percentage information into pounds? Let's say I decided (for purely cosmetic purposes) to reduce to twenty-one percent body fat.

1. I would first multiply my existing weight by my body fat percentage (BFP) to find how many pounds of fat I'm starting with. That's 150 (pounds) × twenty-two percent = 33. So I'm carrying 33 pounds of body fat.

2. I would calculate my lean body mass (LBM) by subtracting my existing 33 pounds of fat from my total weight, or 150 − 33 = 117.

3. If my BFP were 21 percent, the percentage of LBM would be 79 percent, so I could calculate my target weight by dividing 117 (LBM) ÷ 79 percent = 148.

4. By subtracting my target weight from my existing weight, 150 − 148 = 2, I discover that my one percentage point drop in body fat would amount to a two-pound loss on the scale.

The main drawback with the Body Fat Chart, of course, is that it relies exclusively on the measurement of one area of the body—the hips—and does not factor in the *distribution* of fat. If those two pounds I just decided to lose were located in my hips and every other part of my body were exceptionally lean, I not only wouldn't "need" to reduce, but I probably would find it extremely difficult to lose even this small amount of weight. That's because such site-specific fat is often a product of body shape rather than "excess" fat. Which means that even after you know your overall body fat percentage, you need to consider how that mass is "arranged."

Fat Distribution: Waist-to-Hip Ratio

As I mentioned earlier in the book, body fat is not all alike. The fat around the hips and thighs that most women have in abundance is healthy fat, while the waistline fat that men tend to develop is high-risk fat that can contribute to heart disease, stroke, hypertension, and diabetes. Therefore it's not enough to know how much total body fat you have; you need to consider as well how that fat is distributed. The ratio of your waist to your hips (WHR) is the best indicator of body fat distribution. Here's how to calculate:

1. Measure around your waist at the navel. For me, that's 26 inches.

2. Measure around your hips and buttocks at their widest point. For me, 38 inches.

3. Divide the waist measurement by the hip measurement to find your waist-to-hip ratio. For me, 26 ÷ 38 = .68.

For women, a healthy ratio is anything less than .8. This means that the waist measures no more than 80 percent of the hips.

For men, the ratio should be no greater than 1.0. This means the waist should be the same size as or smaller than the hips.

How does this relate to body fat percentage? It means that if your body fat percentage is in the low to mid 20 range and your waist-to-hip ratio is under .8, you don't *need* to lose fat for the sake of your health. Remember, too, that the lower your WHR, the more difficult it may be to lose fat; especially if you are a premenopausal woman, your body will resist losing fat from the hips and thighs even as it readily sheds abdominal fat.

Genetics and Your Family Weight History

After all the calculations are said and done, I would love to tell you that you can be as lean as you want just by eating less fat and exercising more. Unfortunately, for some of us, it's not quite that easy. Genetics do play an important role in determining how fat we are. Most researchers believe that genes bear at least 25 percent of the responsibility in determining our fat levels.

But some studies in which sets of twins have been compared suggest the influence of genes is even greater. At Laval University, researcher Claude Brouchard overfed twelve sets of twins by exactly the same amount and had them follow the same basic daily routine for four months. At the end of the study, some pairs of twins had gained as little as nine pounds, some as much as twenty-eight, but the differences between twins were much smaller than among the different sets of twins. Furthermore, twins seemed to gain in the same ways as their siblings. Some sets of twins were apples, some pears. Some put on the weight entirely as fat, others mostly muscle even though everyone was sedentary throughout the study. Other studies have found that when adopted children grow up they are much more likely to weigh what their natural parents weigh than what their adoptive parents weigh.[1]

The power of genetics seems to increase when there is a family history of obesity. A child with one obese parent has about a 50 percent chance of becoming obese, and with two obese parents the risk jumps to 80 percent. Take heart—this genetic predisposition is not the same as a genetic trait; while you can't change the eye color you inherit, you *can* lower your risk of obesity by staying physically active and by following the low-fat eating principles described in this book.

Still, it's important to work within your genetic reality. If leanness runs in your family you can count your blessings, but if your parents and grandparents were all overweight, then don't beat yourself up over these five extra pounds. You deserve congratulations! And your energy will be much better spent in maintaining your weight than trying to whittle more of it away.

Age and Weight Gain

There is a small increase in body fat that typically occurs with aging. Physiologically and biologically, there is little justification for this increase, but statistically, it's a fact. In most cases, body fat rises as the level of daily activity declines. Both progressions tend to be gradual but consistent. Less time spent physically working and exercising from one decade to the next leads inevitably to a higher percentage of body fat. The majority of this increase in fat can be offset with activity. So, while you may claim a little "grace weight" as you get older, don't use age as an excuse for gaining!

Health and Weight

Sometimes health considerations must be considered when setting an ideal weight. If you have a family history of diabetes or heart disease, for example, your doctor will probably encourage you to maintain a lower than average weight. Likewise, if you suffer from arthritis or back problems you will ease the pain in your joints by staying as lean as possible.

On the other hand, it will do your health no good to be underweight —quite the contrary. The superthin have a lower resistance to many diseases and infections and have inadequate reserves of fat to aid healing in the event of surgery or prolonged illness. The message here is moderation; it can be as unhealthy to be too thin as it is to be overweight, and there's a considerable range in between where you will locate your ideal weight.

Environment and Your Weight

Believe it or not, geography can affect your physical ability to gain or lose pounds. Statistically, people who live in cold climates tend to weigh more than people in warmer locations. There are several fundamental reasons for this.

First, although many popular winter sports such as skiing and snowboarding are terrific fat burners, we rarely engage in these sports on an ongoing or daily basis the way we do warm-weather sports such as jogging, cycling, or swimming. And aside from the hours when Snowbelt residents are skiing or shoveling their driveways, they tend to spend most of their days indoors at sedentary occupations. Of course, many residents of colder climates take advantage of indoor exercise facilities, but many more, it seems, do not. Meanwhile, most Sunbelt residents spend a significant portion of each day outside performing activities that, even if they do not involve exercise per se, likely keep the body in motion.

A second reason we tend to gain more easily in wintry weather is that our bodies try to conserve fat in the cold. Appetite increases for heavier, warmer, richer foods such as stews and meats, and we are far less interested in slimming salads and fresh fruits. Richer foods plus less physical activity naturally results in weight gain, and the reverse is also true. It's not just the threat of the swimsuit that prompts women in the northern part of this country to lose a pound or two as summer approaches.

This does not mean, of course, that you're necessarily heavier if you live in a cold climate, but you do need to recognize that the elements can influence your weight. You may need to work harder than someone who lives in the South to keep yourself physically active, and it may take some extra effort to resist the lure of high-fat foods. Alternatively, you can accept the fact that your weight may climb a couple of pounds when the temperature drops in the fall—and enjoy feeling them evaporate in the summer heat.

Your Activity Habits and Your Ideal Weight

Your weight, your percentage of body fat, and your satisfaction with your body all depend a great deal on your activity level. The more exercise you get, the more likely it is that you are close to your healthiest weight. Studies have shown that, all other things being equal, people who routinely exercise tend to weigh more than twenty pounds less than people who lead sedentary lives!

But gauging activity can be tricky. The experts used to say that the only meaningful exercise was the heavy workout variety; now they say that, while vigorous activity is beneficial, it's not essential. Here, then, are the categories you need to consider when evaluating your activity level:

1. Old-fashioned exercise. You know what I mean: running, cycling, swimming, weight lifting, or playing a high-motion game such as basketball or racquetball. If you work out like this for a half hour to an hour four or more times per week, you are getting a healthy amount of exercise. But that ideally should not be your *only* physical activity.

2. Mandatory motion. Certain occupations make exercise mandatory. Construction workers, postal carriers, flight attendants, gardeners, window washers, and mothers of small children, to name just a few, can have highly physical jobs. While the specific movements may not always build or tone muscles as effectively as an exercise routine or gym workout, they do burn fat and calories. Those whose jobs require them to stay seated do not have this activity advantage—and in today's world that includes more than 90 percent of us!

3. "Local motion." Even people with desk jobs have literally hundreds of opportunities to move each day. Some are minimal, such as fidgeting or pacing. Some require a simple change of habit, such as taking the stairs instead of the elevator or hand washing the car instead of using the car wash. Some forms of "local motion" require more imagination, such as walking instead of driving to the mall or parking at the far instead of the near end of the parking lot. From minimal to maximal, all these motions add up and can dramatically alter body size and shape over time.

4. Recreational activity. Too many Americans equate leisure with movies or television. Leisure can also mean recreation—swimming, sports, games, hikes, camping, or any physical activity that is not performed dutifully for the sake of exercise but enthusiastically for fun. Your body doesn't know you're having fun; it will still burn the same amount of calories or fat as if you hated every minute! And don't overlook opportunities to involve your children, parents, or friends in a ball game or bike ride; exercise can be a social event. (I think TV has such a stranglehold on American life that we sometimes need to remind ourselves that the other Great American Pastimes are still permitted, and are much better for the waistline.)

But perhaps you're getting exercise without even realizing it!
To find out how active you really are, try clocking your activity for a

day or two using the form below. (Lawyers clock their time to keep track of their billable minutes; you can use the same method to keep track of your fitness minutes.) For an accurate reflection of your fitness level, chart your activity on one typical weekday and one typical weekend day. Keep the form or a pad of paper with you throughout the day, and at the end of each hour stop and write down exactly how you've spent that hour. Now tally the minutes when you were moving—walking, stooping, reaching, jumping, or otherwise *working* your body—and enter the total in the column marked "active minutes." Enter the total remaining minutes under "inactive minutes." At the end of the day, add up the number of minutes you were active versus inactive.

Your Lifestyle Activity Schedule

Day of the Week:
Date:

Time Block	Activities	# Active Minutes	# Inactive Minutes
Sample 10:00–11:00 A.M.	Phone: 20 min. Walk to coffee shop: 5 min. Xeroxing, standing: 15 min. Word processing: 20 min.	5	55
6–7 A.M.			
7–8 A.M.			
8–9 A.M.			
9–10 A.M.			
10–11 A.M.			
11 A.M.–12 P.M.			
12–1 P.M.			
1–2 P.M.			

2–3 P.M.			
3–4 P.M.			
4–5 P.M.			
5–6 P.M.			
6–7 P.M.			
7–8 P.M.			
8–9 P.M.			
9–10 P.M.			
10–11 P.M.			
11 P.M.–12 A.M.			
	Total minutes:		

If you have more than 30 active minutes in your day, every day, even without a formal workout session, you are probably moderately fit. If you add a serious workout three or four times per week, you will be *very* fit!

If, on the other hand, you cannot find 30 active minutes in your daily life *and* you do not exercise on a more formal basis, then you need to get moving! This does not mean dropping $70 on a pair of running shoes you use once and toss in your closet. It does not mean joining an aerobics class that is so exhausting you never return. It *does* mean stopping what you're doing for ten minutes and going out for a brisk walk with a friend. Or walking up the stairs to the top of your building on your next coffee break. Or turning on the radio and dancing. Or dusting off your exercise bike and pedaling steadily for ten minutes. Just ten minutes. But make those ten a habit, and then build on them.

Assessing Your Eating Habits

I have positioned this item relatively low on the list to illustrate that it is not necessarily the most important determinant factor in your weight; however, there obviously is a strong connection between your eating habits and your weight. And, as with exercise, the healthier and lower in fat your eating habits, the more likely it is that you're close to your ideal weight.

The guiding principles of eating that I stress are:

1. Low fat
2. High fiber
3. High carbohydrate
4. Nutritional balance and variety

If you already apply these guidelines to your eating *on a consistent basis,* you may already be at your healthiest weight.

Chart Your Personal Weight History

Every one of us has personal high and low weights. As I mentioned at the start of this chapter, my all-time high was 167, my adult low 137 pounds. That thirty-pound "window" represents the outer limits of my weight. At either end are the extremes I achieve during periods of unusual exertion, dietary manipulations, illness, or emotional highs or lows.

Somewhere in the middle is a tighter zone, which I call the target weight zone, where my body settles whenever my life returns to normal. My target zone is between 148 and 152 pounds. When I'm at this weight I feel good, my energy is high, and I find that I'm most productive. Five pounds higher—or lower—and I feel tired, out of sorts, and uncomfortable. Yet occasionally my weight does stray, and that's generally because of upheavals (positive and negative) in my life that affect how I eat and move. It's not always possible to predict how life events will impact my weight. Sometimes when I'm extremely happy I gain, and other times I lose a few pounds without even trying. But when I chart my personal weight history with dates and think about the events that accompanied certain changes, distinct patterns do emerge.

Jamie's Weight Window/Weight History

1. Age 16 (124 lbs.) Flu. My parents separate and divorce. Skipping meals to lose weight.

2. Age 17 (140 lbs.) High school graduation. Hearty eating and plenty of exercise.

3. Age 18 (155 lbs.) College, fast food, alcohol, irregular meals, little exercise.

4. Age 20 (152 lbs.) New boyfriend. Apartment living. Healthier eating but little exercise.

5. Age 21 (137 lbs.) Lowest adult weight. Fasting diets. Breakup with boyfriend. Starting to date again.

6. Age 21 (152 lbs.) College graduation. Dietetic internship. Feeling heavy.

7. Age 23 (157 lbs.) Graduate school. Poor eating habits. High stress. Walking part of daily life.

8. Age 25 (167 lbs.) Highest adult weight. Job in Boston. Loneliness. Boredom. Recreational eating. Too cold to exercise.

9. Age 26 (152 lbs.) More friends and activity, less solitary eating. Walking, jogging, skiing, health club workouts.

10. Age 29 (152 lbs.) Active. Obsessed with calories. Wanted to weigh less.

11. Age 30 (145 lbs.) Move to Nashville. Job at Vanderbilt. Relationship breakup. Increased jogging.

12. Age 31 (157 lbs.) Marriage. Bigger, more frequent meals. More food around the house.

13. Age 32 (152 lbs.) Regular exercise. Low-fat cooking and eating.

14. Age 35 (152 lbs.) Stable life, stable eating and exercise, stable weight.

15. Age 36 (146 lbs.) Divorce, stress, low appetite.

16. Age 37 (150 lbs.) Normalcy, happiness, reduced stress. Restored appetite and exercise habits.

Find Your Weight Window

By charting your weight history you'll discover the patterns that consistently affect your weight and you'll identify the target zone where your weight centers.

To make your own chart you will need a large sheet of graph paper. Using my chart as your guide, list the decades of your life, beginning with your late teens, across the middle. Up the side from that midline, list body weights from your all-time low to your all-time high. Reserve the bottom of the chart to write in what was happening in your life at different points. Now you're ready to graph.

1. Locate the approximate year/age when you reached your all-time low and your all-time high weights and plot them on the graph. At the bottom of the page below each plot point write in what was happening in your life at the time.

2. Now switch gears and think about some of the most dramatic changes in your life: when you graduated from high school or college; the first time you moved away from home; major romances and breakups; marriage; pregnancy; new jobs; promotions; big vacations; important birthdays; serious illnesses or accidents. After you've marked these events in the top section above the associated dates, try to remember your approximate weight at each event, and plot that weight on the chart.

3. Next think back over your past eating and exercise habits. Above the appropriate dates, note any severe diets you've tried—and periods when you know you were overeating; when you started a new exercise regimen—or were not exercising at all. Under each change of habit, plot your approximate weight at the time.

4. You should have quite an extensive picture of your weight history. Now take a colored pen or marker and circle the dates and weights when you remember being happiest (not with your weight but in your life). When you finish that, switch to a different color and circle the dates and weights when you were *least* happy with your life.

5. Sit back and study the results. Is there a particular weight range that corresponds to your happiest periods? What happens to your weight when you are unhappy? What happens to your weight when your life changes dramatically? Where does your weight land when you are eating normally and being moderately active?

6. Identify your target weight zone. If you're like most people this will be a three-to-five-pound range where your weight settles most of the time or most of the time when your life is going well. It's the weight you achieve when you are most happy and active and likely when you're eating healthily and getting adequate exercise, when you are feeling successful and optimistic. *It probably will not reflect your lowest weight.* That's to be expected, and it's okay. If you learn one thing from this book it's that less weight is not necessarily better weight. The ideal weight for you is the weight that suits you physically, emotionally, and psychologically. It's the weight at which your body functions most effectively and you are happiest with your life and yourself *as a whole*.

General Self-esteem: The Weight of Happiness

Study after study has shown a direct connection between low self-esteem and anxiety about weight. I have found this to be true in my weight management groups as well. When I ask participants to name their reasons for wanting to lose weight, they often say that it will help raise their self-esteem and give them a sense of control over their lives. While I agree that losing excess weight can give a psychological boost, I firmly believe that self-esteem is more a *requirement* for change than it is the *result* of change. The chicken-and-egg phenomenon. Losing weight will not help you to value yourself if you don't value yourself to begin with—and if you do not value yourself, you will probably never be content with your weight, whatever the scale says.

As you work toward identifying your personal weight goal, it is imperative that you look at your own sense of self and well-being. If you feel as if your life is out of control, that you have overwhelming problems that you cannot handle, then I honestly would advise you to close this book, forget about your weight, and focus on regaining control, if necessary by seeking professional help to deal with these other problems. It is a mistake even to think about your weight unless you are feeling positive toward yourself as a human being; only then will you be able to view your weight in the context of your life as a whole—and accept the fitness goal that is *realistically* ideal for you.

Get Real! Putting It All Together

As you may have figured out by now, there is no simple formula for calculating the exact number of pounds you should weigh. All the factors we've discussed—genetics, sex, height, bone structure, body composition, fat distribution, personal health and lifestyle—play a role in determining the weight at which you feel and function best. It's not about what size you wear or how closely your body resembles your favorite fashion model's or celebrity's. Ultimately, your recommended weight is the one you naturally achieve through lean and balanced nutrition and regular, consistent activity. Your energy level and your mood, as well as the compliments you receive, will be a better gauge of the magic measure than any standardized weight table or calculation.

When I weigh 150 pounds and am fit and lean, I both look and feel better than when I weigh 145—or even 140—but let myself become a couch potato. The same rule can apply to you.

You know when your body changes, and you notice when you become leaner. You certainly notice when your clothes fit more loosely, and when you have the strength to walk an extra ten minutes or lift a heavier bag of groceries than you used to. In the end, these changes are your best and most cost-effective assessment tools.

You and That Scale

Now. A word of warning. In spite of everything I have said, you may still feel tempted to shoot for a weight that is lower than your body is meant to go. Our cultural worship of thinness is a powerful force, and it's *hard* to stand tall and accept that you will not and should not ever be as thin as those *Vogue* models. I can't stop you from starving yourself in the pursuit of slenderness, nor can I prevent you from overdoing the strategies I offer in the rest of this book. However, you must recognize that this extra measure of leanness requires external vigilance and heroic levels of exercise and dietary control that may be harmful to your physical and emotional well-being. Are those few pounds really worth the sacrifice? I think not.

Therefore, after leading you through all these tests and calculations to determine just how close you really are to your ideal weight, I'm going to propose a really drastic next step.

Throw away your scale!

Ten years ago I would have been horrified by this suggestion. Five years ago I wouldn't have risked it. And to be quite honest, I am still capable of letting a scale ruin my whole day. And that's precisely why I think we should throw the things away. We need to focus on who we are and what we do with our lives instead of what we weigh. We need to get active, eat right, and devote the majority of our time on the people and pursuits that really *deserve* our attention. As for those last five pounds, there are plenty of other, more accurate ways to determine whether we need to lose them—or have already lost them!—than repeatedly weighing ourselves.

The best way to tell if you're the right weight is to take the recommendations of the next chapters to heart. If you eat lean and stay active your body will gravitate to its own perfect weight. And when that happens I hope you will feel so positive about your body and your life that you'll wonder how those last five pounds could ever have seemed so infuriatingly important.

Learning to Eat, Not Diet

Once upon a time nutritious meals were a routine part of daily life and people rarely ate on the run. They did not travel much or have lengthy commutes, so most of their meals were eaten at home at established times and with the entire family. People ate when they were hungry and when they gathered for celebration. They did not persecute themselves or others for eating but viewed food as a normal and natural part of life. They did not eat in hiding, and since they didn't have television sets or Sara Lee cakes or Fritos, they could not combine those elements into an evening of solitary entertainment. For entertainment, they turned to friends and social activities, such as cards, conversation, and dancing.

Does this sound hopelessly old-fashioned? Perhaps it is, but that simply demonstrates how much work we need to do to restore the balance between eating and living. That balance, in combination with a generally leaner diet, is what kept past generations "naturally" fit. It can do the same for us.

Once we stop resenting healthy nutrition we'll be able to bring our weight and eating into a realistic balance. But to do this, we need to develop a new emotional relationship with food as a supportive friend instead of an enemy or a crutch. And we need to quit dieting!

Breaking the Weight Loss Diet Habit

Dieting makes you fat.

There, I've said it. And, strange as it may seem, this statement has been proven to be true.

When researchers tracked a group of 31,000 nurses over eight years they found that the nurses who lost weight near the beginning of the study were *by far* the most likely to gain weight later on. Weight loss not only led to weight gain but it was also the strongest contributing factor to gain, stronger even than individual eating habits.[1] Researchers have also found that, while non-dieters tend to lose weight as they get older, chronic dieters put pounds on.

Why does this happen? Because the typical dieter is preoccupied with calorie restriction. She starves herself. She feels deprived. The whole time she's not eating she obsesses about food. She memorizes calorie counts. She comforts herself with the thought that in just a few days the diet will be over and she can eat everything in sight. She succeeds in losing five pounds, mostly water weight, then goes back to her previous eating patterns and regains those pounds and more within twelve months.

The secret to nondieting is not to eat everything in sight. Well, actually it is. But it's a matter of eating everything in sight in *a healthful balance.* Successful nondieters are flexible and reasonable in their eating. They don't deprive themselves, but they do take their eating cues from actual physical hunger. There is evidence that chronic dieters so confuse their bodies' normal responses that they can't tell when they are hungry. Nondieters don't have this problem; they eat when hungry until they are satisfied, and then they stop.

If you learn to use hunger as your eating guide, you will rarely overeat. But you will occasionally undereat because true hunger is diminished by a wide range of factors, including stress, anxiety, contentment, and distraction. A new love affair, a big project at work, or an engrossing movie can make you forget your hunger and skip dinner; if you're not counting calories you'll hardly notice, and you'll be much less likely to compensate for the skipped meal.

Studies comparing the patterns of dieters and nondieters have found that dieters rarely or never undereat when they're not on a reducing plan. And even when trying to follow a diet, conscientiously counting their calories and fat grams, their caloric estimates tend to be low. Studies released in 1992 found that dieters typically underestimate their calorie and fat consumption by as much as 50 percent. It's not their fault; most popular foods—especially packaged foods and restaurant dishes—are loaded with hidden calories and fat. It's also easy to misjudge portion size. I'm a trained research dietitian and yet in a clinical study a few years back I underestimated my calorie intake by 300 calories per day and my fat intake by more than 10 grams. The key difference between my underestimation and a dieter's underestimation is that I did not use my own low calorie estimates to justify eating *more*, but that is precisely what dieters do.

You know the script: "I've been so good today, and I've only had 1,100 calories, so I'm entitled to a scoop of ice cream. That'll still bring my total in under 1,300 calories." But in reality your intake may be closer to 2,000 calories, plus you're underestimating the content of that full-fat ice cream, so your true total could be even higher, including some 30 grams of fat. And the worst is, you're not really hungry for that ice cream; you're eating it because you've convinced yourself you're entitled to it.

Message: You would have been far better off if you'd listened to your stomach instead of your head, eaten a nourishing range of foods until satisfied, perhaps completing the meal with a low-fat dessert or fruit, then turned your thoughts to something that has nothing to do with eating. Counting (that is, miscounting) calories and fat grams can end up expanding your waistline!

There is another benefit to nondieting that is too often overlooked when talking about weight loss. That's good health. People who are genuinely well nourished are lean and energetic and have a high degree of immunity to infection and illness. Good eating does not make you fat. On the contrary, it gives you the energy you need to stay active, which in turn keeps you fit and reduces your body fat. And there is no way to get this kind of nutrition from any pill, supplement, or meal substitute. You need the real thing. You need food.

Calories and Calories: The Truth about the Bottom Line

Doctors used to say all calories are alike. We now know that's not true; calories come in several different forms, which make a big difference in the way the body processes them. *However,* a calorie remains the basic measure of energy that's consumed and used by the body. We burn calories to live, to eat and digest our food, to move our bodies, and to think. We store surplus calories as fat. And, bottom line, we must take in fewer *usable* calories than we burn up if we are going to lose body fat. So in order to understand the particular balance of foods required to stay fit and lean, we must first look at the body's overall caloric needs.

Resting Metabolic Rate

The resting metabolic rate (RMR) is a minimal count of the calories your body burns to stay alive: to sleep, circulate blood, and breathe. RMR does not take into account the calories used each time you stand up or walk across the room, play with your dog, or make your bed. It reflects the bare minimum number of calories you use each day.

A good estimate for RMR is 10 calories per pound.

Your weight _____ × 10 calories = _____ your RMR.

At my weight, 152 pounds, I should need about 1,520 calories to fuel my body at rest for twenty-four hours.

The ratio of fat to lean body mass skews RMR. If you have a higher than average percentage of lean body mass, your RMR will be higher than the standard estimation. If you have a higher than average percentage of fat body mass, your RMR will be lower. This is because muscle tissue, even at rest, burns three to four times more calories than fat. So, the more muscle you have, the more calories you will burn, pound for pound.

Thermic Response

Above and beyond RMR, you burn calories to digest and process the food you eat. In fact, your energy expenditure jumps measurably after every meal or snack. Approximately 10 percent of the calories you consume are burned away through this process, known as the body's *thermic response.*

But again, this figure is variable. Carbohydrates, which the body breaks down for immediate energy, produce a greater thermic response than do fats, which the body stores largely as is for future energy needs. So the more carbohydrates in your meal, the more calories your body will burn to digest them: more evidence in favor of high-carbohydrate, low-fat eating habits.

Recent studies have also shown that lean people have a significantly higher thermic response than people with a high percentage of body fat. And that difference appears to increase with the size of the meal. Researchers at the University of Vermont found that the thermic response of lean subjects after an 800-calorie meal averaged about 60 calories during the four hours after eating, but the average for obese subjects was just 40 calories.[2] A 20-calorie difference may not sound like much, but over a year those calories will add up to two purely unintentional and unconscious pounds. This helps to explain why people with a high level of body fat seem to gain weight more easily than lean folks. It also gives us yet another good reason to stay lean!

Working Metabolic Rate

So your body burns a certain number of calories at rest, plus a thermic response of about 10 percent of the calories you consume. That gives you a general idea of the calories you burn when you have a cold and spend the whole day in bed with saltines and chicken soup. But normally you use additional calories through activity. As you surely know, the more strenuous exercise you get, the more calories you burn, so precise numbers are difficult to determine without monitoring your movement throughout the day. But to make a general calculation of these "working calories," figure 20 percent of RMR for an inactive day, and up to 50 percent of RMR for an active one.

Your Total Caloric Requirement

Putting these three metabolic calculations together, I calculated my caloric range and found that I should be able to maintain my weight if I keep my caloric intake between 2,024 and 2,480 per day. In fact, these numbers were verified when I spent a night in Vanderbilt's metabolic chamber, a room specially equipped to measure a person's oxygen and carbon dioxide exchange over a twenty-four-hour period to determine exactly how many calories are burned. So, at least for a person of my build and body fat percentage, the calculations are accurate. Here's how I arrived at the final figures:

	1,520	resting metabolic rate
+ 20% of 1,520	304	working calories
+ 10% of the 2,000 cal I ate	200	thermic response
Inactive day's caloric total	2,024	
	1,520	resting metabolic rate
+ 50% of 1,520	760	working calories
+ 10% of 2,000 cal	200	thermic response
Active day's caloric total	2,480	

As you can see, if I eat 2,000 calories, I wind up with a twenty-four-calorie "weight loss" on an inactive day, compared with a 480-calorie loss on the active day. This illustrates how people who eat exactly the same thing day in and day out can see unexpected weight swings. It also explains why so many people with stable eating habits mysteriously gain weight as they get older and stop exercising.

I give this information about caloric consumption not to encourage you to become a calorie-counting fanatic but simply to give you a ballpark idea of the calories your body needs and to demonstrate how critical your activity level is in burning unwanted fat. As I said earlier, there's little use in meticulously comparing the calories you burn with the calories you consume because a) your estimates of caloric intake are likely to be low, and b) all calories are not alike.

If I took my total allotted calories in the form of potato chips and ice cream, my weight would respond in a very different way than if I consumed the same number of calories in bread, fruit, pasta, and vegetables. What makes that difference is the balance—or imbalance—between calories from fat versus carbohydrates or protein.

Breaking the Fat Habit

You may be surprised to learn that lean people may actually eat more food than people with high body fat—in one study, twice as much true food weight. Though this seems to confirm many overweight people's claim that they gain "just by looking at food," surveys have found that most obese people consume a higher percentage of high-fat foods than their leaner counterparts. And the research is now conclusive that our body fat levels are determined less by how much we eat than by how much of what we eat is itself composed of fat.

The importance of fat can be explained in part by simple math. A gram of fat contains 9 calories, and scientists are considering upping its value to 11 calories to reflect more accurately its true impact on the body. By contrast, carbohydrates and protein contain just four calories per gram. Less than half the calories of fat! Furthermore, unlike many high-carbohydrate and lean protein foods, most high-fat foods contain neither fiber nor water. They are less bulky and therefore less filling, so we tend to eat more of them before feeling satisfied.

This inequity has to do with fat's function. Fat is important for healthy cell membranes and nerve sheaths, and also to facilitate the absorption of fat-soluble vitamins such as A, D, E, and K. But fat's primary functions are insulating the body against cold and storing reserve energy. Fat cells are designed to hold as much energy as possible in the most efficient way. Likewise, the body is programmed to hold on to fat for long-term energy and to actively *resist* losing it. Remember, only 3 percent of the calories in fat are burned during the passage from digestion to storage as body fat, compared to 23 percent of the calories in carbohydrates. And the body makes every attempt to use those carbs for immediate energy *instead* of storing them as fat.

Why should the body squander one nutrient and hoard another? Remember, our primitive ancestors had carbohydrates in abundance because they relied on fruit and grain for most of their food, but they had fat only occasionally, through the game they hunted. Their bodies adapted to frequent fat shortage by creating this built-in fat-hoarding mechanism. For better or worse, we must now manufacture a similar shortage of fat in our diets in order to restore the balance our bodies were designed for.

This manufactured "fat shortage" requires far less effort than you might imagine. In a study at the Boston medical center where I worked in the 1980s, my colleague Dr. George Blackburn found that women make an average of twenty to thirty food choices each day. For example, as you stand in front of the bakery case, you choose to have the doughnut instead of the French roll, or for lunch you opt for tuna salad instead of a turkey sandwich. Dr. Blackburn found that when the women in his study switched just seven of those food choices from their customary high-fat selections to low-fat options, the women lost about 5 percent of their original weight. For a 150-pound woman, that's seven and a half pounds!

Another study of some 700 men and women, conducted at Laval University in Canada, found that a 20 percent difference in fat intake caused a ten-pound difference in body weight in women and a twelve-pound difference in men.[3] The high-fat eaters also had proportionally more harmful abdominal body fat than hip and thigh fat. This indicates that, if we reduced the fat in our diet from the American standard of 40 percent to 20 percent, we would be leaner and lighter. Due to the higher percentage of fast-burning carbohydrates, we would have more energy. Due to the lower blood cholesterol that comes with reducing fat, we would remain healthier and more active well into later life. And even while losing weight, we'd actually be eating more!

The 80-20 "Fat-Cat" Rule

You could meticulously cut your fat intake to account for 10 percent of your daily calories and still maintain good health, but you will probably find that it's more realistic to follow what Dr. Martin Katahn and I, here at Vanderbilt, dubbed the 80-20 Rule: a minimum of 80 percent low-fat foods containing less than 3 grams of fat per serving, and a maximum of 20 percent "regular" and "full-fat" foods containing more than 3 grams of fat per serving.

Note that I said "regular" as well as "full-fat." I would not recommend, for example, that you take a fifth of your day's calories in the form of pure butter, cream cheese, or olive oil. These high-octane fats should be used sparingly and preferably not every day. But cheese pizza, a lean burger, or a blueberry muffin would fall into that second, "regular" category. All have other nutritious ingredients, but they also have a considerable fat content. These regular menu items make up some 50 percent of the typical American diet, which is why we have a national weight problem. (It's estimated that 85 percent of American women need to reduce their total fat intake!) Under the 80-20 rule, these regular foods (3–7 grams fat), together with those occasional full-fat treats (7 or more grams), should make up no more than 20 percent of your daily food choices. That means, if you average twenty to thirty food choices total each day, then four to six of those selections may contain more than 3 grams of fat per serving; the rest would be low-fat.

Of course, to observe these limits you need to familiarize yourself with the fat content of the foods you most frequently eat. This does *not* necessarily mean counting daily fat grams but simply knowing whether foods rank as low, moderate (regular), or high in fat (full-fat). I like to call these three groupings the basic Fat-Cats, or Fat Master categories.

Sample "Fat-Cat" Food Choice Chart

"Low" Fat-Cat	*"Regular" Fat-Cat*	*"Full" Fat-Cat*
2 oz. turkey, white meat, skinless	2 oz. roast beef	2 oz. bologna
97% fat-free ham sandwich w/mustard	Grilled chicken sandwich, no mayo	Cheeseburger
1 cup vegetarian chili	1 cup chili w/ beans and lean beef	1 cup beef stroganoff
1 cup broth-based soup	1 cup beef or ham soup	1 cup cream soup
Salad w/non- or low-fat dressing	Salad w/ 2 T. vinaigrette on side	Caesar salad or salad with creamy dressing
Pasta w/marinara sauce	Spaghetti w/ medium meatball	Macaroni and cheese
English muffin	Blueberry muffin	Medium croissant
1/2 cup nonfat frozen yogurt or ice milk	1/2 cup pudding	1/2 cup premium ice cream

To figure out which Fat-Cat a particular food belongs to, simply look at its fat gram count for a standard portion. In general:

• Low Fat-Cat foods will have a fat count of 0–3 grams per serving.
• Regular Fat-Cat foods have a fat count of 3–7 grams per serving.
• Full Fat-Cat foods have a fat count of 7 or more grams per serving.

For quick reference, you will find a listing of common foods with the corresponding portion sizes, divided into Fat-Cats, in the Fat Master Food Guide at the back of the book. Use these listings to familiarize yourself with the broad variety of desirable Low Fat-Cat foods and to check your daily intake against the 80-20 rule.

To give you an idea of how the 80-20 rule works, here's a sample day's food consumption:

80%: Low-Fat Foods (22 food choices)	20%: Regular/Full-fat Foods (6 food choices)
Coffee	With 1 tbsp. whole milk
Whole wheat toast and jam	1 egg scrambled in 1 tsp. butter
Grapefruit juice	
Apple	
Coffee	With 1 tbsp. whole milk
Turkey, lettuce, mustard sandwich	1 slice Swiss cheese
Pretzels	1 chocolate chip cookie
Carrot and celery sticks	
Raisins	
Banana	
Nonfat frozen yogurt	
Skim milk	
Clear broth	
Stir-fry chicken and vegetables	2 tsp. sesame oil
Steamed rice	
Glass of white wine	
Mandarin oranges in syrup	
Fortune cookie	
Air-popped popcorn	
Soda	

Now, this menu lists a lot of food. It should be enough to satisfy you on an ordinary day. But it might seem rather spartan on your birthday or anniversary. What do you do on those special occasions when the meal just doesn't seem complete without a wedge of cake with premium ice cream? By all means, go ahead. A big dessert will not make you fat if you eat it only on your birthday. And a few french fries or a slice of pepperoni pizza won't make you fat if you eat them only a few times a month. Just be careful about *frequency*. Reserve Full Fat-Cat treats for special occasions, and pace yourself so that, *on average,* you observe the 80-20 rule, emphasizing leaner choices.

One of the cardinal laws of weight control is the law of averages. It hardly matters *what* you eat on any single day, but it matters a great deal what you eat over a week, over a month, over a year. It's the average balance of carbohydrate to fat that will make the ultimate difference to your figure. I state the 80-20 rule as a convenience because we tend to think about eating in terms of a single day. But if you have a 40 percent regular/full-fat day on Monday and limit your intake to 10 percent on Tuesday and Wednesday (that's 10 percent of food choices, remember, not 10 percent of calories from fat), you'll still be within the recommended guidelines. Don't agonize over occasional indulgences, just be sure that they really are *occasional.*

In the weight management program follow-up group that I run at Vanderbilt I repeatedly challenge my group to consider the *consistency* of their low-fat food choices and activity patterns. "Well, I did take a long walk last weekend," or "I skipped the cheese on my burger last Tuesday" just won't make the difference unless these choices reflect an ongoing overall pattern of low-fat eating and daily physical activity. Notice that the word is "consistency," though, not "perfection." Having that 20-percent leeway can make all the difference in preventing frustration, deprivation, and regain.

Even "Good Fats" Are Fattening

Some fat, of course, is necessary and permissible within the 80-20 rule for cooking or flavoring food. I recommend that you not exceed 3 teaspoons of added fat a day. But there are so many different kinds of cooking fats: oil, butter, cream, and lard, to name but a few. There are saturated and unsaturated, polyunsaturated, and monounsaturated fatty acids, high-cholesterol and low-cholesterol. The array of fat-related information on food labels can be bewildering, especially when you're trying to make a simple decision between liquid or stick margarine, or one vegetable oil over another. Are they equally unhealthy? Are they equally fattening?

The short answer is that, gram for gram, these products all contain the same amount of fat. So, while the various types of fat have different effects on your blood cholesterol and on your risk of heart disease and cancer, they have the identical effect on your weight and body fat percentage.

To understand the health risks associated with fat, you need to know a little about cholesterol. This fatty substance is produced by our own bodies and is found in food products from animal sources. It is useful in cell maintenance and the production of certain hormones. Excess cholesterol, however, can build up on the inside of arteries and contribute to heart disease.

Since our bodies manufacture all the cholesterol we really need, any cholesterol we take in through diet could be said to be "excess." Yet the greatest dietary impact on blood cholesterol is from saturated fat, the type of fat that is generally hard at room temperature. It is difficult to eliminate such basic foods as butter, cream, milk, cheese, eggs, and meat, which all contain saturated fat and cholesterol. *However,* the lower the fat content, the lower the saturated fat and, with few exceptions, the lower the cholesterol: a cup of whole milk contains a whopping 34 mg. of cholesterol, but skim milk contains just 4 mg. So by switching to nonfat and low-fat dairy products and trimming all visible fat and skin from meat and poultry, we reduce not just calories and total fat but also saturated fat and cholesterol intake.

Products derived exclusively from plants are cholesterol free. Oils, nuts, fruits, vegetables, and grains contain zero cholesterol. However, saturated fats, whether from animal or vegetable sources, can cause trouble by encouraging the body to increase its own production of cholesterol, which may raise blood cholesterol and increase heart disease risk. But researchers now believe that oils such as canola and olive oil, which are rich in monounsaturated fatty acids, can actually *lower* blood cholesterol levels.

If this all seems hopelessly confusing, take heart. If you cut your total fat intake to 20 percent, you really don't need to worry what specific type of fat is used. In our weight loss research groups at Vanderbilt we found a dramatic drop in cholesterol and saturated fats in the diets of those trimming fat *overall,* regardless of the type of oils or spreads people were using. The health benefits remained largely the same as long as the total amount of dietary fat remained low. This means that you needn't spend long hours in the grocery aisle trying to interpret those analyses of fatty acids; buy the oil or spread whose taste you most enjoy, but use it *sparingly* and with plenty of nonfat foods. If your favorite fat is butter, even that's okay within these limits. In terms of weight control, butter and margarine actually have a slight advantage over oils because they contain 100 calories and 11 fat grams per tablespoon, while oils contain 120 calories and 14 fat grams.

Still, if you don't have a personal preference, it's wise to keep animal fats and highly saturated fats such as palm and coconut oil, butter, or lard to a minimum. When you must use fat for cooking, I recommend using oils such as canola or olive oil, which are lowest in saturated fats and highest in monounsaturated fatty acids. Just remember, while these oils and fats may have different effects on your health, they will all have exactly the same effect on your figure, so use no more than 3 teaspoons per day.

Carbohydrates: Discount Calories

Enough about restricting food. Now let's talk about the foods you can and should be eating. First and foremost: complex carbohydrates. You know, bread, pasta, rice, cereal, potatoes, low-fat crackers, and grains. Yes, all those "starches" the diet books of old told us we shouldn't touch. Now, in light of the new nutritional research, these starches have been "rehabilitated" to take their place beside green and yellow vegetables and fruit as the mainstay foods of the fit and lean. Basic recommendation: at *least* half the calories we consume should come from carbohydrates.

That adds up to between six and eleven servings each day. What constitutes a serving? Here are some examples:

I slice bread
1/2 bagel
1/2 cup cooked pasta
I cup cold cereal
1/2 cup cooked cereal
1/2 cup couscous
5 low-fat crackers
I small tortilla

Yielding 4 calories per gram, carbohydrates are the body's energy boosters. The calories in carbohydrates are the first to burn as fuel and the last to be stored as fat. Carbohydrates also contain chemicals that signal the brain to reduce appetite and lift our mood, so they actually help us eat less. Contrary to the negative spin that was popular during the heyday of the fad high-protein diets in the 1970s, carbohydrates are a boon to weight control.

Here is an overview of the key ways the body uses carbohydrates.

• Your muscles rely primarily on carbohydrates for the energy to move. If you eat a peanut butter sandwich and then go to the gym, the first calories you burn off will come from the bread, the last from the peanut butter.

• Your muscles also use carbohydrates in the conversion of fat for energy. So by eating carbohydrates (bread) with higher-fat foods (peanut butter) you make it easier for your body to burn the incoming fat instead of storing it. By eating carbohydrates *without* an accompanying high-fat food, you encourage your body to burn its existing fat. Fat intake, by contrast, does not stimulate oxidation of body fat. If you eat a tablespoon of peanut butter alone (8 grams of fat and 100 calories), then go out and run off 300 calories, your body will pull most of those calories from existing carbohydrate stores; the peanut butter fat will go to your thighs, hips, or belly, joining the rest of the body fat your system is carefully hoarding.

• Your brain requires a minimum of about 400 carbohydrate calories each day to function; the brain uses *only* calories derived from carbohydrates. So while fruit and grains may help you create great thoughts, butter and cream will not.

• The carbohydrate levels in the bloodstream serve to control appetite. When the levels are low, hunger sets in and you become more susceptible to impulse and binge eating. A steady, moderate intake of carbohydrate can minimize hunger.

• Carbohydrates also prompt the brain to produce a chemical called serotonin, which has a calming, soothing effect on mood and may reduce hunger. Thus, carbohydrates help curb anxiety and ward off nervous eating.

• Your muscles can store an average of 400 to 500 carbohydrate calories (100 grams of carbohydrate) for short-term energy use before releasing the surplus to turn into fat. However, the more muscle mass you have, the more carbohydrate calories your body can store in this intermediary form, known as glycogen. Put it another way, the more muscle mass you have, the more carbohydrates you can eat without them turning to fat.

• When the muscle stores for glycogen fill up, the extra carbohydrate calories will be converted and stored as fat. But about one-quarter of the energy contained in carbohydrates is consumed during their conversion to fat. In other words, if you eat a 200-calorie bagel, the most that can possibly stay with you as body fat is 150 calories. This conversion deduction is your "carbohydrate discount." Remember, our fat stores come almost exclusively from the fat in our diets; studies have shown that less than 5 percent of body fat originates from carbohydrates.

The body's specific carbohydrate need is determined by three factors:

1. The amount of lean body mass. Only muscles burn carbohydrates, so the more muscle tissue you have, the more carbohydrates you will burn.

2. The type of activity you perform. Activities that use the body's large muscle groups, such as those found in the thigh, abdominal, and upper body regions, burn more carbohydrates than activities that are concentrated in the smaller muscle groups. Activities that involve muscles in several parts of the body simultaneously burn more carbohydrates than "spot reducing" exercises focused on a single area.

3. The intensity of exercise. Jogging a ten-minute mile burns more carbohydrates than walking a half mile in the same time. The harder you work your muscles the more fuel you will burn. This applies to overall calories and fat, of course, as well as carbohydrates, though, as we'll see later, lower intensity exercise over longer periods can actually boost fat burning.

What About Sugar?

Typically, when people want to lose weight the first thing they cut out are sweets. That's because sugar makes us fat. Doesn't it?

In fact, sugar is no more fattening than any other kind of carbohydrate or than protein, which is to say it contains 4 calories per gram. Sugar, a simple carb (because its molecular structure is simpler than that of complex carbs such as fruit and starch), contains less than half the calories of fat. So a little sugar in your coffee or in the form of hard candies, or nonfat frozen yogurt, or fruit preserves is entirely permissible. It may even help keep you lean by satisfying the craving for sweetness and preventing you from splurging on high-fat treats. Where sugar can get you into trouble is if you eat it in large quantities or in combination with fat.

The problem with sugar in quantity, aside from the cavities it may cause, is that it contains no nutritional components other than calories, and it doesn't fill you up. One Tootsie Roll Pop has the same number of calories as two cups of cantaloupe or three peaches. But the fruit contains fiber and water as well as natural sugar, and so will satisfy your hunger and help curb your appetite longer than the candy will. The fruit also contains essential vitamins and minerals that your body needs for good health.

As I showed you earlier in this chapter, you will burn a certain number of calories based on your resting metabolism and activity level. Out of the foods that provide these calories you also need to get the basic vitamins, minerals, and proteins your body needs. If you get too many of your calories straight from sugar, you will either end up with a poor quality diet or you'll need to take in surplus calories to meet your nutritional quotas. Even with the 23 percent "carbohydrate discount," which applies to sugar just as it does other carbs, the majority of those unused calories will over time wind up as fat.

There is also some evidence that when sugar is eaten together with fat, the combination may be especially likely to wind up around your waist or hips. Recent research from the University of Etsukuba in Japan suggests that sugar stimulates the release of insulin, which in turn encourages fat to be stored. If this is true, then foods such as chocolate bars, doughnuts, pie, and full-fat ice cream may be more fattening than their calories and fat count suggest. They certainly are more fattening than nonfat sweets such as frozen yogurt, jelly beans, gumdrops, or licorice.

Bottom line, there's nothing wrong with a small amount of sugar, even if you have it every day. I would advise you to use sugar substitutes only in moderation because studies have shown that they make little difference on total daily calorie consumption. Many people replace the calories saved with calories from something else. Plus, most sugar substitutes have such heightened sweetness that they set an artificially high taste standard, cuing you to prefer much sweeter foods than you otherwise would. Finally, some artificial sweeteners have been shown to cause possible health problems in some people.

As for desserts, if you have a choice, stick with nonfat sweets, preferably ones such as fruit desserts that have real nutritional value, but remember that even fat-free calories can eventually wind up as body fat.

Miracle Fiber?! What's It Got to Do with Weight Loss?

Another form of carbohydrate that *is* good for fat loss is dietary fiber. Fibers are complex carbohydrates that can't be broken down by enzymes in the human digestive tract. Most commonly found in whole grains, fruits, and vegetables, fiber has acquired a reputation as a kind of miracle cure because of its many health benefits. These include:

• Fiber's laxative effect. Fiber absorbs water inside the intestine, making stools softer and easier to pass and speeding up the process of excretion.
• The water-soluble fibers in fruit, legumes, oats, and carrots have been shown to reduce blood cholesterol levels.
• The fibers in fruit and legumes seem to help control levels of blood sugar and insulin in diabetics.
• The nonsoluble kind of fiber found in whole grains and bran seems to help reduce the risk of intestinal cancer.

If these aren't reasons enough to boost your intake of fruits, vegetables, and whole grains, consider that people who regularly eat high-fiber foods tend to weigh less and have less body fat than people with low-fiber eating habits.

Here's how fiber helps fight fat:

• Off the top, high-fiber foods contain a built-in calorie deduction because the calories contained in the fiber are included in the food's official calorie count but are not usable by the body. As much as 10 percent of a food's calories may be locked up in fiber.
• Fiber binds with small amounts of fat and protein, carrying them out of the body as waste. This reduces the total calories and fat your body absorbs from the food you eat with the fiber.
• Because it absorbs water and swells during digestion, fiber fills you up. You will feel satisfied with fewer calories of a high-fiber meal than you will with a low-fiber meal.
• Fiber takes longer to chew. It slows down the eating process, allowing time for the signal from your digestive tract to reach your brain that you've eaten enough.

The main drawbacks of a high-fiber diet, especially if you increase your fiber intake suddenly, are intestinal gas and discomfort. Women should aim for 20 to 40 grams of fiber a day, men for as much as 50 grams, but if you're not used to whole grains and raw vegetables, don't try to make the conversion overnight. Instead, follow these guide-lines:

Increase your fiber intake gradually. Discomfort, gas, and diarrhea occur when you introduce more fiber than the bacteria in your intestines can easily break down. By increasing your consumption of fiber slowly you give the intestinal bacteria a chance to adapt, thus minimizing discomfort.

Drink lots of fluids. Without enough water, fiber can have a constipating instead of laxative effect.

Don't limit yourself to one type of fiber. If you eat a range of raw foods such as fruits, vegetable, and grains you will get all the health benefits fiber has to offer.

Protein: Building Strong Muscle

Over the past few decades, high-protein diets have been among the most popular fad diets. They have also had some of the highest rates of regain and have done the most harm to dieters' health. Contrary to dieting mythology, protein is neither an appetite suppressant nor a metabolic boon. It *is* an essential nutrient, but most of us eat at least twice as much protein as our bodies really require for good health.

As you probably already realize, proteins contain the basic building blocks, amino acids, that our bodies use to maintain muscle, bone, skin, blood, and other organs. Some proteins, primarily those found in milk, eggs, meat, and other animal sources, are called *complete* proteins because they contain a balance of different amino acids, which the body can apply directly to its own protein needs. A few animal proteins and most proteins derived from vegetable sources contain only certain amino acids and thus are called *incomplete;* you need to eat several different incomplete proteins together for your body to utilize fully the amino acids they contain. Rice and beans together, for example, add up to complete protein. Or corn and lentils.

Virtually every cell in the body contains protein, and young children require a high proportion of protein in the diet so that they will grow strong and healthy. The rest of us also require a steady supply of protein because our bodies cannot store this nutrient for future use. But we require far less than is commonly assumed, and we get protein from far more food sources than most of us realize.

Your need for protein is calculated on the basis of your *ideal* lean weight, because only lean body tissue requires a protein supply.

Assuming you are over nineteen years old and neither pregnant nor nursing, you should figure .36 grams of protein per pound of ideal body weight. (If you are pregnant, your requirement rises to .62 grams per pound; if nursing, to .53 grams per pound. Teenagers require between .39 and .5 grams per pound, and younger children up to .9 grams per pound.)

Your ideal weight _____ × .36 grams = _____ g. protein needed per day.

If I accept 152 pounds as my ideal weight, here's my calculation: 152 lbs. × .36 = 54.72 grams of protein per day.

How does that translate into food? One double cheeseburger contains about 54.72 grams of protein. The problem is, that double cheeseburger also contains 37 grams of fat—which means that in one burger I'd get as much protein and more fat than I need for an entire day! But contrary to popular belief, meat is not our only source of protein, and since it carries such a high fat content it is not even the preferred source. Legumes such as soybeans, chickpeas, brown and black beans, are the richest sources of vegetable protein, with soybeans the closest in quality to animal protein. They are also virtually fat free in their natural form and in many prepared forms. They contain lots of fiber, and they are extremely filling. Dieters traditionally have given legumes a bum rap because of their relatively high caloric content (compared to typical "diet foods" such as carrots and celery), but I have found that these foods are a real boon for fat control and deserve to be on everyone's daily menu.

The table below shows a variety of combinations, including several different types of legumes, that would meet a total day's protein needs and still fit within our 80-20 rule for fat control.

Meeting the Daily Protein Need

To illustrate the variety and the relatively small quantities of food required to fulfill a day's protein needs, I've put together a list of foods that would supply me with all the protein I need for three days. My full day's requirement is 54.72 grams for my ideal weight. Each of these daily food combinations will supply complete protein with a minimum of fat.

Food	*Amount*
DAY ONE	
Shredded wheat	2 biscuits
Skim milk	1 cup
Cream of mushroom soup, made with skim milk	1 cup
Turkey, no skin	3 ounces
Navy beans	1/2 cup
DAY TWO	
Lean ground beef	4 ounces
Lentil soup	1 cup
Bread	2 slices
Banana	1 large
DAY THREE	
Spaghetti	1 cup
All-bean chili	1 cup

Eating a whole day's protein allowance in a single meal does us little good because the body can't assimilate all that protein at one time, nor can it store it for the next day. Spreading protein between meals and snacks throughout the day allows our bodies to obtain the most benefit.

What Happens when We Eat More Protein than We Need?

It's a dieting fallacy that surplus protein simply burns itself off. The truth is that it is either used for energy or turned into fat. Like carbohydrates, protein loses about one-quarter of its caloric value during this conversion process. Unlike carbohydrates, however, excess protein must go through the kidneys, where the nitrogen in the protein molecule is removed for excretion before the rest of the protein can be changed into usable calories or fat. The more protein we eat, the more water we need (up to ten glasses per day) to flush out the kidneys.

But even if you drink enough water, an excessive protein intake places an unnecessary and potentially dangerous burden on the kidneys, particularly if you have a preexisting (and perhaps undiagnosed) kidney condition or are over age sixty. Too much protein can also create a deficit in calcium, which will cause a weakening of bones and teeth. And, I repeat, even if 23 percent of surplus protein is burned up during conversion, you will probably end up wearing the remaining 77 percent as fat.

The secret to fat loss is not to eat high protein but to eat high carbohydrate with just as much protein as your body needs for good health. And that means eating a wide variety of low-fat foods with a moderate protein content rather than those fat-laden meats with soaring protein content that your body doesn't need. As you'll discover throughout the rest of the book, this is neither difficult nor unpleasant, and it means you get to eat *more* and still reduce body fat.

Alcohol: The Good and the Bad

While scientists know that alcohol affects the body differently than most nutrients, they are still learning about this chemical's effect on fat. So far, the news is mixed.

Alcohol contains 7 calories per gram, almost twice as many as carbohydrates or protein and nearly as many as fat. But modest alcohol consumption does not appear to increase body mass. Numerous studies have shown that nondrinkers tend to have significantly greater body mass than moderate drinkers. A study of more than 5,000 young adults conducted at the University of Utah[4] showed that the leanest women, based on body mass and skin fold thickness and waist-to-hip ratio, drank between one and three servings of alcohol per week. The leanest men consumed between two and six drinks per week.

This same study found that certain forms of alcohol, especially beer, seem to increase abdominal fat even if they do not increase total body fat. Across the board—men and women, black and white—the regular beer drinkers in the study really did have larger "beer bellies" than any other group. Hard liquor also shows a slight tendency to increase waist fat. The striking news is that moderate *wine drinkers have lower body mass and lower waist-to-hip ratio* than any other group of drinkers or nondrinkers.

Does this mean you should start guzzling bottles of bordeau and chardonnay for the sake of your weight? Of course not. Look at the number of servings *per week* the thinnest women drank in that Utah study. The key word here is *moderate.* We're talking an average of less than one glass of wine per day. If recent research on the benefits of red wine for the heart is correct, you may want to make that one glass red rather than white. (Red wine contains substances that, in modest doses, may prevent cholesterol from clogging arteries, but this evidence is far from definitive!) The main point is that you needn't deprive yourself of drinking for the sake of your waistline, especially not if you are within five pounds of your ideal weight.

Having said this, I will warn you that, even if alcohol itself isn't fattening, its effect on appetite can be, and this is another reason to drink modestly. Most of us eat more when we drink liquor of any kind. That's because alcohol is what psychologists call a *disinhibitor*. It cuts through our normal inhibitions. We feel less anxious, less cautious, and less restrained when we drink. For many, that's the prime reason *for* drinking. Alcohol gives the sense of reducing stress. But one of the restraints drinking removes is the restraint of appetite. Alcohol weakens restraint and heightens the sensation of hunger. We eat more at parties where we are also drinking. We are more likely to take second helpings at meals while drinking wine—especially if we're on our second or third glass. And we are more likely to reach for the rich, high-fat, high-cholesterol selections that we might resist if not under the influence.

Alcohol also plays tricks with the body's fluid balance. Initially, it has a diuretic effect. If I have a glass or two of wine in the evening, I am often a pound or two lighter the following morning. Alcohol *temporarily* removes water from cells throughout the body and lowers overall body weight. But the cells subsequently retain *more* water than they've lost, so that within a day after drinking that wine my weight will climb up to a pound or two higher than normal. Again, as long as alcohol consumption is limited to an occasional glass of wine, this poses no problem. But if you do drink, you should anticipate these side effects.

Water and Weight

If the five pounds you want to lose are five pounds you never saw before this morning, I have good news! They may be gone by tomorrow without your doing a thing. You guessed it: water weight.

Even without the influence of alcohol, most of us average a daily "swing weight" of two pounds, and we may gain or lose as much as five pounds due to dietary bulk and fluid retention; some studies have shown gains even up to nine pounds in men and the very overweight. Sometimes this water weight shows up as swelling of the breasts (especially premenstrually), fingers and hands, ankles, and abdomen. All this is perfectly normal and has no direct relation to permanent weight gain. But it can be annoying.

Part of the fluctuation is due, quite simply, to the volume of food and water consumed. The reason diet books always tell you to weigh yourself first thing in the morning is that a large mug of black coffee and some juice can put a half pound on you, which you'll see if you weigh right after drinking it. But the chemical content of the food and beverages you consume can also make a big difference.

Carbohydrates and protein have a much higher water content than does fat, and therefore weigh more. Carbohydrates also require more water for digestion and storage as glycogen within the muscles, liver, and, to some extent, in fat cells. In fact, three-fourths of the weight of glycogen is temporary water weight. This is why it's possible to "gain" a pound on the scale by eating just 1,800 calories of pure carbohydrate, while it takes 3,500 calories of fat to cause a one-pound rise. The difference is that the weight increase from carbohydrates consists of less than one-fourth of a pound of actual body mass, while the fat gain is all body mass.

The different effects of fat, carbohydrates, and protein on water weight are responsible for a lot of the mistakes commonly made in dieting. Low-calorie and high-protein diets, for example, produce an impressive and almost immediate weight loss because they're so low in carbohydrates. But most of that loss is water weight, which decreases because the glycogen stores drop to about one-third of normal. When the glycogen stores return to their normal levels after the diet, the weight returns. Studies have shown that dieters on very low-calorie diets can lose up to eleven pounds *without losing any body fat.* This explains why high-protein, low-carbohydrate diets create the illusion of initial success, only to lead inevitably to failure.

On the other hand, a diet low in fat and high in carbohydrates can increase glycogen stores to more than double their normal levels, which in turn causes a water weight gain. If you insist on weighing yourself frequently, this can be discouraging. That's one reason I urge you to get rid of your scale and, instead, use the fit of your clothes and the mirror to measure your progress. The temporary gain in water weight due to high carbohydrate intake often masks an actual *loss* of fat.

This all means that you will likely weigh more the morning after dining on a half pound of vegetarian pasta than you would after eating a half pound of fried clams and onion rings, but a day later the water weight from the pasta will be gone while the fat weight from the fried food has taken up permanent residence on your hips. You tell me which meal is better for your figure.

Another factor that can affect water weight is salt. Normally, the body self-regulates the amount of sodium in the system by taking what it needs from food and excreting the rest. The body uses salt in the fluid that maintains cell function. That fluid contains a precise ratio of salt to water, so if the body is retaining sodium, it must also retain water to keep the ratio in balance. However, sodium retention is quite rare. Less than 10 percent of the population are truly "sodium sensitive" and most of these folks respond to sodium with an increase in blood pressure rather than increased water retention. But salt can cause a *temporary* water weight increase if you're not used to it. Say you rarely eat salt but dine one night at a Japanese restaurant that uses a lot of soy sauce in cooking. Your body may hoard water for a few hours in order to balance this sudden onslaught of sodium. The difference can be as much as a pound or two.

The solution to water retention, ironically, is to drink *more* fluids. The body's response to water is similar to its response to starvation. If it's not getting enough, it automatically goes into conservation mode. When you drink lots of water you send a signal to the cells in your body that it's okay to circulate. In effect, you flush out your system. Contrary to diet mythology, this does not have any affect on fat loss, but it does reduce excess fluid retention and contribute to your overall health. (In California, talk show hosts make jokes about all the health- and weight-conscious women running around with Evian bottles tucked under their belts, but water really is good for you and for your weight.)

Drinking water also helps mitigate against fluid retention caused by hormonal changes during the menstrual cycle and pregnancy. That bloated feeling many of us experience before each period may signal a gain of up to two pounds of water weight. Again, this weight melts away naturally within days. It is no cause for panic!

The Food Pyramid: Mastering the Nutritional Balancing Act

The easiest way to evaluate the nutritional balance of your current eating habits is to use the U.S. Department of Agriculture's Food Guide Pyramid, shown on p. 108. (You might modify the original pyramid slightly to encourage higher consumption of high-protein, zero-fat beans and legumes.) Without going into detailed caloric or fat gram content, the pyramid shows the amounts of different types of food you need to eat each day for optimal health. When used in conjunction with the 80-20 rule, it is also an excellent guide for low-fat eating.

Serving Equivalents

- Fruit: 1 piece raw fruit or 1/2 cup
- Vegetables: 1/2 cup
- Meat/Poultry/Fish: 3 ounces cooked
- Breads: 2-ounce slice or single portion (see pp. 285–86)
- Pasta: 1/2 cup cooked
- Rice: 1/2 cup cooked
- Beans and peas: 1/2 cup cooked
- Cereals: 1-ounce serving, about 1 cup cold cereal, 1/2 cup cooked
- Milk: 1 cup
- Cheese: 1 ounce
- Yogurt: 1 cup

In my weight groups I review my participants' food diaries every few weeks to make sure they are eating a varied, balanced diet with the pyramid as the guiding foundation. I write them notes: "You are averaging only two servings of fruit and vegetables a day." I also offer suggestions for improving the balance, such as keeping fresh fruit at the office, using shredded vegetables or grains in casseroles, or relying on the convenience of frozen vegetables. It is permissible to combine different types of foods and take "credit" on the pyramid for several groups within the same dish. Casseroles, stews, soups, and salads all make excellent multigroup entrees.

The object in using the pyramid is not to compulsively list everything that goes into your mouth but simply to be aware of the general content of your diet, making sure that the emphasis is on starches, fruits, and vegetables, and the *de*emphasis is on fats and high-fat protein sources. It usually requires some adjustment to shift the emphasis of eating away from high-protein foods to carbohydrate sources, but with practice it eventually becomes habit.

To Supplement or Not To Supplement

The Food Guide Pyramid notwithstanding, in my experience and as evidenced by national food consumption surveys, Americans tend to eat plenty, but we also eat poorly. Less than 10 percent of us consume the recommended number of fruit and vegetable servings. Most opt for higher fat, higher sugar, and lower nutrition in the name of convenience. Standard weight loss practices place good nutrition in further jeopardy.

Food Guide Pyramid

A Guide to Daily Food Choices

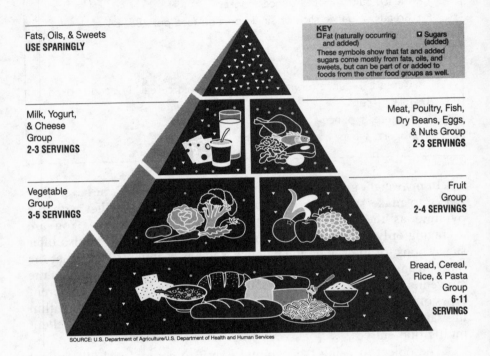

Fats, Oils, & Sweets
USE SPARINGLY

KEY
□ Fat (naturally occurring   ☑ Sugars
and added)   (added)
These symbols show that fat and added
sugars come mostly from fats, oils, and
sweets, but can be part of or added to
foods from the other food groups as well.

Milk, Yogurt,
& Cheese
Group
2-3 SERVINGS

Meat, Poultry, Fish,
Dry Beans, Eggs,
& Nuts Group
2-3 SERVINGS

Vegetable
Group
3-5 SERVINGS

Fruit
Group
2-4 SERVINGS

Bread, Cereal,
Rice, & Pasta
Group
**6-11
SERVINGS**

SOURCE: U.S. Department of Agriculture/U.S. Department of Health and Human Services

Even the best-intentioned weight watchers often end up with dietary inadequacies because they cut out certain food groups altogether. Fat watchers, for example, commonly become vegetarians in an effort to eat lean. But by cutting out all meat, women especially run the risk of not getting enough iron and certain B vitamins. One friend of mine, a vegetarian for twenty-five years, suffered from chronic fatigue, dizziness, heart palpitations. She identified the symptoms of iron deficiency anemia and ended her vegetarian career with a lean steak. After several days of iron-rich foods such as prune juice, raisins, and lentils, in addition to more lean meat, the symptoms disappeared. She now eats lean red meat once or twice a week, has cut the fat in her diet overall, and occasionally takes iron supplements. She has had no recurrence of the anemia symptoms. As this story illustrates, it is neither necessary nor advisable to stop eating meat in order to meet the 80-20 rule, and it is especially *inadvisable* for women, whose iron needs (18 mg. per day) are nearly double those of men (10 mg. per day).

Another food group that fat watchers commonly shortchange is the dairy group. This can lead to inadequate consumption of calcium, which in turn may contribute to osteoporosis and other health problems. There are so many nonfat and reduced-fat milk products these days that there really is no reason to stint on dairy products when cutting fat. Milk, cheese, cottage cheese, and yogurt are all available with little or no fat, and they remain rich in calcium.

It is possible, of course, to take nutritional supplements to boost the vitamin and mineral intake to recommended levels. And given recent evidence of the disease prevention powers of certain vitamins and minerals, such as antioxidants (beta carotene, vitamins C and E), I heartily endorse taking a daily multivitamin-mineral supplement as "insurance" against inadequate intake. I take a generic brand multivitamin-mineral supplement and a calcium supplement each morning with breakfast.

However, it's important for you to understand that nutrients taken in through food are preferable to supplemented nutrients. Many supplements contain excessive and sometimes harmful doses of certain vitamins and minerals. Thus, while you are well advised to take a supplement (as long as it does not exceed the recommended daily allowance, or RDA) every day, the best way to ensure proper nutrition is to eat according to the pyramid.

Allergies, Deficiencies, and Other Nutritional Considerations

While the strategies, menus, and recipes recommended in this book are designed to steer you toward balanced, healthful, and lean eating habits, they are not intended to address special nutritional needs. If you have allergies, chronic health conditions, or other special dietary requirements, or if you wish to limit your diet due to religious beliefs, I strongly recommend that you consult a registered dietitian (R.D.). A qualified dietitian can tailor an individualized eating plan to meet all your nutritional goals. Dietitians can generally be found through your Yellow Pages or through local hospital outpatient services, or, to locate an R.D. for nutritional counseling near you, call the American Dietetic Association (A.D.A.) at 1-800-366-1655.

6

Food to Burn

There's a common misconception that healthy food requires more preparation than fattening food. Nothing could be further from the truth. The main thing so-called convenience foods do for you is to add unnecessary fat. True convenience foods are raw fruits and vegetables, bread, nonfat milk and yogurt, cereal, clear broths, and vegetable soups. All nutritious, nonfattening, and ready to eat at a moment's notice, *these* convenience foods can and should constitute a large portion of your daily consumption. But what about "real meals"? How is it possible to take basic lean ingredients and create a menu that's simple to prepare and as satisfying as Mom's beef stew? That's what this chapter is all about.

Why Plan Meals?

What healthy eating requires is not necessarily more time but, at least initially, more thought. If you are to break the habit of high-fat meals built around entrees such as fried chicken and steak, you'll need to plan out other options. This means familiarizing yourself with new recipes and cooking methods, discovering ways to modify favorite recipes to cut fat content, and experimenting with different combinations of foods. Only by planning meals ahead of time can you make sure that you have the leanest possible ingredients on hand (i.e., that the only food on hand is *not* fried chicken or fish sticks) and that you know what to do with them.

Other benefits of planning menus ahead:

110

• It reduces impulsive high-fat eating. (You'll be less tempted to go out for a drive-through cheeseburger if you already have a lean and healthy meal planned.)

• It saves time and thought over the long run if you know ahead of time what you'll prepare.

• It allows you to test new menu items, adding variety to your meals.

• It allows you to rotate favorite low-fat menu items.

• By preplanning a day's menu, you can check your meals against the U.S.D.A. Food Guide Pyramid to see that you achieve sound nutritional balance and variety.

Plan Around Your Eating Pattern

Eating patterns—what and how much we eat at different times of the day—have been the subject of much debate. While the American standard has always been three meals per day, the modern reality, particularly among women, is that few of us actually eat "normal" meals at regular mealtimes. Instead, we fall into one of three typical categories:

• We graze, eating bits and pieces all day long without sitting down to a real meal until dinner, if then.

• We skip breakfast, eat a substantial restaurant lunch, then snack lightly through the evening.

• We skip or eat a minimal breakfast and lunch, then stuff ourselves at night.

Researchers can't seem to reach agreement about the relative merits of traditional meals versus these disrupted patterns, but there is growing evidence to support the practice of "grazing" on small, frequent snacks throughout the day. One study showed that the "nibbling diet" consisting of seventeen snacks reduced cholesterol and serum insulin levels, thus bolstering the body against heart disease, hypertension, and diabetes. Others have suggested that food is more easily converted to fat if eaten in larger quantities at a time, and also that between-meal hunger triggers overeating at the next meal.

However, other researchers have found that it makes no difference to metabolism, weight, or body fat whether a person eats two large daily meals or several smaller ones. And grazing may permit excessive eating for someone who easily loses track of food intake or who eats mindlessly.

What matters, in the end, is not how much you eat at a sitting or even on a given day, but how much you *average* on an ongoing basis. It is also important to recognize that your eating pattern may be a reflection of your work or lifestyle—and therefore difficult to change. Keep both these points in mind as you play with different menu plans. Plan full meals only when you're accustomed to eating full meals, and plan for snacks at your customary snack times. But do take into account both snacks and meals. The 80-20 rule applies to your *total* daily consumption, wherever and whenever and in whatever increments you do your eating.

Portion Control

I wish I could tell you that you can eat limitless amounts of lean food and still lose weight. With the exceptions of certain vegetables, that simply isn't true. Going back to what I said in the last chapter, our bodies have certain caloric needs, and when you exceed those needs the surplus will be stored as fat. You get "caloric discounts" for carbohydrates and fiber, but it is possible to use up even those discounts and end up with unwanted fat. This is why I warn you not to rely exclusively on the percentage of fat in your diet, but also be sensible in the amount of food you consume.

As a good news–bad news story in this regard, I must tell you about a letter I received from a woman in South Dakota challenging me to explain why, when she had limited her fat intake to 20 grams per day, she was still not losing weight. She'd enclosed a food diary listing everything she'd eaten for a week or so. I was astounded to find that she was consuming 4,000 calories a day! Whole boxes of cereal, whole loaves of bread. Yes, her fat consumption was low, but she was still overfeeding her body so the bad news was that limiting fat was not enough to cause weight loss. The good news, which I actually found to be quite amazing, was that she had not *gained* weight. That's a testimony to the value of high-carbohydrate nutrition.

It's wise to take small or moderate portions, eat slowly, pause frequently, and wait awhile before helping yourself to seconds. As a rule of thumb, it takes about twenty minutes for satiety cues to reach the brain after we eat. This means that, if you are ravenous when you sit down to a meal, you will continue to feel ravenous even after you begin to eat. But you don't really need to eat a huge amount to quell that starved feeling. Whether you eat one modest bowl of spaghetti or three, twenty minutes after you take that first bite your brain will release a signal to stop the hunger. Pacing and portion control can help prevent you from eating more than you need or really want to.

The fact is, your body requires only a certain amount of food and if you give it that amount with the balance tilted heavily toward lean and varied foods, your body will find its lowest natural weight. It is not good to go hungry, but neither is it good for your body or your psychological health to stuff yourself on any food. For example, while zero-fat jelly beans are a fine substitute for fat-dense chocolate, it is not advisable to snack on them all afternoon. Remember, excess calories, even if they come from carbohydrates, can eventually wind up as body fat.

LFP GUIDE TO CONTROLLING QUANTITY

At meals

Be aware of appropriate serving sizes
Prepare only amount needed
Serve yourself only amount needed
Put away leftovers or extra servings as soon as food is served
Serve from kitchen, i.e., don't put food platters on table
Eat on a smaller plate so that amount of food appears larger
Eat slowly; pace yourself; take small bites and chew well
Sip on no-calorie beverages throughout meal
If you go back for seconds, do so for lowest-fat, lowest-calorie options like veggies
Put plate away/scrape leftovers as soon as you have eaten all you want
Don't eat your meals while doing other distracting things like watching TV or
    reading. Focus on the food while you eat your meal

Snacks

Serve yourself the portion desired
Don't snack directly from the box or bag
PREPLAN: have low-fat items available
Have a general idea of your snacking strategy, i.e., timing, choices, fat gram quota,
    quantity, etc.
Buy individual serving sizes of snack items, i.e., 1 oz. bags of pretzels, yogurt bars,
    or preportion snacks in plastic bags

Keep fresh veggies cut up and available in the refrigerator

BE AWARE: watch mindless munching, even on no-fat items

Keep foods out of sight; don't leave out all the time; keep somewhat inaccessible

Don't buy your favorites! (save for special occasions)

Allow urges for unplanned snacks to "stew" for at least 10 minutes (many times the urge will pass)

Chew sugarless gum; drink no-cal beverages, especially hot beverages

Try extremes in flavor, i.e., very sweet, very salty, very spicy — you won't want much!

Parties

Don't go overly hungry; eat a little something before you go

Don't "graze"; fix a plate and enjoy it

Survey the selections before choosing

Be the last through the line; there will be less left and the others will have a head start on you (they'll be finishing their second serving while you are on your first)

Keep your hands occupied

Concentrate on the social aspect and enjoy the company

Stay away from the food table and the bowls of nuts or munchies

Arrive fashionably late

Take low-fat alternatives

Restaurants

Order appropriately (ask questions, request modifications, etc.)

Remove bread/cracker basket from table after serving yourself and others or move out of reach

Order a variety of low-cal beverages

Avoid all-you-can-eat or buffets whenever possible — order from the menu

Decide how much of what you are served you are going to eat before you dig in; actually cut the planned serving with your knife

Ask for a doggie bag — even first thing is okay

Share an entree with a companion

Have the waiter remove your plate promptly when you have had your fill and order a hot beverage to sip on

Eat slowly; pace yourself

Sabotage uneaten (unwanted) food with sweetener, pepper, salt so you won't pick at it

LFP Menu Planning Basics

As you will see, planning a low-fat menu does not require a great deal of time or effort. After you absorb the basic principles, you probably won't even need to write down your plans. Rather, you may find that you map out a week's meals mentally at the same time you make up your grocery list. Then the ingredients you've stocked will dictate the recipes you prepare.

But before low-fat meal planning can become second nature, you have to learn the basics. Here, then, is the checklist against which you should measure each day's menu.

• Does it meet the 80-20 Fat-Cat rule? Each day's menu should include about 80 percent lowfat entries and 20 percent "regular," with only occasional "full-fat" treats. Use the Fat Master Food Guide at the back of this book to check your Fat-Cats.

• Do you include plenty of high-fiber foods? Remember, fiber calories are not absorbed into the body and actually block a small percentage of fat calories from being absorbed. They also help to protect you against a variety of diseases. Your menu should include lots of fiber and lots of different types of fiber.

• Does your plan check out against the U.S.D.A. Food Guide Pyramid? Nutritional variety and balance are your objectives, with the emphasis on grains, fruit, and vegetables.

• Do you control for quantity? Your menu need not break each meal down into actual portion sizes, but you will need some sense of portions when buying ingredients and preparing dishes. As a rule of thumb, plan to use less meat, poultry, and fish (3 ounces per person per meal is nutritionally sufficient—and probably about half what you've been serving) and more vegetables and starches. If you intend to serve an "occasional" high-fat treat, plan to buy only what you need for everyone to have a small helping. That way you won't be faced with tempting leftovers.

• Do the meals and snacks you're planning taste good? Just because you're trying to eat lean does not mean you should eat foods you hate. Now, if the *only* foods you enjoy are high fat, then you will need to experiment to find alternatives. Begin by trying low-fat substitutes for favorites such as cream cheese and sour cream. (See the LFP Guide to Fat Replacements that follows.) Or cut the amount of fats you use (a teaspoon of mayo, say, instead of a tablespoon), gradually weaning yourself until you appreciate the natural flavor of the foods underneath the sauce. Finally, try a wide variety of low-fat recipes, beginning with the ones I will give you in the next chapter. When you find one you particularly enjoy, learn to make it without referring to the recipe, and it will become a regular entry in your menu plan. Remember, if you don't like the food you're eating, you will feel deprived. And if you feel deprived you'll be more likely to slip back to your high-fat habits.

• Are the meals on your menu easy to prepare? If not, you may find yourself making excuses to go out to eat instead of sticking to your plan. Convenience is critical if you are to maintain lean and healthy eating. For this reason, I encourage you to try the many low-fat frozen entrees and dinners now available. If you keep a supply of these in your freezer, you can use them as your fallback on evenings when you come home too late or tired to cook.

• Do you include soup in many or most meals? Recent research has shown that people who routinely begin meals with a bowl of soup tend to be pounds lighter than people who rarely have soup. Homemade or canned soups work equally well (and now, many canned soups are available with lower sodium content for those who must watch their blood pressure). Just make sure that the soups on your menu are vegetable or broth based rather than cream based.

• Does your menu include low-fat versions of old family favorites? Lowering your family's fat intake is no reason to throw out every food you've ever known and loved. Use the tips for recipe modification I give in this chapter to "trim down" your grandmother's chicken fricassee or your uncle's firehouse chili. You can have your favorites *and* less fat.

LFP Guide to Low-fat Replacements

By the year 2000, the food industry tells us, virtually every product now in your grocery store will be available in low- or nonfat versions. The many leaner products already on the market mimic the texture, flavor, color, and odor of the originals. They can have the same "mouth feel" during chewing and swallowing as their higher-fat versions. But the savings in fat grams can be dramatic. Listed below are just a few of the reduced fat products to look for.

Fat Free:
mayonnaise
salad dressings

cheeses
sour cream
ice milks and frozen yogurts
yogurt

Reduced Fat:
luncheon meats
hot dogs (97–98% fat free)
cream soups
cookies and crackers
pastries and cakes
baking mixes

Low Fat:
frozen entrees and meals
cheeses
frozen desserts

Beware, if you have difficulty with overeating or binge eating, that it is easy to consume large quantities of calories with these products, even as you keep your fat count relatively low. Don't use the low-fat labels as an excuse to eat more than is reasonable or necessary to satisfy your appetite.

Entree Fat-Cat Comparisons with Approximate Fat in Grams
(represents standard serving sizes)

Full-fat Entrees
Beef burrito with cheese (37 g.)
Cannelloni, meat-and-cheese (30 g.)
Cheeseburger, regular ground beef and cheese (34 g.)
Chicken breast, fried (20 g.)
Chicken salad, made with regular mayonnaise (22 g.)
Chili, meat, without beans (20 g.)
Eggplant Parmesan, traditional (24 g.)
Lasagne, meat-and-cheese (35 g.)
Meatloaf, traditional (30 g.)
Pizza, cheese and pepperoni (36 g.)
Spaghetti, regular meat sauce (20 g.)
Tuna noodle casserole, traditional (27 g.)

Regular-fat Entrees
Lean-beef burrito with low-fat cheese (16 g.)
Cannelloni, cheese (18 g.)
Cheeseburger, lean ground beef and low-fat cheese (17 g.)
Chicken salad, made with light mayonnaise (12 g.)
Chili, meat and bean (14 g.)
Lasagne, lean meat and low-fat cheese (18 g.)
Meatloaf, made with lean ground beef (15 g.)
Pizza, cheese-and-vegetable (20 g.)
Spaghetti, lean meat sauce (10 g.)
Tuna noodle casserole, with low-fat cheese (17 g.)

Low-fat Entrees
Bean burrito with low-fat cheese or lean-beef burrito without cheese (10 g.)
Cannelloni, spinach and low-fat cheese (8 g.)
Cheeseburger, extra lean ground beef and nonfat cheese (8 g.)
Chicken breast, oven-fried, LFP style (7 g.)
Chicken salad, made with nonfat mayonnaise (4 g.)
Vegetarian chili, LFP style* (4 g.)
Eggplant Parmesan, LFP style* (8 g.)
Lasagna, meatless, with low-fat cheese (9 g.)
Cajun Meat loaf, LFP style* (10 g.)
Pizza, low-fat cheese and vegetable (10 g.)
Spaghetti, meatless sauce (4 g.)
Tuna noodle casserole, with low-fat cream soup and cheese (8 g.)

Customize Your Kitchen

After planning the coming week's menu, the next step is to stock your kitchen so that you will have everything you need to follow that plan. This includes both the ingredients for recipes and a wide variety of low-fat snack items.

The first step toward customizing your kitchen is to take inventory of its current contents. Go through your refrigerator, freezer, and cupboards, and check all labels. (Though this has nothing to do with fat control, you may also want to use this opportunity to get rid of any food that is no longer fresh.) If the product has a high fat content, consider

---

* Recipes included in Chapter 7.

carefully whether you need it in the house. Certain items, such as cooking and salad oils, you will want to keep. Others, such as frozen fried foods, potato or corn chips, high-fat cookies, peanut butter, and full-fat cheese may serve little purpose but to lead you into temptation. My advice is to get rid of them. If not, then at least make a firm commitment to replace these items, when they run out, with lower-fat substitutes. (The challenge of households with children is addressed in Chapter 10.)

Once you know what you have in your kitchen, you can sit down with the chart below and make a shopping list of the items you need. Ideally, after you have stocked up on nonperishable items such as spices and canned goods, you will need to shop only once or, at most, twice a week for fresh fruits, vegetables, dairy products, and meat, poultry, or fish. Review your week's menu plan to determine which of these perishables you will need and how much to buy.

LFP Pantry Supply List

Basic Staples

Applesauce
Bagels
Beans, canned and/or dried, all varieties
Bread, preferably whole grain
Broth—beef, chicken, and vegetable, in cans or bouillon cubes
Plain breadcrumbs
Cereal, high-fiber, low-sugar varieties
Chips, baked instead of fried
Chocolate or cocoa, unsweetened
Clams, canned
Corn, canned or frozen
Cornmeal
Cornstarch
Crackers, low-fat varieties
Egg noodles
English muffins
Flour, white and whole wheat
Fruit, canned and dried, all varieties

LFP Pantry Supply List   *(con't.)*

Basic Staples   *(con't.)*
Fruit preserves
Gelatin, unflavored
Grains, dried, including couscous, barley, bulgur, hominy grits
Honey
Lentils, dried
Maple syrup
Milk, powdered and evaporated nonfat
Molasses
Mushrooms, canned
Mustard, several varieties
Oats, dried
Oil, preferably olive or canola
Pasta, all varieties
Popcorn
Pretzels
Pumpkin, canned
Raisins
Rice, brown and white, all varieties
Salsa, canned and fresh
Shrimp, canned or frozen
Soy sauce
Sugar, brown and white
Tomato paste
Tomato sauces, all varieties except meat
Tomatoes, canned
Tuna, canned, water-pack
Vanilla
Vinegar, all varieties

Reduced-fat refrigerator and pantry basics
Fat-free mayonnaise
Fat-free salad dressings
Fat-free hard cheeses
Fat-free cream cheese and Neufchâtel products
Fat-free cottage cheese
Fat-free yogurt

Fat-free or reduced-fat sour cream
Skim or I percent milk
Reduced-fat and fat-free frozen yogurt and ice milk
Reduced-fat luncheon meats
97 percent fat-free hot dogs
Reduced-fat cream soups
Reduced-fat and fat-free cookies and crackers
Reduced-fat pastries and cakes
Reduced-fat baking mixes
Low-fat frozen entrees and dinners
Low-fat microwave meals

Gourmet Seasonings, Spices, and Secret Ingredients
Capers
Chili pepper, dried
Cinnamon, dried powder and sticks
Extracts of almond, orange, and lemon
Herbs, dried, all varieties
Herbs, fresh, including basil, parsley, dill, tarragon
Sun-dried tomato bits (dried, not in oil)
Water chestnuts
Wheat germ
Wine for cooking: white, red, vermouth, and sherry

Lean Track Shopping Basics

Many people who love to eat high-fat foods get into real trouble when they go to the market. They intend to buy a carton of milk and end up with a full shopping cart of treats. Here, then, are a few tips to help minimize temptation—and safeguard your lean menu plan.

1. Always shop from a list. You have put considerable effort into inventorying your kitchen and figuring out precisely what you need. Rely on the list you made at home. Buy only the items it calls for, and don't let yourself be sidetracked by all the tempting displays your grocery store has set up to sell you fattening new products. If you simply cannot resist, consider phoning in your list to the store and letting them do your shopping for you. Many grocery stores offer this service, and some still deliver; at others, you simply stop in, pay, and pick up your prebagged purchases.

2. Never shop hungry. When you're hungry you are much more susceptible to temptation, and you will tend to stay in the store longer. Shop on a full stomach and you'll be eager to get the job done and move on to other business.

3. Do your shopping at stores that offer variety, quality, and freshness. The higher the quality and freshness of produce, meat, and poultry, the better it will taste and the less it will need to be "doctored" with fattening sauces. A wide variety means that you won't have to go out of your way for special ingredients, and you can vary your menu from week to week.

4. Get to know the layout of your grocery store. Assuming you're shopping from a list, this will cut down on unnecessary roaming. If you know the cereal and canned goods you need are in aisle 4, then you won't need to waste time looking for them—and struggling against temptation—among the pastries in aisle 3. If your store groups lower-fat products together, familiarize yourself with the locations of those displays.

5. Read the nutritional content labels, giving special attention to fat and fiber content. Do not automatically buy products advertised as "lite," "reduced," or "diet." Check the label. Also beware of products advertised as 95 percent—or more—fat free. The fat-free percentage refers to percentage by weight, not percentage of calories. So, for example, a 95 percent fat-free deli meat might actually contain 2 grams of fat per 30-calorie slice, which adds up to 60 percent of the product's total calories. Look instead at the actual gram count of fat and the percentages of other nutrients contained in each serving and check it against the LFP Shopping Guidelines on pp. 124–25. Also check the serving size to make sure it's actually the amount you would eat. If any single serving contains more than 10 grams of fat, see if you can find a similar product with lower fat content.

Translating Label Terminology

Light or Lite: The product has been significantly reduced in fat and calories, or sodium. If "light" in fat, the fat content must be cut by at least 50 percent and caloric content must be cut by at least one-third. If "light" in sodium, salt content must be cut by at least 50 percent.

Fat-free: The product contains less than 0.5 grams of total fat per serving.

Percent (%) Fat-free: The percentage of the product *by weight* that is fat free. Some products, such as milk, must be 99 percent fat free before they are truly low in fat.

Calorie-free: Product contains less than 5 calories per serving.

Cholesterol-free: Product contains less than 2 milligrams of cholesterol *and* 2 grams or less of saturated fatty acids per serving.

Low-fat: Product contains 3 grams or less of total fat per serving.

Reduced-fat: Product contains at least one-third less fat than comparable food item.

Low-calorie: Product contains no more than 40 calories per serving.

Low-cholesterol: Product contains 20 milligrams or less of cholesterol per serving.

Low saturated Fat: Product contains 1 gram or less of saturated fatty acids per serving *and* not more than 15 percent of calories from saturated fatty acids.

6. Keep a mental list of the high-fat products you will buy only on rare occasions, if at all. Once you get out of the habit of buying these, you won't even notice them on the shelves.

High-fat Products to Leave on the Grocery Shelves

Biscuits, any variety
Butter and margarine
Cheese, full-fat varieties
Chips, any fried variety
Cream
Fish, canned in oil
Ice cream, full-fat varieties
Milk, whole or 2% ("low-fat")
Nuts and seeds
Vegetables marinated in oil, canned or fresh

LFP Shopping Guidelines*

Produce
FRUITS

1 gram fat or less per serving (1/2 cup or 140 grams)

VEGETABLES

1 gram fat or less per serving (1/2 cup or 85 grams)

Meats
3 grams fat or less per 1 ounce cooked (less than 9 grams per 3-ounce serving cooked)

Poultry
2 grams fat or less per ounce cooked

Fish
2 grams fat or less per ounce cooked

Breads
LOAF BREADS, VARIETY BREADS, SANDWICH BUNS, ROLLS, ENGLISH MUFFINS

1 gram fat or less per ounce (2 grams fat or less—and 2 or more grams fiber for loaf breads—per standard 2-ounce serving)

Canned Entrees/Main Dishes
8 grams fat or less per 1-cup serving

Soups, Canned and Mixes
3 grams fat or less per 1-cup serving

Sauces and Gravies, Canned, Jarred, Mixes
4 grams fat or less per serving as sauce for main dish (1/2 cup)

2 grams fat or less per serving as sauce for side dish (1/4 cup)

Baking Mixes
4 grams fat or less per serving

Frostings and Toppings
2 grams fat or less per serving (about 2 tablespoons)

Puddings, Pie Fillings, and Gelatins
3 grams fat or less per 1/2-cup serving

Candy
1 gram fat or less per 1-ounce serving

Dairy Foods
MILK

2 grams fat or less per 1 cup (8 ounces) (1% milk)

SOUR CREAM AND CREAM

1 gram fat or less per tablespoon

CHEESES

4 grams fat or less per ounce

YOGURT

2 grams fat or less per cup (8 ounces)

Egg Substitutes
2 grams fat or less per egg equivalent (1/4 cup)

Fats
REDUCED-FAT MARGARINES, BUTTER SUBSTITUTES, AND COOKING SPRAYS

6 grams fat or less per tablespoon

REDUCED-FAT MAYONNAISE AND SALAD DRESSINGS

3 grams fat or less per 2-tablespoon serving

REFRIGERATED AND FROZEN BREADS, BISCUITS,

ROLLS
3 grams fat or less per 2-ounce serving

MUFFINS, PASTRIES, SWEET BREAKFAST BREADS, BREAD MIXES
4 grams fat or less per 2-ounce serving

Pasta/Noodles/Macaroni
(including noodle mixes)
4 grams fat or less per serving (2 ounces dry or 1 cup cooked)

Rice/Rice Mixes
2 grams fat or less per serving (1 ounce dry or 1/2 cup cooked)

Beans and Peas, Canned
2 grams fat or less per 1/2-cup serving

Cereals (with added fiber criterion)
READY-TO-EAT
2 grams fat or less, and more than 2 grams fiber, per 1-ounce serving

COOKED (with water)
2 grams fat or less, and more than 1 gram fiber, per 1-ounce serving (about 2/3 cup)

Crackers, Croutons, Breadsticks
2 grams fat or less per ounce (1 gram fat or less per 1/2-ounce serving)

Cookies
3 grams fat or less per ounce

Packaged Snacks
CHIPS, PRETZELS, POPCORN, RICE CAKES
3 grams fat or less per 1-ounce serving

CAKES AND PASTRIES
4 grams fat or less per 2-ounce serving

Condiments
1 gram fat or less per tablespoon

Frozen Foods
ENTREES
8 grams fat or less per 1-cup serving (minimum 5 ounces)

DINNERS
12 grams fat or less per meal (minimum 10 ounces)

SIDE DISHES/POTATOES
3 grams fat or less per serving (1/2 cup)

DESSERTS
4 grams fat or less per serving (1/2 cup or 2-ounce slice)

Miscellaneous (jellies, jams, syrups, pickles; hot cocoa mixes)
0 gram fat per serving for jellies, jams, syrups, pickles
$\leq$1 gram fat per cup serving (8 ounces) for hot cocoa mixes

*Taken from *The Low Fat Supermarket Shopper's Guide*, by Jamie Pope, M.S., R.D., and Martin

7. Familiarize yourself with the leanest varieties of meat, poultry, and fish—and avoid their higher-fat counterparts.

LFP Guide to Low-fat Meat Selection

USE	*INSTEAD OF*
Lean, well-trimmed cuts of meat with < 15 percent fat (flank steak, round tip, top round, eye of round, top loin, tenderloin, top sirloin)	Higher-fat, marbled meats, greater than 15 percent fat
Extra lean ground beef, ground turkey	Regular ground beef
Pork tenderloin, leanest pork loin, lean ham	Other cuts of pork
Skinless poultry	Poultry with skin
Fresh or smoked turkey	Self-basting turkey
U.S.D.A. "Select" cuts of meat	U.S.D.A. "Prime" or "Choice" cuts of meat
3-4 ounce servings of meats (about size of a deck of cards)	Larger servings of meat
Lower fat preparation methods: broil, grill, bake, roasted on a rack, microwave, poach	Higher-fat methods like frying or cooking in own fat
Canadian bacon, breakfast ham	Bacon, sausage as breakfast meat
Lean, unprocessed, deli-type meats like roast beef, turkey breast, chicken breast, boiled ham	Higher-fat packaged, processed meats
Low-fat packaged luncheon meats, hot dogs, and sausage (>90% fat free)	Regular higher-fat packaged luncheon meats, hot dogs, and sausage
Water-packed tuna or other canned fish	Fish canned in oil
Fresh or frozen fish	Fried fish, breaded frozen fish
Meatless meals (beans, legumes, grains) at least once or twice per week	Meat at all meals

LFP Cooking Basics

Here's the bottom line: Get the most flavor with the least amount of fat. Never before has this goal been so attainable. Now, with the vast array of available reduced-fat foods and fat replacements, it is possible to slash the fat content of everything from macaroni and cheese to chocolate layer cake. In the next chapter I will offer specific recipes that do just that. But first I want to introduce you to the basic principles of low-fat cooking so that you can create or convert your own recipes as well.

There's a lot of material here, and it may seem a bit overwhelming at first. I suggest you read through these suggestions several times. You may find you're already using many of these low-fat cooking techniques without even realizing they help keep you lean. If they seem unfamiliar, try copying the charts and posting them in your kitchen for quick reference during meal preparation. After just a week or two of consistent use, these methods will become second nature.

LOW-FAT COOKING AND BAKING TIPS

Meats
- Select the leanest cuts of meat
  Beef: tenderloin, eye of round, top round, round tip, top loin, sirloin
  Pork: tenderloin, center loin, leg (fresh ham), shoulder
  Lamb: leg of lamb, shoulder, loin
  Veal: cutlets, sirloin, shoulder, loin
- Always trim meats of excess fat prior to cooking.
- Keep portion sizes to 3 ounces (about the size of a deck of cards).
- Remove skin from poultry prior to cooking (to prevent becoming too dry, reduce recipe temperature slightly and avoid overcooking).
- If possible, make soups, stews, and stocks ahead of time and chill in refrigerator for several hours or overnight. Skim off hardened fat and reheat.
- Purchase a "fat skimmer" to remove fat from meat drippings.
- Purchase ground meats that contain less than 10% fat by weight (i.e., are at least 90 percent fat free).
- Don't add additional fat to the skillet when browning. Transfer to a colander to drain excess fat.
- Bake, broil, grill, or poach rather than fry or roast in own juices.
- It is best to cook lean cuts of meat at low temperatures to avoid drying out.
- Roast on a broiler rack to allow fat to drip away.

- "Oven fry" by coating small to medium pieces of lean meat, skinless poultry, or fish with egg white, plain yogurt, or buttermilk. Then dip in breadcrumbs, flour, or cornmeal. On a foil-lined baking sheet that has been sprayed with nonstick cooking spray cook at 400 to 500 degrees. Turn after 5 to 7 minutes, then continue cooking until done (fish requires the least amount of cooking time).
- Marinate in fat-free marinades to tenderize and enhance flavor. Include flavored vinegar, wine, or citrus juices with other low-fat ingredients and seasonings. Discard marinade after removing the meat for cooking.

Baked Goods and Desserts

- Coat baking pans with nonstick cooking sprays or baking sprays rather than "greasing." Flour as you normally would. For chocolate baked goods, trying "flouring" with cocoa powder.
- Use egg whites (2) or egg substitute (1/4 cup) for one egg in recipes. It is not always necessary or advisable to replace all the eggs called for in a recipe—for example, when a recipe calls for four eggs, try two whole eggs and a substitute for the remaining eggs.
- Use skim or 1 percent milk for any milk the recipe calls for.
- Replace cream with canned evaporated skimmed milk.
- Reduced-fat margarines have a higher water content and were designed as spreads rather than for baking.
- For most baked goods, reducing the fat the recipe calls for by 1/3 to 1/2 will not alter the quality of the product.
- Replace all or part of the fat in baked goods with fruit purees or "butters" (see below), applesauce, mashed bananas, plain yogurt or yogurt cheese, or reduced-fat mayonnaise. Replace in equal amounts (i.e., if a recipe calls for 1 cup butter or margarine, try using 1/3 cup butter or margarine and 2/3 cup fruit puree).

> prune or date "butter" 1 1/3 cup prunes or dates
> 1/3 cup water
> 1. Combine in a food processor.
> 2. Puree, occasionally scraping sides, until smooth.
> Makes one cup "butter" to replace one cup real butter or shortening

- Cookies are not as adaptable to sugar and fat reductions as are most other baked goods. They become less tender and crisp. However, prune or date butter can be used to replace up to 3/4 of the fat in cookies with very good results!

- Try a small amount of butter extract to add butter flavor to puddings, cakes, and other cooked desserts.
- Replace sour cream or cream cheese with yogurt cheese. To make 1 cup, invert 16 ounces of plain, nonfat yogurt in a small colander lined with cheesecloth or coffee filters. Place over a bowl, cover with plastic wrap, and place in refrigerator overnight. Discard excess liquid. If using yogurt cheese in place of cream cheese in a recipe that calls for an electric mixer, beat all other ingredients together, then fold in the yogurt cheese with a spatula.
- When a recipe calls for nuts, reduce the amount by half or, as a topping, replace with Grapenuts cereal (to retain crunchiness, sprinkle on a cookie sheet and bake for 10 minutes at 375 degrees).
- Replace unsweetened baking chocolate with cocoa powder (1 ounce chocolate = 3 tablespoons cocoa powder plus 1 tablespoon liquid). For semisweet chocolate, add 3 tablespoons of sugar.
- Chocolate syrup contains only 1–2 grams of fat per two tablespoon serving. Use this instead of fudge sauce or other chocolate topping.
- In place of a pastry crust, try a meringue pie shell, philo dough, or a crumb pie shell made with graham crackers, lower fat cookies, cereal (like cornflakes), or even pretzels. Honey makes a good "binder" for crumb crusts in place of some of the fat (1 1/2 cups crumbs, 2 table-spoons of honey, and 1 tablespoon of oil or melted margarine makes one pie crust).
- As a whipped topping, partially freeze 6 ounces (1/2 can) of evaporated skim milk in a mixing bowl. Add one tablespoon of sugar and whip till soft peaks form.
- To increase fiber and heartiness, replace up to 1/3 all-purpose flour with whole grain flour.
- Remember these desserts that are already naturally low in fat: angel food cake, sherbet, fruit ices, frozen yogurts, ice milks, puddings made with low-fat milk, and, of course, fresh fruit!

Vegetables and Salads

- For sautéing, use a nonstick skillet with minimal or no added fat. Make use of nonstick cooking sprays (try the olive oil or butter flavored varieties) or use some broth or water to prevent sticking.
- Experiment with herbs and seasonings. Try fresh herbs (1 teaspoon dried = ~1 tablespoon fresh, finely crushed herb).
- For those Southern-style vegetables, use an ounce or two of lean ham, beef broth, or smoke flavoring in preparation.
- For butter taste, use butter sprinkles or reduced- or no-fat margarine.

- Let family and friends add butter or margarine at the table if desired.
- Use low- or no-fat salad dressings instead of regular salad dressings (0–2 grams of fat compared to 6–10 grams of fat for regular dressings).

Miscellaneous (Casseroles, Sandwiches, Etc.)

- Because of the higher water content of many reduced- and no-fat products, baked casserole dishes may appear watery. To remedy, stir in beaten egg whites or a tablespoon or two of cornstarch into the mixture before baking to bind the excess water.
- Replace regular canned cream soups with reduced-fat cream soups.
- Select cheeses that contain less than 4 grams of fat per ounce. If you choose fat-free cheeses, it is better to mix them into the dish than to use as a topping (they do not always melt as well but give good flavor within the dish).
- If using full-fat cheese, cut amount recipe calls for by 1/3 to 1/2. A few tablespoons of a strongly flavored cheese go as far as much more of a milder cheese, for example, sharp cheddar rather than mild.
- Use reduced-fat sour cream in place of regular sour cream in recipes.
- Use flavored mustards or reduced- or no-fat mayonnaise in place of regular mayonnaise, which contains 11 grams of fat per tablespoon!
- On toast, bagels, or muffins use jelly and jams (no fat!) or make use of the reduced- and no-fat margarines.

SUBSTITUTIONS TO TRIM FAT AND CALORIES

Use	Instead of
Skim or 1% milk	Whole or 2% milk
Evaporated skim milk (canned)	Cream, whipping cream, coffee creamers
Evaporated skim milk (canned) with added sugar	Sweetened condensed milk
Nonfat dry milk	Whole or 2% milk, coffee whiteners or creamers
Plain nonfat yogurt	Sour cream, mayonnaise, whole-milk yogurt
Nonfat or low-fat yogurt "cheese" (made by draining liquid from yogurt)	Sour cream, cream cheese
Fat-free cream cheese	Regular cream cheese
Nonfat or "light" sour cream alternative	Sour cream
Reduced-fat, "light," or fat-free cheeses	Regular cheeses

Use	Instead of
1–2% fat cottage cheese, skim or "lite" ricotta	4% fat cottage cheese, whole-milk ricotta
Part-skim cheeses in moderate quantities, farmer, sapsago, other cheeses with < 4 g. fat/oz.	Regular whole-milk cheese
Extra sharp cheeses in smaller quantities	Regular, milder cheeses
Reduced-calorie or fat-free mayonnaise	Regular mayonnaise, part of fat in baked recipes
Mustard, ketchup as condiment	Mayonnaise
Reduced-calorie margarine	Margarine, butter, shortening
1/3 to 1/2 less fat and/or oil in recipes	Amount original recipe calls for
Applesauce, mashed bananas, fruit juice or puree	Part of fat called for in muffins or baked goods
Prune "butter" (puree)	Fat in cookies or other baked goods
Nonstick cooking spray	Oil, shortening, butter, other fat
Butter-flavored sprinkles or sprays	Margarine, butter to flavor
No- or low-fat salad dressings	Regular salad dressings
2 egg whites or 1/4 cup egg substitute	Whole egg
Cocoa powder (3 tbsp. + 1 tbsp. liquid)	Chocolate in recipes (= 1 ounce)
Sherbet, low-fat frozen yogurt, ice milk, "light" ice creams (< 4 grams per 4 ounce)	Ice cream
Popsicles, fruit bars, "diet" ice cream bars	Ice cream bars
Angel cake, "light" cake mixes	Higher fat cakes
Seven-minute frosting, "light" frostings	Regular frostings
Lower-fat cookies (gingersnaps, fig bars, rice cereal bars, graham crackers, devil's food cake bars, animal crackers, molasses cookies)	Higher-fat cookies, chocolate or chocolate-coated cookies
Puddings made with skim milk	Pudding with whole milk
Graham cracker or cornflake crumb crust (1 1/2 cup crumbs, 2 tbsp. honey, 1 tbsp. oil)	Pastry crust
Jelly or jams on toast or breads	Margarine, butter
FRESH FRUIT	Other desserts

SUBSTITUTIONS TO TRIM FAT AND CALORIES   *(con't.)*

Use	Instead of
Bagels, English muffins, raisin bread	Croissants, biscuits, pastries
Pretzels, unbuttered popcorn, no-oil bagel chips, no-oil tortilla chips, rice cakes	Chips, nuts, buttered snacks or popcorn
Lowfat crackers with < 3 grams fat per ounce (matzos, crisp breads, saltines, melba toast, flat breads, rice cakes)	Higher-fat crackers, chips
Toasted Grapenuts cereal	Nuts as dessert topping
No added fat to packaged rice, pasta, or cereals	Added fat in directions
Chopped water chestnuts	Chopped nuts in vegetable casseroles
Broth-based soups	Cream or cheese soups
Reduced-fat cream soups	Regular cream soups
Steamed vegetables seasoned with herbs, spices, lemon juice, boullion, low-fat sauces	Vegetables seasoned with margarine/ butter, oil or meat fat, in cheese sauce, fried vegetables
Frozen entrees with < 8 grams fat/ serving	Higher-fat frozen entrees
Frozen dinners with < 12 grams fat/ serving	Higher-fat frozen dinners

Planned Snacking

The most important thing to remember about snacking is that there is nothing *wrong* with it. Most of us snack between meals, and healthy snacking can help maintain a higher level of nutrition and energy than eating larger, less frequent meals. The main problems with this plan are that Americans' most popular snack foods also happen to be among the highest in fat content, and it's easy to lose track of what and how much we actually consume when snacking. In certain "high-risk" situations, we tend to eat more than we really desire. For instance:

• Eating alone. Even if we don't binge, many of us eat more alone than we do around others. Solo snacking also tends to be the least conscious snacking, which means that little attention is paid to the selection of food or quantities consumed. Because of this tendency toward unconscious snacking, we often underestimate the real amount of fat we've eaten.

• Finger foods. Bite-sized servings are so easy to swallow and dismiss. Who among us knows how many potato chips we *really* eat at a time? The more readily available and easy a food is to eat the more it invites unconscious snacking.

• Car food. We found in our weight management groups at Vanderbilt that being alone in the car commonly prompted higher-fat, higher-calorie snacking. Drive-through restaurants coupled with long commutes and crammed schedules have encouraged this tendency. Unless you brown-bag your car food, the snacks you tend to pick up along the road are likely to be full-meal fare such as burgers, fries, and shakes. These may be easy to eat as you drive, but they will also drive your fat consumption out of sight.

• The power of temptation. Some people are easily "turned on" by the sight or smell of food—especially high-fat, sweet foods. These folks cannot pass a bakery or candy store without stopping in. They have trouble getting through the supermarket without loading up on packaged cookies and chips, and they generally start munching before they reach the checkout line. Unfortunately, temptation has a way of overruling moderation.

• Snack times. Two to four hours after your last meal, particularly if you're not busy, you get hungry. Most people tend to do the heaviest snacking between four and six in the afternoon, and between eight and ten in the evening. Sometimes the catalyst is genuine hunger, but more often it's boredom or loneliness. Why is it that cakes, cookies, and ice cream make better substitutes for human companionship than do apples, popcorn, and bagels? Or do they, *really?*

Knowing when and where you're most likely to snack is half the battle. Now you can *plan* for these situations. The idea is to satisfy the urge to eat when it strikes, but at the same time, to subvert the habit of snacking on fat.

Here, then, are the basic principles of planned snacking:

• Feed your hunger. When your stomach is growling or you feel lightheaded, don't delay. Your body is telling you it needs fuel. Even if you know you'll be having lunch in an hour, have a small *lean* snack now to tide you over. Otherwise you'll be so ravenous at lunch that you'll eat everything in sight. I tell my weight management groups that if they routinely get hungry at a particular time, such as midafternoon, they should plan to snack—not try to resist in the hope of eating less. Then they come up with two or three alternatives that are available, appealing, and low in fat. I encourage them to take preferred snacks to work, such as pretzels or fruit, so they won't be tempted by vending machine fare.

• Make a habit of low-fat snack foods. The main reason we eat so much fattening snack food is that we're accustomed to snacking on these products. But we can just as easily become accustomed to snacking on pretzels, fresh fruit, low-fat crackers, air-popped popcorn, and dried fruit. If you stock only low-fat snack items in your kitchen, you'll quickly get into the habit. The chart below offers some suggestions for leaner snacking when you're away from home.

Impulse Junk Food Substitutions

Impulse Choice (fat grams)	Better Choice (fat grams)	Fat gram savings
Convenience Store		
Chocolate doughnut (21 g.)	Cinnamon raisin bagel (1 g.)	20 g.
Coffee w/2 tbsp. cream (5.5 g.)	Coffee w/2 tbsp. milk (1 g.)	4.5 g.
Footlong hot dog (27 g.)	Ham sandwich, no mayo (6 g.)	21 g.
Hostess apple pie (19 g.)	Large apple (0 g.)	19 g.
Airport		
1 oz. bag peanuts (14 g.)	Bag pretzels (1 g.)	13 g.
Gourmet chocolate chip cookie (16 g.)	Soft pretzel w/mustard (3 g.)	13 g.
Mall		
Large cinnamon bun w/icing (34 g.)	Cinnamon raisin bagel (1 g.)	33 g.
Nacho plate w/sour cream (35 g.)	Plain baked potato (0 g.)	35 g.
Movie Theater		
Small buttered popcorn (50 g.)	Med. box Jujyfruits or Dots (0 g.)	50 g.

• Snack in limited portions. You may have unrestricted numbers of portions, but make yourself work for each one. Take a single handful of pretzels and leave the kitchen to eat it instead of taking the whole bag with you. Serve yourself a modest bowl of frozen yogurt instead of eating out of the container. Or buy individual-sized servings of frozen desserts such as Popsicles or reduced-fat ice milk bars. Portion eating accomplishes two goals. First, it makes you conscious of how much you are eating, so that quantity becomes a decision rather than something that "just happens." Second, it stretches the process of snacking, giving your digestive tract time to relay the signal of satiation to your brain. Even when you go back for multiple portions, you'll end up eating less.

• Move to safer snacking grounds. In other words, protect yourself against temptation. Customize your kitchen. Shop at grocery stores that stock lots of tasty low-fat snack foods. Seek out movie theaters that offer air-popped popcorn (saving 16 grams of fat on a small unbuttered serving). Frequent restaurants that offer leaner menu items—and get used to ordering them. Instead of treating yourself to a trip to the pastry shop, enjoy an outing to the local fruit and vegetable market.

• Travel with safe snacks. If you spend long hours in the car or on the train or plane, take along a supply of low-fat snacks in case you get hungry. You may not need them, but having them will safeguard you against the more fattening temptations of the road.

• Wait out the urge to snack. The sight and smell of food give almost all of us the urge to eat; if we acted on these urges every time, we'd be worrying about the last fifty pounds instead of the last five! Impulse eating generally involves a narrow window between sighting the temptation and giving in to it. If you wait a few moments and think about it, you may decide that sugared doughnut isn't worth the fat grams, or that it's probably stale and can't possibly taste as good as it looks, or that you're really not all that hungry anyway. Give yourself permission to come back in five or ten minutes if you still want that doughnut—but you'll often find the temptation evaporates within this time. What if it doesn't? Well, enjoy the doughnut as long as it lives up to your expectations. Remember that you're entitled to an *occasional* treat. But if the doughnut does turn out to be stale and tasteless, don't hesitate to throw it away!

• Enjoy occasional treats in smaller portions. Many of my weight management group members feel that once they "give in" to that cookie or candy bar they've "already blown it, and might as well blow it big." We spend at least a couple of sessions learning to eat *reasonable* portions of even problem foods. Research shows that we get the most enjoyment from the first two or three bites, with diminishing returns thereafter. Thus, if we really have to have that Snickers bar, it's okay to go ahead and buy it, but we only need a third or half to satisfy the urge, so the secret is to *throw away the rest* before leaving the store. By slowly eating and savoring the smaller portion we satisfy the craving without loading up on fat.

• Freeze restricted snack foods. There's nothing like leftover birthday cake sitting on the counter to force your hand. It's there, it's delicious, and it's bound to go stale if you don't eat it right now! But in the freezer, that same cake is out of sight, out of mind—and too much trouble to eat. It's a sneaky tactic, but it helps.

• Don't confuse snacking with R and R. Snacking is not particularly restful, and it's a poor substitute for true recreation.

• Stay busy! Surround yourself with work, friends, hobbies. Get out of the house on your days off. By minimizing aimless hours you minimize the urge to snack—and the tendency to gain weight.

7

LFP Fat Master Menus and Recipes

One of the first requests I receive from people looking for help in their weight management efforts is for menus. And I've planned more than my share in my career, including those that appear in my colleague Dr. Katahn's latest best-sellers. "Could you give me some menus I could follow to lose weight?" they'll ask. I very rarely grant their request; rather, I encourage them to monitor their own food choices and eating patterns for a week or so. I then look over their written food record and make recommendations to improve overall nutrition, balance, and timing of meals or snacks. However, since I can't provide this personalized service for each of you, I've tried to provide the ammunition you need to evaluate your own diet and fat intake.* Armed with the U.S.D.A. Food Guide Pyramid as a guide to daily food choices (p. 108), your basic calorie needs (pp. 87–88), the 80-20 rule with the Fat-Cats (p. 90), and the menus and recipes that follow, you can be well on your way to maximizing nutrition and minimizing fat.

As I mentioned above, I feel that it is very important that you examine your own eating style and food choices with fat intake and nutritional balance in mind. Menus certainly don't conform to everyone's lifestyle or food preferences, but they can be used as a guide or model of a healthful, varied diet. We don't always do such a great job on our own, considering that fewer than 10 percent of Americans take in the four to five recommended servings of fruits and vegetables each day

---

*For personalized evaluation of your diet and recommendations, I suggest you obtain the services of a Registered Dietitian (see p. 109 for information on finding an R.D. in your area).

and that women consume less than half of the recommended intake of calcium. I don't necessarily recommend that you follow these menus to the letter. You may choose to; some find it helpful as a way to gear up for change or to try to overcome some less than positive eating practices. However, at the least you can use the menus as a basis for ideas for meal choices, to introduce new recipes, and to determine "appropriate" portion sizes.

The fourteen days average 22 grams of fat and about 1,500 calories (1,460 to be exact).* This brings the daily percentage of calories from fat to less than 15 percent; however, as I'll explain, these menus serve only as a core for your overall day. *Your own additions, combined with how easy it is to underestimate hidden fats in food,* will likely be somewhat higher, but still comprise an overall low fat diet. This is a level conducive not only to loss of excess body fat but also to disease prevention. As you'll recall from previous chapters, Americans average around 40 percent calories from fat, and major health organizations recommend that we need to reduce fat intake to less than 30 percent of total calories. The 15 percent that these menus represent and that the LFP approach teaches is considered by the majority of health experts to be an optimal level for achieving your personal best weight and overall health. The menus average 27 grams of dietary fiber by emphasizing whole grain breads and cereals, fruits, and vegetables. Americans typically consume only about 10 grams, and we need well over 20 grams per day! In addition, the average of the fourteen days meets at least 75 percent of, and in most cases exceeds, the recommended dietary allowances (RDA) for more than twenty-five vitamins and minerals.

Feel free to trade meals around within the menus. Trade one breakfast for another, Day 2 lunch for Day 11, and so on. There is no magic in the combination of foods or meals. I have specified fruits and vegetables with the meals, but go ahead and interchange another fruit or vegetable when convenience dictates. Vegetables are prepared within the menus without added fat unless otherwise noted. Try to emphasize whole grain, higher fiber breads, grains, and cereals. I've included in the menus many of the LFP recipes that appear later in this chapter. I hope you'll try them!

I hope you don't have to ask, after reading the previous chapters, why the basic menus are 1,500 calories instead of the restrictive 1,000–1,200 calorie plans you're used to seeing in "diet" books. Remember,

---

*I analyzed the menus and recipes that appear in this book using Food Processor III Nutrition and Diet Analysis System from ESHA Research.

"livability" is the goal. These menus serve as the core to which, according to your activity level and calorie needs, you can (and should!) add snacks, additional desserts, and a moderate amount of alcohol. In addition, the menus include one teaspoon of added fat in the form of light margarine. This is certainly on the conservative side, so there is room to choose regular butter or margarine instead or add an extra teaspoon. Or you may wish to avoid added fats altogether in favor of choosing a higher fat food now and then. It's up to you!

I've listed some possible snack suggestions on p. 146 that contain less than 3 grams of fat and less than 200 calories. Note that most of the snacks include milk or a milk product; that's because the basic menus contain an average of 900 mg. of calcium. Women's needs are at minimum 800 mg. per day (the menus have that covered), but for many of you the recommended intake is 1,200 mg.. If you don't like milk, can't digest it easily, or aren't including at least three servings per day (and most of us don't!), it's advisable to supplement your diet with calcium. You can do so through one of the chewable antacids that contain calcium (such as Tums), a calcium supplement (they range from 200 to 600 mg. per tablet), or another food product that's been fortified with calcium (like some brands of orange juice).

Whether you choose to follow my menus or simply use them for ideas, the important things to keep in mind for your own menus are choosing a wide variety of foods, emphasizing low-fat foods (from the Low Fat-Cat), and planning ahead. You can't expect everything to fall in place without some preplanning, which involves strategies like stocking a low-fat kitchen, having the foods you need on hand, packing your lunch a few days a week, and choosing weight-friendly restaurants.

LFP MENUS

DAY 1

Breakfast
1 toasted bagel or English muffin; 2 tablespoons fat-free cream cheese; jelly or jam; 1 cup skim or 1 percent milk; 1 cup berries or other fresh fruit; coffee or tea

Lunch
2 ounces lean ham with 2 pineapple slices on whole grain pita bread; alfalfa sprouts; mustard or fat-free mayonnaise; 1 ounce pretzels; no-cal beverage

Dinner
1 serving Chicken Picante*; 1/2 cup brown or wild rice; 1/2 cup black beans or canned refried beans; 1 cup broccoli; 1 piece Corn Bread* with 1 teaspoon light margarine (or 2 corn tortillas); no-cal beverage

Total for Day 1: 18 grams fat (12%); 1,420 calories; 25 grams fiber

DAY 2

Breakfast
1 ounce ready-to-eat cereal; banana, sliced; 1 cup skim or 1 percent milk; 1 slice whole grain toast; 1 teaspoon light margarine; jelly or jam; coffee or tea

Lunch
Spinach salad: fresh spinach, sliced fresh mushrooms, 1/2 hard-boiled egg, 1 ounce no- or reduced-fat cheese, chopped red onion, 3 tablespoons fat-free salad dressing; Hummingbird Muffin* or other low-fat muffin; orange; no-cal beverage

Dinner
1 serving Beef Goulash* over 1/2 cup cubed potatoes; 1 cup asparagus; tossed vegetable salad; 3 tablespoons fat-free salad dressing; whole grain roll; 1 serving Gingerbread*; no-cal beverage

Total for Day 2: 25 grams fat (13%); 1,540 calories; 30 grams fiber

DAY 3

Breakfast
Refrigerator Bran Muffin*; 1 cup nonfat yogurt (plain or 100 calorie variety); grapefruit; coffee or tea

Lunch
Fast-food restaurant broiled chicken sandwich (hold the mayo!) with lettuce, tomato, mustard or barbecue sauce; 1 ounce pretzels; small side salad; fat-free salad dressing; no-cal beverage

Dinner
1 serving Eggplant Parmesan*; 1 cup pasta of choice; 1 slice garlic toast (Italian or other bread broiled with 1 teaspoon light margarine and garlic powder); 2 pineapple slices; no-cal beverage

Total for Day 3: 24 grams fat (15%); 1,400 calories; 20 grams fiber

---

* These recipes appear in the recipe section that follows. Serving sizes are as noted in recipe.

DAY 4

Breakfast
1 ounce ready-to-eat cereal; sliced peaches or other seasonal fruit; 1 cup skim or
1 percent milk; 1 slice whole grain toast; 1 teaspoon light margarine; jelly or
jam; coffee or tea

Lunch
Baked potato stuffed with 1/2 cup no- or low-fat cottage cheese, chopped green
onions, chopped tomatoes, and salsa; apple; no-cal beverage

Dinner
1 serving Fish Casserole*; 1/2 cup brown or wild rice; 1 cup green beans; Potato
Roll*; tossed vegetable salad; 3 tablespoons fat-free salad dressing; citrus fruit
cup; no-cal beverage

Total for Day 4: 17 grams fat (11%); 1,380 calories; 27 grams fiber

DAY 5

Breakfast
1 slice Brenda's Banana Bread*; 2 teaspoons apple butter; 1 cup melon or other
seasonal fruit; 1 cup nonfat yogurt (plain or 100 calorie variety); coffee or tea

Lunch
1 cup September Chowder* or broth-based soup; 1 ounce low-fat crackers;
assorted raw vegetables; 2 plums; no-cal beverage

Dinner
1 Tarragon Chicken Patty*; whole grain hamburger bun; lettuce, tomato, onion,
mustard, or fat-free mayo toppings; 1 serving Spicy Oven Fries*; 1/2 cup
applesauce; 2 reduced-fat cookies; no-cal beverage

Total for Day 5: 23 grams fat (13%); 1,440 calories; 21 grams fiber

DAY 6

Breakfast
1 ounce ready-to-eat cereal; 2 tablespoons raisins; 1 cup skim or 1 percent milk;
1 slice whole grain toast; 1 teaspoon light margarine; jelly or jam; coffee or tea

---

* These recipes appear in the recipe section that follows. Serving sizes are as noted in recipe.

Lunch

Tomato stuffed with 1/2 cup tuna salad (made with water-packed tuna, fat-free mayo, pickles, chopped onion); 1 ounce breadsticks or low-fat crackers; grapes; no-cal beverage

Dinner

1 serving Cilantro Pesto with Pasta*; whole grain roll; tossed vegetable salad; 3 tablespoons fat-free salad dressing; 1/2 cup low-fat frozen yogurt with sliced strawberries; no-cal beverage

Total for Day 6: 20 grams fat (13%); 1,380 calories; 27 grams fiber

DAY 7

Breakfast

1 serving Raspberry Pancakes*; 3 tablespoons light syrup; 1 ounce reduced-fat sausage (≤ 3 grams fat) or 1 ounce Canadian bacon; 1 cup skim or 1 percent milk; coffee or tea

Lunch

2 ounces sliced turkey or chicken on 6″ sub roll; lettuce, tomato, mustard, or fat-free mayo; 1 ounce pretzels; banana; no-cal beverage

Dinner

1 serving Savory Vegetable Beef Soup*; 1 Sour Cream Biscuit*; tossed vegetable salad; 3 tablespoons fat-free salad dressing; 1 serving Peach Cobbler* (or angel cake with sliced peaches); no-cal beverage

Total for Day 7: 21 grams fat (12%); 1,660 calories; 25 grams fiber

Average for Week 1/Days 1–7: 21 grams fat (14%); 1,465 calories; 25 grams fiber

DAY 8

Breakfast

1 ounce ready-to-eat cereal; fresh berries of choice; 1 cup skim or 1 percent milk; 1 slice whole grain toast; 1 teaspoon light margarine; jelly or jam; coffee or tea

Lunch

1/2 cup canned refried beans (spice them up as desired!); 2 medium soft flour tortillas; shredded lettuce, chopped tomatoes, chopped onion, salsa; orange; no-cal beverage

---

* These recipes appear in the recipe section that follows. Serving sizes are as noted in recipe.

Dinner
1 serving Raspberry Chicken*; 1/2 cup serving brown or wild rice; 1 cup Brussels sprouts; whole grain roll; tossed vegetable salad; 3 tablespoons fat-free salad dressing; fruit of choice; no-cal beverage

Total for Day 8: 20 grams fat (12%); 1,540 calories; 45 grams fiber

DAY 9

Breakfast
1 bagel or English muffin; 2 tablespoons fat-free cream cheese; jelly or jam; 1 cup nonfat yogurt (plain or 100 calorie variety); 1 tangerine; coffee or tea

Lunch
2 ounces turkey on 2 slices whole grain bread with 1/4 cup cranberry sauce and alfalfa sprouts; 1 ounce pretzels or no-oil tortilla chips; grapes; no-cal beverage

Dinner
1 serving Cajun Meat Loaf*; baked potato; cauliflower, broccoli, and carrot medley; whole grain roll; tossed vegetable salad; 3 tablespoons fat-free salad dressing; 2 reduced-fat cookies; coffee or tea

Total for Day 9: 21 grams fat (12%); 1,570 calories; 24 grams fiber

DAY 10

Breakfast
1 serving Mixed-Grain Cereal*; 1 cup skim or 1 percent milk; 1 sliced whole grain toast; 1 teaspoon light margarine; jelly or jam; coffee or tea

Lunch
1 serving leftover Cajun Meat Loaf* on sandwich roll; lettuce, tomato slices; 1 ounce pretzels or no-oil tortilla chips; pear or peach; no-cal beverage

Dinner
1 serving Quick Tuna Noodle Casserole*; 1 slice Oatmeal Molasses Bread*; tossed vegetable salad; 3 tablespoons fat-free salad dressing; citrus fruit of choice; no-cal beverage

Total for Day 10: 23 grams fat (15%); 1,400 calories; 27 grams fiber

---

* These recipes appear in the recipe section that follows. Serving sizes are as noted in recipe.

DAY 11

Breakfast
1 serving Apricot Coffee Cake*; 1 cup nonfat yogurt (plain or 100 calorie variety); 1/2 cup orange or other juice; coffee or tea

Lunch
Small fast-food hamburger or lean roast beef sandwich (no mayo!); small side salad with fat-free dressing or broth-based soup; no-cal beverage

Dinner
1 serving Champ Beans* or other beans of choice; 1/2 cup brown or wild rice; 1 cup asparagus; Whole Grain Muffin*; tossed vegetable salad; 3 tablespoons fat-free salad dressing; 2 slices pineapple; no-cal beverage

Total for Day 11: 24 grams fat (14%); 1,510 calories; 17 grams fiber

DAY 12

Breakfast
1 ounce ready-to-eat cereal; sliced banana; 1 cup skim or 1 percent milk; 1 slice whole grain toast; 1 teaspoon light margarine; jelly or jam; coffee or tea

Lunch
1 cup nonfat yogurt (plain or 100 calorie variety); 1 slice Carrot-Pineapple Bread*; grapes; no-cal beverage

Dinner
3 ounces grilled flank or round steak; 1 baked potato; 1 cup broccoli; 1 slice whole grain bread; tossed vegetable salad; 3 tablespoons fat-free salad dressing; citrus fruit cup; 2 reduced-fat cookies; no-cal beverage

Total for Day 12: 22 grams fat (13%); 1,480 calories; 25 grams fiber

DAY 13

Breakfast
1 serving Breakfast Casserole*; 1 cup skim or 1 percent milk; grapefruit; coffee or tea

---

* These recipes appear in the recipe section that follows. Serving sizes are as noted in recipe.

Lunch

Chef salad: assorted raw vegetables, 2 ounces lean ham or turkey breast, 1/2 ounce shredded reduced-fat cheese, 1/4 cup croutons; 3 tablespoons fat-free salad dressing; 1/2 ounce low-fat crackers; apple; no-cal beverage

Dinner

1 serving Spinach Lasagne*; 1 cup carrots; 1 whole grain roll; 1 piece New York Style Cheesecake* with sliced strawberries; no-cal beverage

Total for Day 13: 26 grams fat (16%); 1,450 calories; 27 grams fiber

DAY 14

Breakfast

Whole Wheat Waffles or Pancakes*; 3 tablespoons light syrup; sliced fruit; 1 ounce reduced-fat sausage or 1 ounce Canadian bacon; 1 cup skim or 1 percent milk; coffee or tea

Lunch

1 serving Wheat Berry Minestrone Soup* or other broth-based soup; 1 bagel; seasonal fruit; no-cal beverage

Dinner

1 serving Fragrant Pork (or beef) Roast*; 1 serving Citrus Rice*; 1 cup green beans; 1 whole grain roll; tossed vegetable salad; 3 tablespoons fat-free salad dressing; orange; no-cal beverage

Total for Day 14: 21 grams fat (13%); 1,400 calories; 27 grams fiber

Average for Week 2/Days 7–14: 22 grams fat (13%); 1,480 calories; 27 grams fiber

Average for both weeks, Days 1–14: 21 grams fat (12%); 1,460 calories; 26 grams fiber

---

* These recipes appear in the recipe section that follows. Serving sizes are as noted in recipe.

LFP SNACK IDEAS

The following snack ideas contain less than 3 grams of fat and 200 calories. Add these to LFP menus when you're hungry between meals or have a snack planned. When you just want a nibble, remember that *fresh fruit* is always a great snack, which you can eat virtually anytime without any fat and fewer than 100 calories!

- 1 ounce ready-to-eat cereal; 1 cup skim or 1 percent milk; sliced fruit
- 1 cup nonfat yogurt (plain or 100 calorie variety); sliced fruit; 2 graham crackers
- 4 cups air-popped popcorn; fresh fruit
- 1 1/2 cups Tropical Fruit Smoothie (p. 203)
- 2 fat-free cookies; 1 cup skim or 1 percent milk
- 1 cup frozen low-fat yogurt; sliced fruit
- 1 cup plain, nonfat yogurt; 1 ounce ready-to-eat cereal; sliced fruit
- 1 slice Brenda's Banana Bread (p. 161); 1 cup skim or 1 percent milk
- 1 Refrigerator Bran Muffin (p. 160); 1 cup skim or 1 percent milk
- 1 English muffin toasted with tomato sauce and 1/2 ounce reduced-fat cheese
- 1 ounce low-fat crackers; 1/4 cup Dill Vegetable Dip (p. 168)
- 1 ounce no-oil tortilla chips; 1/2 cup nonfat sour cream; Salsa Verde (p. 201)
- 1 cup broth-based soup; 1/2 ounce low-fat crackers
- 1 ounce pretzels; fresh fruit
- 1 soft pretzel; mustard
- 1/2 sandwich; 1 slice whole grain bread; 1 ounce lean luncheon meat; mustard or fat-free mayonnaise; tomato slice, pickles, and lettuce
- 1 medium bagel
- 1/2 bagel; 1 tablespoon fat-free cream cheese; jelly or jam
- Milk shake: 1/2 cup frozen yogurt; 1/2 cup skim or 1 percent milk; 1 tablespoon chocolate syrup; chipped ice (whip in blender till smooth)
- 3 rice cakes; 1/2 cup low- or no-fat cottage cheese with diced tomatoes
- 1/3 cup dried fruit of choice
- 1 slice angel food cake (~1/16 cake); sliced fruit
- 6 ounces "diet" hot cocoa (from mix); 10 mini marshmallows; 1 fat-free cookie
- Reduced-calorie frozen dessert bar (for example, Weight Watchers brand)

LFP RECIPES

I've chosen over eighty recipes across all the food categories. They include many of my personal favorites along with specialties from some of my friends and weight management group participants. Some of the recipes were chosen for convenience, while others are a bit more time consuming for a weekend dinner or special meal. I wanted to include a sampling of "down-home," "everyday" recipes that we all grew up on and inevitably turn back to, as well as some new and different recipes. I hope you'll find something that suits your taste, time, and mood.

Each recipe lists the ingredients in common household measures with step-by-step instructions. At the end of each recipe you'll find a computer software–generated nutritional profile that includes total fat in grams, percentage of calories from fat in parentheses, total calories, dietary fiber in grams, and sodium in milligrams (mg.). Whenever the ingredient listing says "or," for example, "1 whole egg or 2 egg whites," I have analyzed for the first ingredient listed, in this case, the whole egg. Unless otherwise specified, I used canola oil in the analysis when a recipe calls for oil. If an ingredient is listed as "optional," then it is not included in the nutritional analysis. Likewise for any suggested variation for the recipe.

Some of the recipes may appear to be rather high in sodium. If you have been advised by your physician to limit your intake of sodium or salt, you can omit any added salt in most of the recipes without adverse effect. However, for most of us, the amount of sodium in any of the recipes can easily be incorporated into your overall diet.

I encourage you to try several of the recipes from this book, not only to discover some new additions to your repertoire but also to try for yourself some of the low-fat cooking principles that I covered in Chapter 6. Pay attention to the techniques used in the recipes to translate to your favorite recipes. For example, is it necessary to use those 3 tablespoons of butter to sauté the vegetables for Aunt Emma's famous casserole? No—use nonstick cooking spray or minimal added fat and save 30 grams of fat! Or couldn't you substitute a low-fat cream soup, sour cream, or cheese for the full-fat version your regular recipes call for?

You don't have to rush out and replace your cookbooks with low-fat versions. Once you learn low-fat cooking fundamentals you can adapt or modify virtually any recipe to be lower in fat. Not "no" fat—that's not the goal—just lower in fat. A woman in one of my weight management groups several years ago went through her entire Betty Crocker cookbook with a red pencil, making recipe modifications a constructive pastime as she watched television. Of course, there are some wonderful low-fat cookbooks and magazines on the market. Put a title or subscription request on your birthday wish list!

BREAKFAST FOODS

The most common breakfast foods certainly don't require a recipe. Cereal, toast, bagels, commercial pastries, juice, milk, and coffee are the mainstays for most morning meals. Breakfast fuels your morning and can give you a nutritional advantage. Breakfast eaters, especially those who regularly include ready-to-eat cereals, consume less fat, less cholesterol, more fiber, and more essential vitamins and minerals overall. Use breakfast selections like high-fiber cereals, whole grains, and citrus fruits or juices as a vehicle to boost the quality of your diet for the day.

I've selected a few recipes for special breakfast fare including coffee cakes, pancakes, hot cereals, and a breakfast skillet dish. If you'd like a breakfast meat with your pancakes, try lean ham, Canadian bacon, or a reduced-fat sausage (less than 3 grams fat per ounce). Many of the bread and muffin recipes that follow are also super choices for breakfast. And of course, there's no rule against less-than-traditional breakfast foods (leftovers, for example).

APRICOT COFFEE CAKE

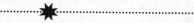

1 cup all-purpose flour
1/2 teaspoon baking powder
1/4 teaspoon salt
1 cup apricot preserves, divided (other flavors may be substituted)
2 large eggs, lightly beaten

1/2 cup granulated sugar
1 teaspoon vanilla extract
1/4 cup sliced almonds or other chopped nuts
1/4 cup packed light brown sugar

1. Preheat the oven to 350 degrees. Coat a 9-inch cake pan with vegetable oil cooking spray.

2. In a large bowl, whisk together the flour, baking powder, and salt. In a separate bowl, beat together 1/3 cup of the preserves, the eggs, granulated sugar, and vanilla. Add to the flour mixture and stir just until evenly blended. Spoon into the prepared pan. Drop the remaining 2/3 cup preserves by spoonfuls evenly over the batter. Sprinkle with nuts and brown sugar.

3. Bake for 40 minutes or until golden brown. Serve while warm.

❖ Makes 8 servings. Per serving: 3.0 grams fat (12%); 222 calories; 1 gram fiber; 135 mg. sodium

CEA'S COFFEE CAKE

GETS BETTER WITH EVERY BITE!

*2 cups plus 2 tablespoons
  all-purpose flour*
3/4 cup granulated sugar
1 tablespoon baking powder
1/2 teaspoon salt
2 tablespoons vegetable oil
1/4 cup applesauce

*1 whole egg or 2 egg whites,
  lightly beaten*
1 1/2 teaspoons vanilla extract
1/2 cup packed brown sugar
2 teaspoons cinnamon
1/2 cup raisins (if desired)

1. Combine 2 cups of flour, the granulated sugar, baking powder, and salt in a mixing bowl. Stir in the oil, applesauce, egg, and vanilla until just combined (do not overmix).

2. Pour half the mixture into a 9-inch cake pan that has been coated with vegetable oil cooking spray.

3. Mix together the brown sugar, cinnamon, and raisins and sprinkle this mixture over the batter.

5. Pour the remaining batter into the pan, spreading with a spatula.

6. Bake at 375 degrees for 35 to 40 minutes or until golden brown.

❖ Makes 8 servings. Per serving (with whole egg): 4.3 grams fat (17%); 233 calories; 1 gram fiber 328 mg. sodium

RASPBERRY PANCAKES

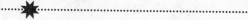

2/3 cup all-purpose flour
1 tablespoon sugar
1 teaspoon baking powder
3/4 teaspoon baking soda
1/3 cup plain nonfat yogurt

1 large egg, lightly beaten
1/2 cup skim milk
*1 cup fresh raspberries (or
  thawed and drained frozen
  berries)*

1. In a bowl, whisk together the flour, sugar, baking powder, and baking soda. Combine the yogurt, egg, and milk in another bowl and slowly stir into the dry ingredients just until combined. The batter should be lumpy. Gently fold in raspberries.

2. Coat a griddle with vegetable oil cooking spray and heat over moderate heat until a drop of cold water dances on the surface. Drop the batter by scant 1/4 cupfuls onto the griddle and cook the pancakes until bubbles form on the surface. Turn carefully and brown on flip side.

3. Serve with maple syrup.

❖ Makes about eight 4-inch pancakes. Per serving of 4 pancakes: 3.4 grams fat (11%); 287 calories; 4 grams fiber; 668 mg. sodium

OATMEAL PANCAKES

1 cup rolled oats
1 cup low-fat buttermilk
1 large egg, lightly beaten
1/4 cup all-purpose flour

1 1/2 teaspoons sugar
1/2 teaspoon baking powder
1/2 teaspoon baking soda

1. Pour the buttermilk over the oats in a medium bowl and let stand at least 5 minutes. Stir in the egg. In a separate bowl, whisk together the flour, sugar, baking powder, and baking soda. Add to the buttermilk mixture and stir just until combined. The batter should be lumpy.

2. Coat a griddle with vegetable oil cooking spray and heat over moderate heat until a drop of water dances on the surface. Drop the batter by 1/4 cupfuls onto the griddle and cook the pancakes until bubbles form over the surface; turn carefully and brown the other side.

❖ Makes about eight 4-inch pancakes. Per serving of 4 pancakes: 6.3 grams fat (18%); 312 calories; 5 grams fiber; 321 mg. sodium

WHOLE WHEAT PANCAKES

AN EXCELLENT BASIC PANCAKE BATTER RECIPE. THIS WILL
KEEP IN THE REFRIGERATOR FOR A FEW DAYS; ADD MORE
LIQUID AND STIR BEFORE USING.

1 cup whole wheat flour
1 cup all-purpose flour
1/2 teaspoon salt
1 tablespoon baking powder
1 teaspoon baking soda

1 whole egg and 2 egg whites,
   lightly beaten
2 tablespoons applesauce
2 1/2 cups buttermilk

1. In a bowl or wide-mouthed pitcher, whisk together the flours, salt, baking powder, and baking soda. Add the eggs, applesauce, and buttermilk and stir just until blended. The batter should be lumpy.

2. Drop by approximately 1/4 cupfuls onto a hot griddle. When the edges of the pancakes begin to brown and bubbles appear in the center, turn carefully and brown the other side.

3. Serve with fruit topping or syrup.

❖ Makes 6 servings. Per serving: 2.0 grams fat (9%); 190 calories; 3 grams fiber; 656 mg. sodium

Whole Wheat Waffles
Preheat a waffle iron according to the manufacturer's directions. Pour batter onto the hot iron as directed and bake until the steaming stops and the waffle is golden brown and crisp.

BAKED SKIERS' FRENCH TOAST

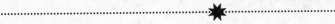

THIS DISH IS ASSEMBLED THE NIGHT BEFORE AND POPPED
IN THE OVEN THE NEXT MORNING.

2 tablespoons corn syrup
1 teaspoon butter-flavored
* sprinkles*
1 cup packed brown sugar
12 slices whole grain bread
1 1/4 cups egg substitute

2 egg whites
1 1/2 cups skim or 1 percent
* milk*
1 teaspoon vanilla extract
1/4 teaspoon salt

1. In a small saucepan, combine the corn syrup, butter flavor, brown sugar, and 2 tablespoons of water. Bring to a boil, reduce the heat, and simmer until the sugar is dissolved. Pour this mixture over the bottom of a 9 × 13-inch baking dish.

2. Arrange the bread slices over the sugar mixture in the dish.

3. In a bowl, beat together the egg substitute, egg whites, milk, vanilla, and salt. Pour over the bread. Cover the dish with foil and refrigerate overnight.

4. Remove the dish from the refrigerator and preheat the oven to 350 degrees. Bake, uncovered, 45 minutes or until browned and puffy. Serve hot.

❖ Makes 6 servings. Per serving: 3.0 grams fat (8%); 339 calories; 5 grams fiber; 527 mg. sodium

FRUITY BREAKFAST BARLEY

1 cup orange juice
1/4 cup chopped dried apricots
Dash of ground cloves

1 cup quick-cooking barley
1 tablespoon honey

1. In a medium saucepan combine the orange juice, apricots, and cloves with 1 1/2 cups of water. Bring to a boil. Stir in the barley. Cover and simmer for 12 to 15 minutes or until the barley is tender. Stir in the honey. Serve with skim milk, if desired.

❖ Makes 4 servings. Per serving: 0.4 grams fat (2%); 165 calories; 5 grams fiber; 54 mg. sodium

MIXED-GRAIN CEREAL

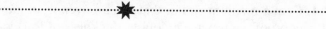

A WHOLESOME HOT CEREAL THAT COMBINES OATS,
BARLEY, AND BULGUR.

1 cup regular rolled oats
1 cup quick-cooking barley
1 cup cracked wheat (bulgur)

1 cup raisins
1/2 cup millet

1. Combine oats, barley, cracked wheat, raisins, and millet in an airtight storage container.
2. To make 4 servings: In a saucepan, bring 1 1/3 cups water to a boil. Stir in 3/4 cup of the cereal mixture. Cover, reduce the heat, and simmer for 12 to 15 minutes or until the cereal has the desired consistency. Serve with skim milk and honey, if desired.

❖ Mix makes 4 1/2 cups (24 servings). Per serving: 0.7 grams fat (6%); 104 calories; 3 grams fiber; 23 mg. sodium

POTATO AND SAUSAGE FRITTATA

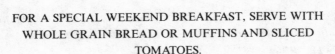

FOR A SPECIAL WEEKEND BREAKFAST, SERVE WITH
WHOLE GRAIN BREAD OR MUFFINS AND SLICED
TOMATOES.

1 teaspoon olive oil
1 small onion, chopped fine
1 small green bell pepper,
  seeded and chopped fine
1 teaspoon minced jalapeño
  pepper
4 ounces 90 percent lean
  kielbasa or smoked cooked
  sausage, sliced thin and
  halved

1 medium boiled potato,
  peeled and sliced thin
2 whole eggs
4 egg whites (or 1/2 cup egg
  substitute)
1/4 teaspoon salt
1/2 teaspoon Tabasco
1 tablespoon chopped cilantro
  (optional)

1. Coat a medium skillet that has an ovenproof handle (if handle is not ovenproof, wrap with a double thickness of foil) with vegetable oil cooking spray. Heat the olive oil over moderate heat and add the onion, green pepper, and jalapeño. Sauté until tender, about 5 minutes, while stirring. Add the sausage and sauté for 2 minutes. Layer the potato slices over the sausage mixture.

2. In a medium bowl, beat together the eggs, egg whites, salt, and Tabasco, and pour over potatoes. Sprinkle with cilantro. Reduce the heat to low and let the mixture cook until the edges begin to set.

3. Place the skillet under the broiler until the top of the mixture begins to brown and bubble.

4. To serve, loosen the edges of the frittata with a spatula. Place a large plate over the skillet on top of the frittata and invert.

❖ Makes 4 servings. Per serving: 8.0 grams fat (46%); 163 calories; 1 gram fiber; 423 mg. sodium

BREADS, MUFFINS, AND ROLLS

I love bread! And for that reason here are eleven wonderful low-fat, high-nutrition recipes for you to try at breakfast, with lunch or dinner, or as a snack.

NO-KNEAD BREAD
✷

1 package active dry yeast
  (1 scant tablespoon)
1/4 cup warm water
2 tablespoons sugar
1 teaspoon salt
1/2 teaspoon baking soda

1 cup reduced-fat sour cream
1 egg, lightly beaten, or
  1/4 cup egg substitute
3/4 cup whole wheat flour
1 3/4 cups all-purpose flour,
  divided

1. In the large bowl of an electric mixer, stir the yeast and 1 teaspoon of sugar into the warm water and let stand until foamy, about 10 minutes. Add the remaining sugar, the salt, soda, sour cream, egg, whole wheat flour, and 3/4 cup of the all-purpose flour.

2. Beat on medium speed with mixer until thoroughly blended. Continue to mix on high for 2 1/2 minutes. Stir in the remaining 3/4 cup of flour until it is thoroughly incorporated.

3. Transfer the dough to a medium loaf pan that has been coated with vegetable oil cooking spray.

4. Cover lightly with a kitchen towel and let rise in a warm place until doubled, about 1 hour.

5. Bake in a preheated 350 degree oven for 45 to 50 minutes, or until the loaf is golden brown and sounds hollow when thumped. Remove from the pan and cool on a wire rack.

❖ Makes 16 servings. Per serving (with egg): 1.5 grams fat (14%); 95 calories; 2 grams fiber; 172 mg. sodium

No-Knead Rolls
Follow the above recipe through step 2. Coat two 8-cup muffin tins lightly with vegetable oil cooking spray. Turn the dough out onto a floured surface and roll with floured hands into a cylinder. Cut with a floured knife into 16 pieces and transfer them to the muffin pans.

Cover lightly with a kitchen towel and let rise until doubled, about 1 hour. Bake at 350 degrees for 25 to 30 minutes, or until golden brown. Remove from pans and cool on a wire rack.

OATMEAL MOLASSES BREAD

✳

2 cups boiling water
1 1/2 cups old-fashioned or
   quick-cooking oatmeal
1/4 teaspoon sugar
1 1/2 packages (scant 4
   teaspoons) active dry yeast

1 1/2 teaspoons vegetable
   shortening
1 1/2 teaspoons salt
1/2 cup dark molasses
4 1/2 to 5 cups all-purpose
   flour, or as needed

1. In a large bowl, pour the boiling water over the oatmeal and let stand for 1 hour.

2. In a small bowl, sprinkle sugar and yeast over 1/3 cup lukewarm water, stir to dissolve, and let stand until foamy, about 10 minutes. Stir the yeast mixture into the oatmeal with the shortening, salt, and molasses. Add 4 cups of the flour, 1 cup at a time, beating well after each addition. Turn the dough out onto a floured surface and knead, adding a little more flour at a time, to form a soft but slightly sticky dough. Form the dough into a ball, put it in a lightly buttered bowl, and turn it to coat with the butter. Cover the bowl with plastic wrap and a kitchen towel and let the dough rise in a warm place for about 1 hour, or until doubled in size.

3. Punch down the dough, knead it for 3 to 5 minutes, and form into 2 loaves. Place the loaves in two medium loaf pans that have been coated with vegetable oil cooking spray. Cover lightly with the towel and let rise for 45 minutes, or until doubled.

4. Bake in a preheated 375 degree oven for 1 hour, or until the loaves are browned and sound hollow when tapped. Remove from pans and cool on the rack.

❖ Makes 2 loaves (16 slices per loaf). Per slice: 0.6 grams fat (6%); 95 calories; 1 gram fiber; 102 mg. sodium

POTATO ROLLS

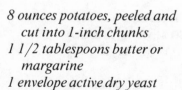

8 ounces potatoes, peeled and
   cut into 1-inch chunks
1 1/2 tablespoons butter or
   margarine
1 envelope active dry yeast
   (1 scant tablespoon)

2 tablespoons plus
   1/2 teaspoon sugar, divided
1 egg, lightly beaten
2 teaspoons salt
5 1/2 cups all-purpose flour,
   or as needed

1. Place potatoes in medium saucepan. Add cold water to cover, bring to a boil, and simmer until very tender, about 20 minutes. Drain potatoes, reserving 1/4 cup cooking liquid. Place potatoes in the large bowl of an electric mixer. Add butter and beat until smooth. Add reserved cooking liquid, 1 tablespoon at a time, beating until potatoes are fluffy. Cool potatoes to lukewarm.

2. Sprinkle yeast and 1/4 teaspoon sugar over 1 cup warm water in a small bowl; stir to dissolve. Let yeast mixture stand 10 minutes or until foamy.

3. Stir the egg, 2 tablespoons sugar, and salt into the mashed potatoes. Add the yeast mixture and 2 cups of flour. Stir vigorously with a wooden spoon until smooth, about 3 minutes. Mix in enough flour, 1/2 cup at a time, to form a soft, slightly sticky dough. Knead on a lightly floured surface until smooth and elastic, adding more flour if necessary, for about 8 minutes (the dough will be somewhat sticky).

4. Butter a large bowl. Add the dough, turning to coat the entire surface. Cover the bowl with plastic wrap. Let the dough rise in a warm area until doubled, 45 minutes or longer.

5. Turn the dough out onto a floured surface and divide in half. With floured hands, roll each half into a cylinder. Cut each cylinder into 15 pieces.

6. Lightly spray two 9-inch round or square cake pans with vegetable oil cooking spray. Flour hands and form the dough into balls, arranging 15 in each pan. Cover lightly with a kitchen towel and let rise in a warm place until doubled, about 1/2 hour or longer.

7. Preheat the oven to 375 degrees. Bake the rolls about 20 minutes, or until golden brown. Turn out of pans and cool on a rack.

NOTE: The rolls may also be frozen after they are shaped into balls. Allow several hours for them to thaw and rise.

❖ Makes 30 rolls. Per roll: 1.0 gram fat (9%); 94 calories; 1 gram fiber; 151 mg. sodium

SOUR CREAM BISCUITS

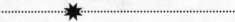

GREAT FOR BREAKFAST WITH JELLY OR JAM.
THIS BISCUIT DOUGH ALSO MAKES A GOOD
LOW-FAT PIE CRUST ALTERNATIVE.

1 cup all-purpose flour   *1/2 teaspoon salt*
1 teaspoon sugar   *1/2 cup light sour cream*
2 teaspoons baking powder   *1/4 cup evaporated skim milk*
1/2 teaspoon baking soda

1. Preheat the oven to 425 degrees. Lightly coat a cookie sheet with vegetable oil cooking spray.

2. Combine the flour, sugar, baking powder, soda, and salt in a medium mixing bowl and whisk to blend thoroughly. Combine the sour cream and evaporated milk and stir into the dry ingredients just until blended. Do not overmix.

3. Turn the dough out onto a floured board and roll or pat out to approximately 1/2 inch thickness. Cut with a biscuit cutter into 8 rounds (or cut with a knife into 8 squares). Place on the prepared cookie sheet.

4. Bake approximately 8 minutes, or until browned.

❖ Makes 8 biscuits. Per biscuit: 2.0 grams fat (21%); 86 calories; 0 grams fiber; 333 mg. sodium

CORN BREAD

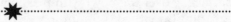

THIS TASTY GOLDEN BREAD GOES WELL WITH SOUPS,
STEWS, OR ANY MEAL.

2 cups self-rising cornmeal   *3/4 cup buttermilk*
1/2 cup light sour cream   *2 egg whites, lightly beaten*
1 (15-ounce) can cream-style
* corn*

1. Preheat the oven to 375 degrees. Coat an 8-inch baking pan with vegetable oil cooking spray.

2. Combine all the ingredients in a medium mixing bowl, stirring just until blended.

3. Pour the batter into the prepared baking pan.

4. Bake 25 to 30 minutes, or until the top is lightly browned and the bread pulls slightly from the edge of the pan.

❖ Makes 9 servings. Per serving: 2.5 grams fat (13%); 173 calories; 2 grams fiber; 586 mg. sodium

Skillet Corn Bread

Heat 1 tablespoon vegetable oil in a heavy iron skillet in the oven. Turn the batter into the skillet and bake for 25 to 30 minutes or until lightly browned and firm to the touch.

❖ (Per serving: 4 grams fat; 186 calories)

WHOLE GRAIN MUFFINS

3/4 cup skim milk
3/4 cup bran cereal
1 egg, lightly beaten
1/4 cup applesauce
1/2 cup molasses or honey

1 cup rolled oats
2/3 cup all-purpose flour
1 tablespoon baking powder
1/4 teaspoon salt

OPTIONAL: Add 1/2 cup raisins, blueberries, chopped dates, or chopped apple to the dry ingredients and toss to coat.

1. Preheat the oven to 400 degrees. Spray the bottoms (not the sides) of two 6-cup muffin tins with vegetable oil cooking spray (or line with paper liners).

2. Combine the milk and bran cereal in a mixing bowl. Add the egg, applesauce, and molasses. Mix well.

3. Combine the oats, flour, baking powder, and salt in a separate bowl. Stir into the cereal mixture just until the dry ingredients are moistened.

4. Fill the muffin cups 2/3 full. Bake 20 to 25 minutes, or until lightly browned and springy to the touch.

❖ Makes 12 muffins. Per muffin: 1.1 grams fat (8%); 115 calories; 3 grams fiber; 247 mg. sodium

HUMMINGBIRD MUFFINS

3/4 cup all-purpose flour
3/4 cup whole wheat flour
2/3 cup sugar
1/4 cup toasted wheat germ
1/2 teaspoon baking soda
1/2 teaspoon salt
1/2 teaspoon ground cinnamon

1/4 teaspoon grated nutmeg
2 large eggs, lightly beaten
1 teaspoon vanilla extract
2 large ripe bananas, mashed
  (about 1 cup)
1 (8-ounce) can unsweetened
  crushed pineapple, with juice

1. Preheat the oven to 350 degrees. Coat the bottoms (not the sides) of two 6-cup muffin pans with vegetable oil cooking spray.

2. In a large bowl, stir together flours, sugar, wheat germ, baking soda, salt, cinnamon, and nutmeg. Add the eggs and vanilla, stirring until blended. Fold in bananas and pineapple.

3. Pour the batter evenly into 12 muffin cups, filling them 2/3 full. Bake for about 25 minutes, or until lightly browned and springy to the touch.

❖ Makes 12 muffins. Per muffin: 1.4 grams fat (8%); 146 calories; 2 grams fiber; 135 mg. sodium

REFRIGERATOR BRAN MUFFINS

A GREAT WAY TO HAVE FRESH HOT MUFFINS ANY TIME.
THE BATTER, STORED IN THE REFRIGERATOR AND
TIGHTLY COVERED, WILL KEEP FOR SEVERAL WEEKS.

5 cups all-purpose flour (or 3
  cups all-purpose and 2 cups
  whole wheat flour)
1 teaspoon salt
4 teaspoons ground cinnamon
5 teaspoons baking soda
3 cups sugar
2 cups rolled oats

1 (15-ounce) box raisin bran
  cereal
1 pound raisins
1 (22-ounce) jar applesauce
1/4 cup vegetable oil
4 eggs, lightly beaten
1 quart buttermilk

1. In a very large mixing bowl, whisk together the flour, salt, cinnamon, soda, sugar, and rolled oats. Add the bran cereal and the raisins and stir to combine.

2. In a separate bowl, combine the applesauce, oil, eggs, and buttermilk and mix thoroughly. Add to the dry ingredients; stir well, and transfer to a large airtight storage container.

3. Refrigerate. Prepare muffins as needed by filling oiled or paper-lined muffin cups 2/3 full. Bake at 400 degrees for 15–20 minutes, or until the muffins are lightly browned and springy to the touch.

❖ Makes 72 medium muffins. Per muffin: 1.5 grams fat (10%); 130 calories; 2 grams fiber; 138 mg sodium

BRENDA'S BANANA BREAD

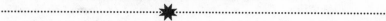

THIS MOIST AND SWEET RECIPE USES PRUNE PASTE,
AN EXCELLENT SUBSTITUTE FOR BUTTER, MARGARINE,
OR OIL IN BAKED GOODS OR COOKIES (USE IN
EQUAL MEASURES).

2 cups sugar	3–4 ripe bananas, mashed
1 cup prune paste (see Note below) or applesauce	3 1/3 cups all-purpose flour
	1 1/2 teaspoons salt
2 whole eggs	2 teaspoons ground cinnamon
4 egg whites	2 teaspoons baking soda

1. Preheat the oven to 350 degrees. Lightly coat 2 loaf pans with vegetable oil cooking spray.

2. In a large mixing bowl, combine the sugar, prune paste, eggs, egg whites, and mashed bananas. Add 2/3 cup of water and stir until thoroughly combined. In another bowl, whisk together the flour, salt, cinnamon, and soda. Stir into banana mixture.

3. Divide the batter between the 2 pans, smoothing the top with a spatula. Bake for 60 to 70 minutes, or until the loaves shrink slightly from the pans. Let the bread cool in the pans on a wire rack for 15 minutes, then remove from the pans to the rack and cool completely.

NOTE: To make prune paste, put prunes in a blender with a little water and blend until puréed. Store, covered, in the refrigerator.

❖ Makes 2 loaves. Per serving (1/16 loaf): 0.6 grams fat (3%); 143 calories; 2 grams fiber; 163 mg. sodium

CARROT-PINEAPPLE BREAD

REMINISCENT OF CARROT CAKE, THIS BREAD IS
WONDERFUL AS A DESSERT BREAD, A SNACK WITH
COFFEE, OR A BREAKFAST BREAD. OR SERVE IT WITH
FRUIT SALAD AND COTTAGE CHEESE FOR LUNCH.

1 3/4 cups sugar
1 1/4 cups applesauce
2 tablespoons vegetable oil
2 teaspoons vanilla extract
4 whole eggs or 1 cup egg
  substitute
1 1/2 cups whole wheat flour
1 1/2 cups all-purpose flour

1 tablespoon baking powder
1 teaspoon baking soda
1 teaspoon salt
1 tablespoon ground cinnamon
2 1/2 cups shredded raw carrots
1 (8-ounce) can crushed
  pineapple with juice

1. Preheat the oven to 350 degrees. Spray 2 loaf pans with vegetable oil cooking spray.

2. Combine the sugar, applesauce, oil, and vanilla in a large mixing bowl. Beat by hand or with an electric mixer on medium speed until well blended. Beat in the eggs one at a time.

3. In a separate bowl, combine the flours, baking powder, soda, salt, and cinnamon; whisk thoroughly. Stir into the applesauce mixture just until combined—do not overmix. Fold in carrots and pineapple.

4. Divide the batter between the baking pans and smooth the tops with a spatula. Bake for 50 minutes, or until the bread shrinks slightly from the side of the pan. Allow to cool in the pans for 15 minutes, then remove from the pans to cool on a rack.

❖ Makes 2 loaves (12 slices per loaf). Per slice: 2.2 grams fat (13%); 150 calories; 2 grams fiber; 112 mg. sodium

DATE-BRAN BREAD

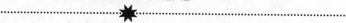

A HIGH-FIBER, LOW-FAT BREAD FOR BREAKFAST OR A
SNACK. THIS IS ALSO GREAT TO SLICE AND TAKE TO WORK.

1 cup all-purpose flour
1 cup whole wheat flour
1 1/2 cups all-bran cereal
2 teaspoons baking powder
1/2 teaspoon baking soda
1 teaspoon salt
1/2 cup molasses

1 1/2 cups skim or 1 percent
  milk
1 egg, lightly beaten
1/4 cup applesauce
1 cup finely chopped pitted
  dates

1. Preheat the oven to 350 degrees. Lightly coat a 9 × 5 × 3-inch
loaf pan with vegetable oil cooking spray.

2. In a large mixing bowl, whisk together the flours, bran, baking
powder, soda, and salt. In a separate bowl combine the molasses, milk,
egg, and applesauce; add to the dry ingredients. Stir just until combined
—do not overmix.

3. Pour into the prepared pan and bake about 1 hour, or until the
loaf shrinks slightly from the side of the pan. Cool in the pan for 15
minutes, then turn out of the pan and cool on a rack completely before
cutting.

❖ Makes 6 servings. Per serving: 0.8 grams fat (4%); 146 calories; 5 grams fiber; 330 mg. sodium

SOUPS

Soups are a great way to start a meal. With a good bread and a salad, a hearty soup can make a satisfying main course. I've included five soups that are delicious and distinctively different!

SAVORY VEGETABLE BEEF SOUP

1 pound soup bones, with all visible fat removed
1/2 cup dried split peas
Salt
1 pound eye of round beef, cut into 1/2-inch cubes
1/4 medium head of cabbage, chopped fine
1 large onion, chopped
3 carrots, peeled and sliced thin
2 (14-ounce) cans tomatoes, chopped
1 (10-ounce) package frozen mixed vegetables
2 medium potatoes, peeled and diced

1 bay leaf
6 peppercorns
1/2 teaspoon dried basil
1/2 teaspoon dried oregano
1/4 teaspoon chili powder
1/4 teaspoon dried thyme
1/8 teaspoon dried rosemary
1/8 teaspoon dried marjoram
1/8 teaspoon ground cloves
1/4 teaspoon freshly ground pepper
1/4 cup barley
1 teaspoon Maggi seasoning (optional)
1 1/2 teaspoons sugar
2 tablespoons flour

1. In a large pot, cover the soup bones with 7 cups of cold water. Bring to a boil, lower the heat, and allow to simmer for 10 to 15 minutes, skimming off impurities as they rise to the surface. When thoroughly skimmed, add the split peas and 2 teaspoons of salt and cook over medium heat for 30 minutes. Add the beef, cabbage, onion, carrots, and tomatoes and return to a boil. Reduce heat and simmer 30 minutes. Remove soup bones. Add the mixed vegetables, potatoes, and spices, and simmer for 1 hour. Stir in the remaining ingredients except flour.

2. Place flour into small bowl and gradually thin with 2/3 cup of cold water, stirring in 1 tablespoon at a time, using a small whisk if necessary to remove lumps. When smooth, stir into the soup and cook 15 minutes to thicken slightly.

❖ Makes 8 servings. Per serving: 3.3 grams fat (12%); 243 calories; 7.5 grams fiber; 663 mg. sodium

WHEAT BERRY MINESTRONE SOUP

WHEAT BERRIES MAKE THIS SOUP UNIQUE AND
DELICIOUS.

1/2 cup wheat berries
1 (15-ounce) can Great
  Northern beans, drained
1 1/2 cups beef broth
1 cup canned tomatoes, crushed
1 cup loose-pack frozen mixed
  vegetables (carrots,
  cauliflower, green beans,
  zucchini, and butter beans)

1/2 cup chopped onion
2 tablespoons parsley flakes
1 teaspoon dried basil
1 clove garlic, minced
Grated Parmesan cheese
  (fat-free) for topping
  (optional)

1. In a saucepan combine wheat berries with 3 1/2 cups of cold water. Bring to a boil, reduce the heat, and simmer, covered, for 1 hour.

2. Add the beans, beef broth, undrained tomatoes, frozen vegetables, onion, parsley, basil, and garlic. Return to a boil, reduce the heat, and simmer, covered, for 15 to 20 minutes or until vegetables are tender.

❖ Makes 8 servings. Per serving: 1.0 grams fat (8%); 107 calories; 5 grams fiber; 235 mg. sodium

SEPTEMBER CHOWDER

2 teaspoons butter or
  margarine
1/2 cup chopped onion
1 stalk celery, chopped
1 carrot, peeled and sliced thin
2 fresh tomatoes, seeded and
  chopped
2 medium potatoes, peeled
  and diced

1 teaspoon salt
1/4 teaspoon ground red pepper
3 cups chicken stock
2 cups fresh or frozen corn
  kernels
1 cup evaporated skim milk
1/2 cup chopped fresh basil

1. Coat the bottom of a 5-quart pot with vegetable oil cooking spray and melt the butter over moderate heat. Sauté the onion, celery, and carrot until the onion is limp, about 5 minutes. Add the tomatoes, potatoes, red pepper, salt, chicken stock, and corn to the pot.

2. Simmer the mixture for 25 minutes, or until the potatoes are tender (do not overcook or potatoes will be mushy). Add the milk and chopped basil and heat for 2 or 3 minutes or until piping hot. Serve immediately.

❖ Makes 6 servings. Per servings: 2.9 grams fat (15%); 167 calories; 4 grams fiber; 829 mg. sodium

WHITE CHILI

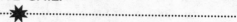

4 boneless chicken breast
   halves, skins removed
1 teaspoon olive oil
1 onion, chopped
1 garlic clove, minced
2 (9-ounce) packages frozen
   white shoe-peg corn
2 (4-ounce) cans diced green
   chiles

2 teaspoons powdered cumin
Juice of 1 lime
2 (15-ounce) cans Great
   Northern beans, drained
Salsa Verde (page 200)
1 cup crushed no-oil tortilla
   chips

1. In a saucepan, cover the chicken breasts with 2 1/2 cups of water and bring to a boil. Reduce the heat, cover, and simmer about 25 minutes, or until done. Drain (reserving stock for another use) and set chicken aside to cool.

2. Coat the bottom of a large pot with vegetable oil cooking spray and heat the olive oil over medium heat. Sauté the onion until tender; add the garlic and cook for 1 minute. Add the corn, chiles, cumin, lime juice, and beans. Cut the chicken into 1/2-inch pieces and add to pot. Continue cooking until thoroughly heated and flavors are blended.

3. Serve with salsa verde or commercial green salsa and top with crushed tortilla chips.

❖ Makes 6 servings. Per serving: 2.6 grams fat (6%); 349 calories; 12 grams fiber; 70 mg. sodium

SUMMER MELON SOUP

REFRESHING AND DELICIOUS!

1 large ripe cantaloupe, peeled
  and cubed (about 4 1/2 cups)
3 tablespoons slivered
  crystallized ginger
1 1/2 teaspoons grated orange
  zest

1 teaspoon honey
1 cup plain nonfat yogurt
2/3 cup fresh orange juice
1 tablespoon fresh lemon juice

1. Place the cantaloupe, ginger, orange zest, and honey in a food processor or blender and purée. Add the yogurt, orange juice, and lemon juice and blend until smooth.
2. Transfer to a bowl or large jar, cover, and refrigerate until chilled, at least 3 hours.

❖ Makes 4 servings. Per serving: 0.7 grams fat (5%); 124 calories; 1 gram fiber; 65 mg. sodium

BROCCAMOLI DIP

*1 (10-ounce) package frozen
  chopped broccoli*
*1/2 teaspoon minced dried
  onion*
1/2 cup nonfat sour cream
1 tablespoon lemon juice

1 tablespoon chunky salsa
*1 teaspoon Worcestershire
  sauce*
1/4 teaspoon ground coriander
1/8 teaspoon ground red pepper

1. Cook the broccoli with the onion according to broccoli package directions, adding 2 to 3 minutes to the cooking time; drain.

2. Place the broccoli, sour cream, lemon juice, salsa, Worcestershire, coriander, and red pepper in a blender or food processor. Blend until smooth. Turn into a serving bowl and cover with plastic wrap. Chill at least 1 hour.

3. Stir the dip before serving. Serve with raw vegetables or low-fat crackers or pretzel chips.

❖ Makes about 1 3/4 cups. Per 1/4 cup serving: 0.1 grams fat (2%); 23 calories; 1 gram fiber, 37 mg. sodium

DILL VEGETABLE DIP

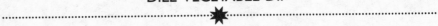

SERVE WITH ASSORTED RAW VEGETABLES—OR SOME OF
THE NEW FAT-FREE POTATO CHIPS.

1 cup fat-free sour cream
1 cup fat-free mayonnaise
1 tablespoon parsley flakes
*1 tablespoon dried minced
  onion*

1 tablespoon dried dill weed
1/4 teaspoon garlic powder

Combine all ingredients. Chill in refrigerator at least 1 hour. Sprinkle with paprika if desired and serve.

❖ Makes 2 cups. Per 1/4 cup: 0 fat (0%); 41 calories; 0 fiber; 359 mg. sodium

VEGGIE SANDWICH SPREAD

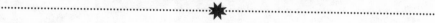

THIS FLAVORFUL LOW-FAT SPREAD IS GREAT ON BAGELS,
WHOLE GRAIN BREADS, OR PITA. SERVE WITH SOUP AND
FRUIT TO ROUND OUT AN EASY MEAL.

*1/2 cup diced vegetables (try
a combination of carrots,
green onions, broccoli,
mushrooms, and zucchini)*

*1 cup light ricotta cheese
2 teaspoons Dijon or spicy
mustard*

Blend the combination of finely diced vegetables with ricotta and
mustard. Keep refrigerated (use original ricotta container for leftovers).

❖ Makes 1 1/2 cups. Per 1/4 cup serving: 0.4 grams fat (8%); 45 calories; 1 gram fiber; 164 mg. sodium

NO-FAT COLESLAW

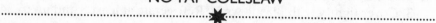

THIS GOES WELL WITH PORK BARBECUE OR BURGERS.
STORED IN THE REFRIGERATOR, IT KEEPS FOR
SEVERAL WEEKS.

*1 cup vinegar
1/2 teaspoon turmeric
1/2 teaspoon salt
1 teaspoon mustard seeds
Nutrasweet to equal 1/2 cup
sugar, or 1/2 cup sugar*

*1 medium head of cabbage,
shredded
1/2 large onion, chopped fine
1 bell pepper, seeded and
chopped fine*

1. In a small skillet, combine the vinegar, turmeric, salt, mustard
seeds, and 1/2 cup water. Bring to a boil on top of the stove or in the
microwave. Remove from the heat, cool the mixture, and stir in
Nutrasweet.

2. Combine the cabbage, onion, and pepper in a large bowl; pour
vinegar mixture over the vegetables, stirring well. Refrigerate for several
hours before serving.

❖ Makes 4 cups. Per 1/2 cup serving: 0.1 gram fat (4%); 25 calories; 1 gram fiber; 140 mg. sodium

SEVEN-LAYER SALAD

1 head of iceberg lettuce,
chopped
1 cup chopped celery
1/2 cup chopped onion
1/2 cup chopped green bell
pepper
1 (10-ounce) package frozen
peas (do not defrost)

2 cups fat-free mayonnaise
mixed with 2 tablespoons
sugar
1/2 jar imitation bacon bits
(3 ounces)
1/2 cup shredded reduced-fat
sharp Cheddar cheese

1. Line the bottom of a 9 × 13-inch glass casserole dish with chopped lettuce. Spread the celery in a layer over the lettuce, sprinkle evenly with the onion, then with the green pepper, and top with a layer of peas.

2. "Frost" with the mayonnaise dressing, spreading with a spatula to the edges. Sprinkle with bacon bits and cheese.

3. Cover tightly with plastic wrap. Refrigerate at least 8 and up to 24 hours before serving.

❖ Makes 8 servings. Per serving: 3.5 grams fat (20%); 152 calories; 4 grams fiber; 1,019 mg. sodium

VEGETABLE SALAD

1 (14-ounce) can white
whole-kernel corn, drained
1 (14-ounce) can small peas,
drained
1 (14-ounce) can French-style
green beans, drained
1 small onion, chopped
1 green bell pepper, seeded
and chopped (or use

1/2 green and 1/2 red
pepper for added color)
3/4 cup vinegar
3/4 cup sugar
2 tablespoons olive or canola oil
1 teaspoon salt
1/2 teaspoon freshly ground
pepper

1. Place the corn, peas, green beans, onion, and chopped pepper in a serving bowl. Toss lightly.

2. In a small saucepan, combine the vinegar, sugar, oil, salt, and pepper. Add 2 tablespoons of water and bring to a boil. Pour over the vegetables. Mix well, cover with plastic wrap, and refrigerate for at least several hours. The salad will keep up to 2 weeks.

❖ Makes 12 servings. Per serving: 2.6 grams fat (17%); 129 calories; 3 grams fiber; 423 mg. sodium

SHRIMP–SNOW PEA SALAD

1 tablespoon vegetable oil   *Dash of pepper*
1 tablespoon apple juice   *6 ounces fresh snow peas*
2 tablespoons Dijon mustard   *10 ounces frozen cooked salad*
2 tablespoons fresh lemon juice   *shrimp*
1/2 teaspoon celery seed   *6 cups torn mixed salad greens*

1. Combine oil, apple juice, mustard, lemon juice, celery seed, and pepper. Mix well. Chill in a covered container.

2. Remove strings from snow peas and place in a small saucepan with 2 tablespoons of water. Cover and steam over high heat for 2 to 3 minutes or until crisp tender. Chill.

4. Thaw shrimp by rinsing under cold water. Drain well.

5. To serve, place greens in a large bowl; add shrimp and peas. Shake dressing; pour over salad. Toss to coat.

❖ Makes 6 servings. Per serving: 3.2 grams fat (30%); 95 calories; 2 grams fiber; 186 mg. sodium

SPINACH WITH HEARTS OF PALM SALAD

1/2 pound fresh spinach,   *2 navel oranges, peeled and*
washed, stemmed, and dried   *sectioned or sliced*
1 (14-ounce) can hearts of   *1 small red onion, peeled and*
palm, drained and sliced   *sliced thin*

In a large bowl, combine the spinach, hearts of palm, oranges, and onion. Toss gently with Strawberry-Peppercorn Vinaigrette (see recipe below).

❖ Makes 4 servings. Per serving: 0.5 grams fat (3%); 123 calories; 5 grams fiber; 55 mg. sodium

STRAWBERRY-PEPPERCORN VINAIGRETTE

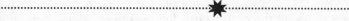

*1 cup cut-up fresh
    strawberries or frozen
    strawberries, thawed
2 tablespoons balsamic vinegar*

*1/2 teaspoon honey
1/8 teaspoon whole black
    peppercorns or coarse
    ground red pepper*

Combine the strawberries, vinegar, honey, and peppercorns in a blender or food processor. Cover and blend until smooth.

❖ Makes about 1 cup. Per 1/4 cup serving: 0.1 gram fat (6%); 15 calories; 1 gram fiber; < 5 mg. sodium

FROSTED APRICOT SALAD

THIS MAKES A DELICIOUS SWEET SALAD
OR A FRUITY DESSERT.

*2 cups boiling water
1 package (6 ounces)
    apricot-flavored gelatin
1 can (16 ounces) "lite"
    apricot halves
1 can (8 ounces) crushed
    pineapple in its own juice
2 large bananas, sliced
1 cup "lite" whipped topping*

*1/2 cup fat-free sour cream
4 ounces fat-free cream
    cheese, at room temperature
3 tablespoons confectioner's
    sugar
1/2 teaspoon almond extract
1 tablespoon flaked or
    shredded coconut (optional)*

1. Pour boiling water over gelatin in a mixing bowl; stir until gelatin is dissolved. Stir in apricots (with syrup), and pineapple (with juice). Refrigerate until slightly thickened, about 1 1/2 hours.

2. Fold the bananas into the gelatin mixture. Pour the mixture into a 9 × 9 × 2-inch pan. Refrigerate until firm, at least 4 hours.

3. Beat together the whipped topping, sour cream, cream cheese, sugar, and almond extract until smooth. Spread over gelatin; sprinkle with coconut, if desired.

❖ Makes 8 servings. Per serving: 1.6 grams fat (7%); 196 calories; 2 grams fiber; 151 mg. sodium

APRICOT NECTAR DRESSING*

1 tablespoon brown sugar
1/2 cup plain nonfat yogurt
1/2 cup apricot nectar

1/8 teaspoon ground cinnamon
Dash of grated nutmeg

Stir brown sugar into yogurt. Add the apricot nectar, cinnamon, and nutmeg and mix until smooth.

❖ Makes about 1 cup. Per 1/4 cup serving: 0.1 gram fat (2%); 43 calories; 0 fiber; 25 mg. sodium

FAT-FREE HONEY MUSTARD DRESSING

1 cup fat-free mayonnaise
1/3 cup honey
3 tablespoons Dijon mustard
1/8 teaspoon garlic powder

1/8 teaspoon onion powder
1 teaspoon dried mustard
Dash of white pepper (to taste)

Combine all the ingredients in a blender or food processor. Add 1/4 cup of water and mix until well blended. Store in the refrigerator in airtight container. Keeps for several weeks.

❖ Makes 1 3/4 cups dressing. Per 2 tablespoon serving: 0.2 grams fat (3%); 39 calories; 0 fiber; 235 mg. sodium

---

*This makes a great sweet salad dressing, especially good with spinach salad. Or, you can use it as a fresh fruit topping.

CAJUN MEAT LOAF

1/2 small onion, chopped fine
1/2 cup finely chopped green
  bell pepper
1 pound extra-lean ground beef
1/4 cup egg substitute or 2
  egg whites
1/2 cup dry bread crumbs
1 teaspoon Worcestershire
  sauce

1/2 teaspoon salt
1/4 teaspoon cayenne pepper
1/2 teaspoon dried thyme,
  crumbled
1/4 teaspoon freshly ground
  black pepper
1/4 teaspoon ground cumin
1/2 cup ketchup, divided

1. In a small microwave-proof container, combine the onion and bell pepper with 1 tablespoon of water; cover and microwave on High for 3 minutes. Remove cover, and cool. (Or steam the vegetables in the water in a small covered saucepan for 5 to 6 minutes, or until tender.)

2. Combine cooked vegetables with the beef, egg, bread crumbs, seasonings, and 1/4 cup of the ketchup. Mix well.

3. Turn the mixture into a loaf pan that has been coated with vegetable oil cooking spray, spreading it evenly in the pan.

4. Bake in a preheated 375 degree oven for 40 minutes. Spread the top with the remaining ketchup and bake an additional 15 minutes.

❖ Makes 4 servings. Per serving: 9.4 grams fat (31%); 277 calories; 2 grams fiber 850 mg. sodium

BEEF GOULASH

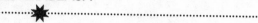

THIS IS PARTICULARLY SATISFYING SERVED OVER
BOILED CUBED POTATOES, BUT IT'S ALSO GOOD
OVER RICE OR NOODLES.

1 teaspoon olive oil
1 small onion, chopped
1/2 medium green bell
  pepper, chopped
1 garlic clove, minced
1/2 pound eye of round steak,
  cut in 1/2-inch cubes
1/2 teaspoon dried marjoram
1 teaspoon paprika
1/4 teaspoon caraway seed
1/4 teaspoon dried dillweed
1/2 teaspoon salt
1/4 teaspoon pepper

1 tablespoon flour
2 tablespoons Burgundy or
  other dry red wine
1 cup finely chopped fresh
  mushrooms
2/3 cup canned tomatoes,
  chopped (juice included)
2/3 cup beef stock or beef
  bouillon
1/3 cup plain nonfat yogurt
2 tablespoons chopped fresh
  parsley

1. Coat a medium nonstick skillet with vegetable oil cooking spray and heat the olive oil over moderate heat. Add the onion and bell pepper and sauté until softened, about 5 minutes. Stir in the garlic and cook for 1 minute. Add the beef and cook, stirring, until it loses its red color. Add the marjoram, paprika, caraway, dill, salt, pepper, and flour and stir to blend. Add the wine and cook for 2 minutes, reducing heat to low.

2. Stir in the mushrooms, tomatoes, and beef stock; cover and simmer for 30 to 45 minutes, or until beef is tender.

3. Stir in yogurt and fresh parsley and heat through. Serve immediately.

❖ Makes 3 servings. Per serving: 9.4 grams fat (28%); 310 calories; 2 grams fiber; 1,027 mg. sodium

INDIAN KHEEMA

1 pound extra-lean ground beef
1 medium onion, chopped fine
2 teaspoons curry powder
3/4 teaspoon turmeric
1/2 teaspoon salt
1/2 teaspoon garlic powder
1/4 teaspoon ground cayenne
    powder

1/4 teaspoon ground ginger
1/4 teaspoon black pepper
1 large potato, peeled and cut
    into 1/2-inch cubes
1 cup canned tomatoes,
    chopped, with their juice
1 (10-ounce) package frozen
    English peas

1. Cook ground beef and onion in a skillet coated with vegetable oil cooking spray until browned, stirring frequently. Add the curry powder, turmeric, salt, garlic powder, cayenne, ginger, and pepper. Stir in the potato, tomatoes, peas, and 1 1/2 cups water.

2. Bring to a boil, reduce the heat, and simmer, covered, for 20 to 25 minutes or until potatoes are tender. Serve over rice.

❖ Makes 4 servings. Per serving: 10.5 grams fat (31%); 307 calories; 5 grams fiber; 528 mg. sodium

BRENDA'S SWEET AND SOUR MEATBALLS

SERVE OVER RICE OR NOODLES FOR A MAIN DISH
OR ALONE FOR A COCKTAIL SUPPER.

2 pounds extra-lean ground
    beef or ground turkey
Garlic powder to taste
2 egg whites
1 cup skim or 1 percent milk
1 1/2 cups fat-free cracker
    crumbs or rolled oats
1/3 cup sugar

1 tablespoon cornstarch
1/4 cup soy sauce
1/3 cup apple juice
1 15-ounce can tomato sauce
1/4 cup barbecue sauce
1/2 cup finely chopped onion
1/2 green bell pepper,
    chopped fine

1. Combine the ground beef, garlic powder, egg whites, milk, and cracker crumbs and mix until well combined. Form into 1 1/2 inch balls. Arrange in shallow microwave-safe dish, cover with waxed paper, and brown on High about 20 minutes (turn after 10 minutes). Drain well on paper towels and reserve.

2. Combine the sugar and cornstarch in a large saucepan. Gradually stir in the soy sauce, apple juice, and 2/3 cup water. Bring to a simmer over low heat, stirring frequently.

3. Add the tomato sauce, barbecue sauce, onion, and green pepper. Simmer until onion and green pepper are tender, then add the meatballs and simmer another 15 minutes.

❖ Makes 8 servings. Per serving (without rice): 11.0 grams fat (29%); 347 calories; 3 grams fiber; 1,012 mg. sodium

CRANBERRY BRAISED BEEF

THIS RECIPE GOT RAVE REVIEWS. SERVE OVER NOODLES.

*1 pound lean beef cubes
   (stewing beef)
1 (6-ounce) can mushroom
   slices, undrained
1 1/2 cups beef broth*

*1/2 cup cranberry cocktail
Pepper to taste
Garlic powder to taste
1 teaspoon Worcestershire
   sauce*

1. Place the beef in a heavy skillet and add the mushrooms, beef broth, cranberry cocktail, pepper, garlic powder, and Worcestershire.

2. Bring to a boil over medium heat, then reduce heat, cover, and simmer for 1 1/2 to 2 hours over low heat. Add water as needed if liquid boils dry.

❖ Makes 4 servings. Per serving (with 1/2 cup egg noodles): 8.9 grams fat (39%); 210 calories; 1 gram fiber; 559 mg. sodium

NOTE: For a thicker gravy, stir 1 to 2 tablespoons of cornstarch into 1/4 cup of cold water and add with the beef broth.

FRAGRANT PORK ROAST

THIS IS VERY TENDER, MOIST, AND REDOLENT
OF THE HERBS THAT FLAVOR IT. IT SMELLS WONDERFUL
WHILE IT ROASTS.

1 pound pork tenderloin
1 stalk leafy celery, sliced
1/2 small onion, sliced
1 small garlic clove, slivered
1 sprig rosemary, or 1/4
  teaspoon dried
3 sage leaves, or 1/4 teaspoon
  dried

1 sprig thyme, or 1/4
  teaspoon dried
1 teaspoon Dijon mustard
Freshly ground black pepper
  to taste

1. Preheat the oven to 300 degrees.

2. Place the pork tenderloin on a piece of aluminum foil that is a few inches longer than the length of the meat. Separate the tenderloin into 2 lengthwise sections. (This has probably already been done by the butcher; if not, simply cut it right down the middle, lengthwise.)

3. In a small bowl, combine the celery, onion, garlic, rosemary, sage, and thyme; mix well.

4. Spread the flat side of both halves with mustard. Place one half flat side up, sprinkle with pepper, and top with an even layer of the vegetable mixture. Press the flat side of the remaining tenderloin half against the first so that the roast is reassembled with vegetables and herbs sandwiched between the 2 halves. Wrap foil snugly around the roast and fold ends over tightly to seal.

5. Bake for 2 hours. Remove foil and let stand 5 minutes before serving.

❖ Makes 4 servings. Per serving: 5.5 grams fat (27%); 192 calories; 0 fiber; 89 mg. sodium

PORK BARBECUE

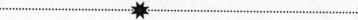

A LOW-FAT VERSION OF A SOUTHERN FAVORITE.

1 pound pork tenderloin
2 tablespoons white vinegar
1 teaspoon liquid smoke
1/4 teaspoon salt

1/8 teaspoon ground cloves
1 small onion, quartered
1 bay leaf

1. Cut the pork loin crosswise into 2 or 3 pieces so that it will fit into a 1-quart slow cooker (crockpot), standing pieces on end if necessary.

2. In a small bowl, mix together vinegar, liquid smoke, salt, and cloves. Pour over meat. Tuck the onion and bay leaf in among the meat and cook over low heat for 8-10 hours or until meat is tender.

3. Remove the pork from the cooker; let stand 5 minutes. Shred the meat, using 2 forks, and serve on hamburger buns with barbecue sauce and no-fat coleslaw (page 169).

Recipe may be doubled if you have a large slow cooker.

❖ Makes 4 servings. Per serving (without bun): 4.8 grams fat (27%); 167 calories; 0 grams fiber; 235 mg. sodium

PORK CHOPS WITH APPLES

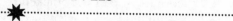

A SUPER COMBINATION!

4 apples, Rome or other
   cooking variety
4 loin pork chops, cut 1 inch
   thick, well trimmed

1/2 cup packed brown sugar
1 teaspoon ground cinnamon

1. Brown the chops in a nonstick skillet coated with vegetable oil cooking spray.

2. Peel, core, and slice the apples thin. Place in the bottom of a baking dish large enough to hold the chops in one layer.

3. Pour 1 cup water over the apples. Sprinkle with brown sugar and cinnamon.

4. Arrange browned pork chops over apples.

5. Cover and bake 1 to 1 1/2 hours at 375 degrees.

❖ Makes 4 servings. Per serving: 5.4 grams fat (18%); 273 calories; 3 grams fiber; 48 mg sodium

REBA McINTIRE'S BEST YOGURT CHICKEN

BEING FROM NASHVILLE AND A COUNTRY MUSIC FAN,
I COULDN'T LEAVE OUT A FAVORITE FROM
ONE OF COUNTRY'S FEMALE LEGENDS.

1 cup plain nonfat yogurt
1/2 cup fresh lemon juice
1 teaspoon curry powder
1 teaspoon ground cumin

1 teaspoon ground cinnamon
1 to 2 garlic cloves, minced
4 large boneless skinless
* chicken breast halves*

1. In a small bowl, combine the yogurt, lemon juice, curry powder, cinnamon, and garlic. Mix well.

2. Score the top of the chicken by making 2 or 3 shallow cuts, about 1/8 to 1/4 inch deep, on each piece. Place in a zipper-topped plastic bag and add the yogurt mixture. Gently shake the bag until the chicken is coated. Let stand at room temperature for 15 minutes.

3. Spray a broiler pan with vegetable oil cooking spray. Arrange the chicken pieces on the pan and brush with the yogurt mixture. Broil 4 to 6 inches from the heat for 6 to 8 minutes. Turn the chicken; brush with mixture. Broil an additional 7 to 9 minutes, or until chicken is fork tender and juices run clear. Discard any remaining yogurt.

❖ Makes 4 servings. Per serving: 3 grams fat (18%); 150 calories; 0 fiber; 70 mg. sodium

CHICKEN PICANTE

1/2 cup medium-chunky taco
* sauce*
1/4 cup Dijon mustard
6 tablespoons plain low-fat
* yogurt*
2 tablespoons fresh lime juice

6 chicken breast halves,
* skinned and boned*
1 teaspoon olive oil
1 lime, cut into 6 slices
Chopped fresh cilantro
* (optional)*

1. In a large bowl, make a marinade by mixing taco sauce, mustard, yogurt, and lime juice. Add the chicken, turning to coat. Cover and refrigerate at least 30 minutes.

2. Coat a large nonstick skillet with vegetable oil cooking spray and heat olive oil over moderate heat. Remove the chicken from the marinade and place in the skillet. Cook 5 minutes on each side.

3. Add the marinade to the skillet and cook about 5 minutes more, until a fork can be inserted in the chicken with ease and the liquid is slightly reduced.

4. Remove the chicken to warmed serving platter. Raise the heat to high and boil the marinade 1 minute; pour over chicken. Garnish with lime slices and cilantro.

❖ Makes 6 servings. Per serving: 3.4 grams fat (19%); 165 calories; 1 gram fiber; 271 mg. sodium

OVEN-FRIED CHICKEN

3/4 cup wheat germ
1 teaspoon paprika
2 teaspoons dried parsley
1 teaspoon dried minced onion
1/2 teaspoon garlic salt

3/4 teaspoon ground sage
6 skinless chicken breasts
(bone in or boneless)
1/2 cup buttermilk
Butter-flavored cooking spray

1. In a bowl, mix the wheat germ with the paprika, parsley, onion, garlic salt, and sage. Dip the chicken pieces in buttermilk, then roll in the crumb mixture. Arrange in a 13 × 9-inch baking pan. Sprinkle with any remaining crumb mixture. Spray each piece with flavored cooking spray.

2. Bake, uncovered, at 375 degrees about 45 minutes to 1 hour.

❖ Makes 6 servings. Per serving: 3.2 grams fat (15%); 191 calories; 2 grams fiber; 187 mg. sodium

TARRAGON CHICKEN PATTIES

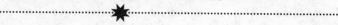

THESE ARE GREAT SERVED ON HAMBURGER BUNS.

1 pound raw boneless chicken breast
1/4 cup chopped onion
1/4 cup fine dry bread crumbs
2 tablespoons chopped fresh parsley
1/2 teaspoon dried thyme leaves

1/2 teaspoon pepper
1/4 teaspoon salt
1 egg white
1/4 cup all-purpose flour
1 teaspoon olive oil
1/2 cup dry white wine
1/2 teaspoon dried tarragon leaves

1. Cut the chicken into 1-inch cubes and place in a food processor. Pulse approximately a dozen times, or until the chicken is about the consistency of ground turkey. Transfer the ground chicken to a bowl and add the onion, bread crumbs, parsley, thyme, pepper, salt, and egg white. Stir well. Divide the mixture into 4 equal portions, shaping each into a 3/4-inch-thick patty.

2. Place the flour in a shallow dish. Dip the patties in flour, one at a time, to coat both sides.

3. Coat a nonstick skillet with vegetable oil cooking spray, add the olive oil, and place over moderate heat. Add the patties; cook 3 minutes on each side. Cover and cook an additional 3 minutes or until done. Remove from the skillet and keep warm.

4. Add the wine and tarragon to the skillet; scrape the bottom of the skillet to loosen any browned bits. Cook 1 minute, or until the wine is reduced by half. Spoon the wine mixture over the patties and serve hot.

❖ Makes 4 servings. Per serving: 3.0 grams fat (14%); 215 calories; 1 gram fiber; 277 mg. sodium

ZULA'S CHICKEN SALAD PIE

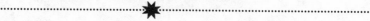

MAKES 2 DELICIOUS "PIES." FREEZE ONE (UNBAKED)
FOR A BUSY WEEKEND LUNCH. DOUBLE
SOUR CREAM BISCUITS RECIPE (SEE PAGE 158)

3 cups cubed cooked chicken
Whites of 2 hard-boiled eggs,
  chopped
1 cup chopped celery
1 small can water chestnuts,
  drained and chopped
1/2 cup fat-free mayonnaise
1 (10-ounce) can low-fat
  cream of chicken soup

1 tablespoon lemon juice
Pepper to taste
1 cup shredded fat-free or
  "lite" Cheddar cheese
6 ounces crushed pretzels or
  fat-free potato chips

1. Preheat the oven to 350 degrees. Coat two 9-inch pie pans with vegetable oil cooking spray.

2. Divide the biscuit dough in half and roll out on a floured surface into two circles, 1/8 inch thick.

3. Fit the pastry into the pans and cut away excess. Pinch all along the edges to crimp.

4. In a medium mixing bowl, combine the chicken, egg whites, celery, water chestnuts, mayonnaise, cream of chicken soup, lemon juice, and pepper. Mix well.

5. Fill each pie shell with half the filling. Top with the cheese and crushed pretzels.

6. Bake for 30 minutes. Cover the pies with foil after 15 minutes to prevent overbrowning.

❖ Makes 6 servings per pie. Per serving: 5.6 grams fat (18%); 276 calories; 1 gram fiber; 1,080 mg sodium

RASPBERRY CHICKEN

GREAT WITH CITRUS RICE (PAGE 194)
AND GREEN VEGETABLES.

*4 boneless, skinless chicken
  breast halves
Pepper to taste
1 (10-ounce) package frozen
  raspberries, thawed*

*1 tablespoon cornstarch
1/4 teaspoon ground cinnamon
1 tablespoon honey
1 teaspoon lemon juice*

1. Place the chicken breasts on a broiler pan or cookie sheet lined with foil. Sprinkle with pepper. Broil 6 inches from the heat for 10 minutes. Turn and broil on the other side for 10 minutes. Transfer to a shallow ovenproof serving dish and keep warm.

2. Drain the berries, reserving syrup. In a saucepan, blend together the syrup, cornstarch, cinnamon, and honey. Cook over medium heat until bubbly.

3. Add the lemon juice and stir. If desired, add water to make a thinner sauce.

4. Gently stir the berries into the sauce and pour over the chicken. Place the dish in the turned-off oven and let sit for 10 minutes for the flavors to mellow.

❖ Makes 4 servings. Per serving: 3.1 grams fat (12%); 239 calories; 3 grams fiber; 65 mg. sodium

ITALIAN FISH FILLETS

*2 whole tomatoes, chopped
1/2 cup chopped onion
Italian seasoning to taste
Garlic powder to taste
Salt and pepper to taste*

*3 tablespoons tarragon
  vinegar or wine vinegar
4 fish fillets (about
  1 1/2 pounds)*

1. Combine the tomatoes, onion, seasonings, and vinegar in a nonstick skillet. Bring to a boil, reduce the heat, and simmer until the onion is tender. Add 1/4 cup water. Cover and cook 3 or 4 minutes.

2. Arrange the fish fillets over the tomato mixture. Cover and simmer 4 or 5 minutes, then flip. Continue to cook another 5 to 8 minutes, or until done. Add more water if necessary.

❖ Makes 4 servings. Per serving: 4.2 grams fat (18%); 209 calories; 1 gram fiber; 200 mg. sodium

FISH CASSEROLE

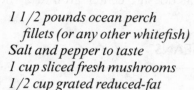

1 1/2 pounds ocean perch
  fillets (or any other whitefish)
Salt and pepper to taste
1 cup sliced fresh mushrooms
1/2 cup grated reduced-fat
  mozzarella cheese

2 scallions, sliced
2 stalks celery, chopped
Chopped parsley
Paprika

1. Arrange fish in an ovenproof casserole dish that has been lightly coated with vegetable oil cooking spray. Sprinkle with salt and pepper. Layer the mushrooms, cheese, scallions, celery, and parsley on top of the fish. Sprinkle with paprika.

2. Bake at 350 degrees for 30 minutes.

❖ Makes 4 servings. Per serving: 5.3 grams fat (23%); 210 calories; 1 gram fiber; 397 mg. sodium

QUICK TUNA NOODLE CASSEROLE

8 ounces uncooked egg noodles
1 can reduced-fat cream of
  mushroom (or celery) soup
3/4 cup skim or 1 percent milk
1 tablespoon minced onion
1 (10-ounce) package frozen
  peas

1/4 teaspoon freshly ground
  pepper
2 (6-ounce) cans water-packed
  tuna, drained
2 ounces reduced-fat cheese
  (shredded variety)

1. Cook noodles according to package directions. Drain and set aside.

2. In a medium saucepan, combine the soup, milk, onion, peas, and pepper. Cook over medium heat until hot (not boiling), stirring occasionally. Reduce the heat, stir in the flaked tuna and cheese, and simmer 10 more minutes.

3. Serve over or toss with the hot noodles.

❖ Makes 6 servings. Per serving: 3.2 grams (10%); 289 calories; 5 grams fiber; 495 mg. sodium

MEATLESS MEALS

Include at least one meal a week that doesn't center around a meat entree. Here are four super options!

CHAMP BEANS

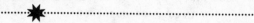

2 cups assorted dried beans
(like pinto, black, kidney)
6 cups soup stock (or 6 cups
water with 6 teaspoons
instant bouillon)
2 bay leaves
1 teaspoon ground sage
1 teaspoon thyme
1 teaspoon rosemary
1 teaspoon dried savory

4 dried hot red peppers or
1/2 teaspoon Tabasco (or
more to taste)
1 cup chopped onion
2 large garlic cloves, minced
1 green bell pepper, seeded
and chopped
2 large carrots, diced
4 stalks celery, diced
Salt and pepper to taste

1. Rinse and pick over the beans thoroughly and place in a large bowl with the stock, bay leaves, herbs, and dried peppers. Cover and refrigerate overnight.

2. The next day, transfer the mixture to a large pot and add the onion, garlic, green pepper, carrots, and celery. Bring to a boil, reduce the heat, and simmer for at least 3 hours, stirring occasionally. Season with salt and pepper during the last half hour of cooking. Serve plain, over rice, or over a baked potato with a salad.

❖ Makes 8 servings. Per serving: 0.9 grams fat (4%); 205 calories; 8 grams fiber; 605 mg. sodium (with bouillon)

LOW-CAL VEGETARIAN CHILI

2 cups diced yellow onions
1 cup diced peeled carrot
1 cup diced (cored and
seeded) green bell pepper
1 cup chopped mushrooms
1 cup chopped celery

2 (14 1/2-ounce) cans
chopped tomatoes with juice
2 tablespoons chili powder (or
to taste)
2 teaspoons ground cumin
1/8 teaspoon cayenne pepper

1 cup cooked and drained
   black beans
1 cup canned whole-kernel
   corn, drained, or frozen
   corn, thawed

2 cloves garlic, peeled and
   minced
1/2 teaspoon salt

1. In heavy 6-quart Dutch oven or saucepan, combine the onions, carrot, green pepper, mushrooms, and celery. Simmer in just enough water to cover until soft. Add the beans, corn, tomatoes, chili powder, cumin, cayenne, garlic, and salt. Stir until mixed.

2. Cover and simmer for about 30 minutes.

3. Taste and add seasonings as needed. Serve as is or over rice. This may be topped with nonfat yogurt or low-fat sour cream and fresh chopped cilantro.

❖ Makes about 2 to 2 1/2 quarts. Per 1 cup serving; 0.8 grams fat (6%); 103 calories; 5 grams fiber; 326 mg. sodium

EGGPLANT PARMESAN

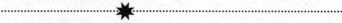

THIS IS ONE OF MY RECIPES THAT ALSO APPEARED IN
DR. KATAHN'S *T-FACTOR DIET*. TRADITIONAL EGGPLANT
PARMESAN IS QUITE HIGH IN FAT BECAUSE THE EGGPLANT
IS BREADED AND FRIED IN OIL—AND EGGPLANT ABSORBS
A LOT OF OIL! THE FAT IN THIS BAKED VERSION IS EVEN A
LITTLE LOWER WITH THE NEW LIGHT MOZZARELLA
CHEESES NOW AVAILABLE.

1 large eggplant
2 egg whites
2 tablespoons skim or
   1 percent milk
1/4 cup wheat germ
1/2 cup bread crumbs
2 tablespoons grated
   Parmesan cheese (fat free if
   you have it)

2 cups Traditional Tomato
   Sauce (pp. 200–01) or
   meatless tomato sauce
3/4 cup shredded
   reduced-fat/light mozzarella
   cheese

1. Preheat the oven to 350 degrees. Spray a foil-lined baking sheet with vegetable oil cooking spray.

2. Peel the eggplant and cut into 1/2-inch-thick slices.

3. Beat together the egg and milk in a shallow bowl.

4. In another bowl, combine the wheat germ, bread crumbs, and Parmesan cheese.

5. Dip the eggplant slices into the egg mixture, coating well. Then dip into the bread crumb mixture and place on the prepared baking sheet. Bake for 15 minutes; turn slices over and bake for 10 more minutes.

6. Line the bottom of a lightly oiled ovenproof casserole dish with the eggplant slices. Top with half the tomato sauce, then with half the mozzarella cheese. Repeat the layers.

6. Cover and bake covered for 25 minutes, then uncover and bake an additional 15 minutes.

❖ Makes 4 servings. Per serving: 6.7 grams fat (25%); 235 calories; 7 grams fiber; 583 mg. sodium

NO-FRY FALAFEL

THIS IS AN INSPIRED ALTERNATIVE TO TRADITOINAL
DEEP-FRIED FALAFEL. SERVE IN WHOLE WHEAT PITA
POCKETS WITH TAHINI MIXED WITH NONFAT PLAIN
YOGURT AND SOME LEMON JUICE.

*1 cup mashed potatoes
   (leftover or instant)*
*3 (15-ounce cans) garbanzo
   beans (chick-peas), drained
   and mashed*
*2 tablespoons regular or
   toasted tahini (sesame paste)*
*2 tablespoons plain nonfat
   yogurt*
*3/4 cup bread crumbs,
   preferably whole wheat*

*2/3 cup finely chopped red
   onion*
2 garlic cloves, minced
1 tablespoon ground cumin
2 teaspoons paprika
1/4 teaspoon cayenne pepper
1/2 teaspoon salt
1/4 cup minced fresh cilantro

1. In a large bowl, combine the potatoes, mashed beans, tahini, yogurt, and bread crumbs. Add the onion, garlic, cumin, paprika, cayenne, salt, and cilantro and mix well.

2. Shape into 6 patties and arrange on an aluminum-foil–lined cookie sheet that has been sprayed with vegetable oil cooking spray.

3. Bake for 10 minutes at 450 degrees, turn and continue baking until browned.

❖ Serves 6. Per serving (with one 6″ whole wheat pita): 6.0 grams fat (14%); 375 calories; 14 grams fiber; 932 mg. sodium

CHICKEN AND VEGETABLES ALFREDO

8 ounces uncooked linguine
2 cups chopped broccoli
2 cups thinly sliced carrots
1 cup sliced mushrooms
1 chicken bouillon cube
1/2 cup chopped onion
1 to 2 garlic cloves, minced
3 tablespoons flour
1/4 teaspoon freshly ground
   pepper

1 (12-ounce) can evaporated
   skim milk
1 1/2 cups cubed cooked
   chicken
1 (8-ounce) container reduced
   or nonfat sour cream
1/3 cup grated Parmesan
   cheese

1. Cook linguine according to package directions. Drain and set aside.

2. Meanwhile, in a medium saucepan combine the broccoli, carrots, mushrooms, and enough water to cover the vegetables. Bring to a boil, reduce the heat, and cook about 5 minutes until just tender. Drain, reserving 1/4 cup of the liquid. Set the vegetables aside.

3. Spray a large nonstick saucepan with cooking spray. Dissolve the chicken bouillon cube in the reserved liquid over medium-high heat. Add the onion and garlic, and cook until onion is tender.

4. Stir in the flour and pepper. Gradually stir in the evaporated milk. Cook until the sauce boils and thickens, stirring constantly.

5. Stir in the vegetables, chicken, sour cream, and 1/4 cup of the Parmesan cheese. Heat throughly *without* boiling. Add hot linguini, tossing to mix. Place on a serving platter and sprinkle with remaining Parmesan cheese.

❖ Makes 6 servings. Per serving: 4.4 grams fat (11%); 345 calories; 5 grams fiber; 442 mg. sodium

SPINACH LASAGNE

THIS RECIPE IS A FAVORITE WITH MY
WEIGHT-MANAGEMENT PARTICIPANTS. IT'S GREAT FOR A
DINNER WITH FRIENDS (LEFTOVERS ARE GREAT, TOO).

1/2 pound lasagne noodles
1 medium onion, chopped
2 garlic cloves, minced
1 teaspoon olive oil
16 ounces "light" ricotta or
nonfat cottage cheese
1/4 cup grated Parmesan
cheese (fat-free if you've got
it)
1 1/2 pounds fresh spinach,
washed and chopped (about
2 cups packed) or 1
(10-ounce) package frozen

chopped spinach, thawed
and drained
2 egg whites, beaten
1/4 teaspoon freshly ground
pepper
2 to 3 tablespoons chopped
fresh parsley
6 cups Traditional Tomato
Sauce (page 200–01) or
other meatless tomato sauce
8 ounces reduced-fat/light
mozzarella, grated

1. Spray a 9 × 13-inch casserole dish with vegetable oil cooking spray. Preheat the oven to 350 degrees.

2. Cook the lasagne noodles according to package directions.

3. While the noodles are cooking, sauté the onion and garlic in the olive oil in a nonstick skillet (add water if necessary to prevent sticking).

4. Combine the ricotta, Parmesan, spinach, egg whites, pepper, parsley, and sautéed onion and garlic, mixing well.

5. Spread 1/4 of the tomato sauce (1 1/2 cups) over the bottom of the prepared casserole dish. Arrange 1/3 of the noodles over the sauce, top with 1/3 of the ricotta-spinach mixture, sprinkle with 1/3 of the mozzarella, and top with more tomato sauce. Repeat layers twice more, ending with the sauce.

6. Cover the dish with aluminum foil, crimping edges tightly. Bake for 40 minutes; remove foil and bake 10 to 15 minutes more.

❖ Makes 12 servings. Per serving: 5.6 grams fat (22%); 229 calories; 4 grams fiber; 633 mg. sodium

SPAGHETTI PIE

DESTINED TO BE A FAMILY FAVORITE.

1 (6-ounce) package spaghetti
1 tablespoon reduced-fat
　margarine
1/2 cup fat-free Parmesan
　cheese
1 egg, beaten
1 pound extra-lean ground
　beef or ground turkey
1/2 cup chopped onion

1/4 cup chopped green pepper
1 cup crushed canned tomatoes
1 (6-ounce) can tomato paste
1 teaspoon sugar
1 teaspoon dried oregano
1/2 teaspoon garlic salt
1 cup fat-free cottage cheese
1/2 cup shredded part skim
　or "light" mozzarella cheese

1. Cook spaghetti according to package directions and drain. Stir in the margarine, egg, Parmesan cheese, and 1 tablespoon of water. Form the spaghetti into a crust in a 10-inch pie plate.

2. In a skillet, cook the beef, onion, and green pepper, while stirring, until the meat is browned and the vegetables are tender. Drain off excess fat. Stir in the crushed tomatoes, tomato paste, sugar, oregano, and garlic salt. Heat thoroughly (do not boil).

3. Spread the cottage cheese over the spaghetti crust. Fill the pie with the meat mixture. Bake uncovered in a preheated 350-degree oven for 20 minutes. Sprinkle mozzarella on top and bake 5 minutes more. Let stand 15 minutes before cutting.

❖ Makes 6 servings. Per serving: 10.2 grams fat (27%); 337 calories; 4 grams fiber; 58 mg. sodium

PASTA WITH CILANTRO PESTO

1 cup plain nonfat yogurt
1/2 cup chopped fresh cilantro
1/4 cup chopped fresh parsley
1/4 cup chopped fresh spinach
1/4 cup grated Parmesan
　cheese
2 tablespoons pine nuts,
　toasted lightly
3 garlic cloves, peeled and
　chopped

2 tablespoons olive oil
1/4 teaspoon salt
1/8 teaspoon ground black
　pepper
12 ounces dry pasta
　(cappellini is good)
Other additions: roasted or
　grilled chicken; whole
　kernel corn, drained; or
　cooked black beans, drained

1. In a blender or food processor, combine the yogurt, cilantro, parsley, spinach, Parmesan, pine nuts, olive oil, salt, and pepper. Cover and process about 1 minute. Scrape the sides of the container and process the pesto again until smooth.

2. Cook and drain the pasta according to package directions. Place the pasta in a large bowl and toss gently with the pesto.

3. Serve while hot.

❖ Makes 8 servings. Per serving (without additions): 7.8 grams fat (27%); 255 calories; 3 grams fiber, 225 mg. sodium

SUMMERTIME ROTINI

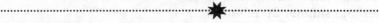

1 teaspoon olive oil	*packed in brine (not oil),*
1 red bell pepper, seeded and	*drained and halved*
chopped fine	*Salt and pepper to taste*
1 cup sliced fresh mushrooms	*6 ounces rotini, gemelli, or*
2 cups puréed fresh tomatoes	*other spiral-shaped pasta,*
1/4 cup chopped fresh basil	*cooked and drained*
1 small jar artichoke hearts	*2 ounces feta cheese, crumbled*

1. Coat a medium skillet with vegetable oil cooking spray and heat the olive oil over moderate heat. Sauté the bell pepper 5 minutes, add the mushrooms and cook 2 more minutes. Stir in the tomatoes and cook 3 minutes; add artichokes and cook 2 more minutes. Season with salt and pepper and remove from the heat.

2. Pour the sauce over the hot pasta and sprinkle with feta cheese.

❖ Makes 4 servings. Per serving: 5.3 grams fat (19%); 247 calories; 6 grams fiber; 267 mg. sodium

CITRUS RICE

A REFRESHING VARIATION FOR RICE, THIS IS EXCELLENT
WITH PORK OR CHICKEN.

1 cup converted rice
1 teaspoon salt
1/4 cup orange juice
concentrate

1/4 cup chopped water
chestnuts
2 to 3 tablespoons raisins
(optional)

1. Bring 2 cups of water to a boil in a medium saucepan. Add the rice, salt, orange juice, water chestnuts, and raisins (if desired).
2. Cover and simmer 20 minutes.
3. Remove from the heat and let stand until all the water is absorbed.

❖ Makes 4 servings. Per serving: 0.1 grams fat (1%); 104 calories; 1 gram fiber; 537 mg sodium

SPINACH AND WILD RICE CASSEROLE

1 (6-ounce) package
long-grain and wild rice
2 (10-ounce) packages frozen
spinach, thawed

4 ounces "light" or no-fat
cheese, shredded (1/2 cup)
1 tablespoon minced onion
Pepper to taste

1. Cook rice according to package directions but excluding margarine.
2. Press moisture from the spinach with paper towels.
3. Combine the cooked rice, spinach, onion, and pepper. Mix well.
4. Transfer the mixture to a 1-quart casserole dish that has been coated with vegetable oil cooking spray. Bake 35 minutes at 350 degrees.

❖ Makes 6 servings. Per serving: 2.6 grams fat (13%); 182 calories; 3 grams fiber; 320 mg. sodium

VEGETABLE SIDE DISHES

MARINATED CARROTS

1 can tomato soup
1/4 cup olive or canola oil
1 cup sugar
3/4 cup vinegar
1 teaspoon prepared mustard
1 teaspoon Worcestershire
   sauce
1 teaspoon salt

1 teaspoon pepper
15 carrots, sliced, cooked, and
   drained (or 2 pounds frozen
   carrots)
1 medium red onion, cut into
   rings
1 green bell pepper, cut into
   thin rings

1. Make a marinade by combining the tomato soup, oil, sugar, vinegar, mustard, Worcestershire, salt, and pepper. Pour over the carrots, onion, and green pepper.

2. Marinate overnight. Drain off the liquid before serving.

❖ Makes 12 servings. Per serving: 2.9 grams fat (17%); 147 calories; 3 grams fiber; 396 mg. sodium

BAVARIAN RED CABBAGE

THIS KEEPS WELL—IN FACT, THE FLAVOR IS EVEN BETTER
AFTER A DAY OR TWO. REGRIGERATE,
THEN REHEAT SLOWLY.

2 teaspoons butter or
   margarine
1 tablespoon honey
1 small onion, minced
1 large Granny Smith or
   other tart apple, peeled,
   cored, and chopped coarse
1 pound red cabbage, cored
   and coarsely shredded

1 bay leaf
1 teaspoon soy sauce
2 tablespoons cider vinegar
1/2 cup beef or chicken broth
1 tablespoon flour
1/2 cup cranberry cocktail
1 tablespoon red currant jelly

1. Coat a large nonstick skillet with vegetable oil cooking spray and melt the butter over medium heat. Stir in the honey until well blended.

Add the onion and apple and sauté for about 5 minutes, until limp and golden. Add the cabbage and sauté for 5 minutes or until glazed. Add the bay leaf, soy sauce, vinegar, and half the broth; allow to come to a slow simmer.

2. Cover the skillet and simmer 20 to 25 minutes, or until the cabbage is just tender. Sprinkle the flour over the cabbage and toss well. Add the cranberry cocktail and remaining broth. Stir gently and heat for 5 minutes, until liquids thicken.

3. Remove and discard the bay leaf. Add the jelly and toss lightly to mix. Warm another 5 minutes and serve.

❖ Makes 6 servings. Per serving: 1.6 grams fat (15%); 88 calories; 3 grams fiber; 146 mg. sodium

STUFFED PEPPERS

6 medium-size green bell
  peppers
1 cup cooked rice, preferably
  brown
1 cup canned whole-kernel
  corn, drained (or frozen
  corn, thawed)
1 cup chopped mushrooms
2 teaspoons Italian seasoning

1 cup (4 ounces) reduced-fat
  Parmesan cheese
1/2 cup diced celery
1/2 cup diced onion
1 (16-ounce) can diced
  tomatoes with juice
1 garlic clove, peeled and
  minced
Salt and pepper to taste

1. Cut the tops off the peppers and remove the seeds and membrane (dice the tops and reserve for the sauce).

2. Cook the peppers in boiling water for about 5 minutes, just to soften them. Drain and set aside.

3. In a medium bowl, combine the rice, corn, mushrooms, Italian seasoning, and cheese.

4. Spoon the rice mixture evenly into the peppers and place into a shallow baking pan. Pour hot water into the pan to a depth of 1/2 inch. Cover and bake in a preheated 350 degree oven for 25 to 30 minutes. Remove from the pan and arrange the peppers on a serving dish.

5. Meanwhile, in a medium saucepan combine the pepper tops, celery, onion, tomatoes, garlic, salt, and pepper. Simmer until the vegetables are soft. Pour the sauce over the cooked stuffed peppers.

❖ Makes 6 servings. Per serving: 3.2 grams fat (19%); 140 calories; 4 grams fiber; 366 mg. sodium

SWEET POTATO–PINEAPPLE CASSEROLE

*1 (40-ounce) can sweet
   potatoes in light syrup or
   2–3 boiled and peeled
   sweet potatoes
1 tablespoon butter-flavored
   sprinkles
2 eggs*

*1 teaspoon dried orange peel,
   minced
1 teaspoon ground cinnamon
1 teaspoon grated nutmeg
1/2 teaspoon salt
1 (8-ounce) can crushed
   pineapple in juice*

1. Preheat the oven to 350 degrees. Spray a 1 1/2-quart casserole dish with vegetable oil cooking spray.

2. Drain and mash the sweet potatoes. Beat in the butter sprinkles, eggs, orange peel, cinnamon, nutmeg, and salt. Stir in the pineapple.

3. Turn into the prepared casserole dish, cover, and bake for about 45 minutes.

❖ Makes 8 servings. Per serving: 1.6 grams fat (8%); 165 calories; 3 grams fiber; 224 mg. sodium

SPICY OVEN FRIES

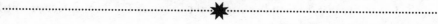

CRISPY AND DELICIOUS! YOU'LL NEVER MISS
FRIED POTATOES AGAIN.

*1 teaspoon olive oil
2 large Yukon gold or baking
   potatoes, scrubbed*

*1 1/2 teaspoons Herb Salt
   (p. 201) or commercial
   Cajun seasoning*

1. Coat a large baking sheet (with sides) with vegetable oil cooking spray and add the olive oil. Place in the oven and turn it on to 450 degrees.

2. While the oven is heating, cut potatoes (do not peel) into 1/2-inch slices.

3. Remove the baking sheet from the oven (it will be very hot) and use a spatula to spread the heated oil so that it coats the entire sheet. Distribute potato slices in an even layer on the sheet. Sprinkle with 3/4 teaspoon Herb Salt.

4. Bake 15 minutes. Using tongs, turn the potato slices individually so that browned side is now up. Sprinkle with remaining 3/4 teaspoon Herb Salt, return to the oven, and continue baking until tender and brown, about 10 minutes. Serve immediately.

❖ Makes 4 servings. Per serving: 1.2 grams fat (9%); 120 calories; 2 grams fiber; 275 mg. sodium

POTATOES AU GRATIN

3 1/2 cups peeled, finely
  chopped potatoes
1/2 cup nonfat cottage cheese
1/2 cup buttermilk
1 tablespoon chopped fresh
  chives
1 tablespoon chopped fresh
  parsley

2 teaspoons cornstarch
1/2 teaspoon salt
1/4 teaspoon pepper
1/4 cup (1 ounce) reduced-fat
  Cheddar cheese
1/8 teaspoon paprika

1. Preheat the oven to 350 degrees. Coat a 1 1/2-quart casserole with vegetable oil cooking spray.

2. Cook the potatoes in boiling water to cover for 8 minutes, or until just tender. Drain and set aside.

3. Combine the cottage cheese and buttermilk in a food processor or electric blender; process until smooth. Transfer to a large bowl; stir in the potatoes, chives, parsley, cornstarch, salt, and pepper. Spoon into the prepared casserole.

4. Bake uncovered for 20 minutes. Sprinkle with cheese and paprika and bake an additional 5 minutes.

❖ Makes 6 servings. Per serving: 0.6 grams fat (5%); 110 calories; 2 grams fiber; 342 mg. sodium

CHEESY SPINACH CASSEROLE

*1 (10-ounce) package frozen
  chopped spinach*
1 cup nonfat cottage cheese
1 whole egg and 2 egg whites
*1 teaspoon caraway seeds
  (optional)*
1 teaspoon seasoned salt

1/4 teaspoon pepper
Dash of nutmeg
*1 teaspoon butter-flavored
  sprinkles*
*2 tablespoons Parmesan
  cheese (preferably fat-free)*
Paprika to taste

1. Cook the spinach according to package directions and drain well. Combine with the cottage cheese, eggs, caraway, salt, pepper, nutmeg, and butter sprinkles. Transfer to a small shallow casserole or 8-inch pie pan that has been coated with vegetable oil cooking spray. Top with Parmesan cheese, then sprinkle with paprika.

2. Bake for 20 minutes at 350 degrees.

❖ Makes 4 servings. Per serving: 2.0 grams fat (20%); 88 calories; 2 grams fiber; 602 mg. sodium

SAUCES AND SEASONINGS

ORANGE SAUCE

THIS SAUCE IS EXCELLENT WITH CHICKEN OR PORK.
IT WILL KEEP FOR SEVERAL DAYS IN REFRIGERATOR.

1/4 cup orange juice
1/4 cup chicken broth (or
1/4 cup water with 1
instant chicken bouillon
cube)

2 tablespoons honey
1/4 teaspoon grated orange peel
1 teaspoon ground ginger

Combine all ingredients and beat with a wire whisk.

❖ Makes 1/2 cup. Per 2 tablespoons: 0.1 gram fat (2%); 42 calories; 0 fiber; 49 mg. sodium

SALSA VERDE

2 cups coarsely chopped fresh
tomatillos or drained
canned tomatoes
1/2 cup chopped onion
1/2 cup chopped fresh cilantro

1 fresh or pickled jalapeño
pepper, seeded and minced
1 garlic clove, minced
1/2 teaspoon dried oregano
Juice of 1 lime

Combine all the ingredients in a bowl or jar and refrigerate for at least 30 minutes. Keeps for 1 week.

❖ Makes 3 cups. Per 1/2 cup serving: 0.3 grams fat (9%); 21 calories; 1 gram fiber; 48 mg. sodium

TRADITIONAL TOMATO SAUCE

YOU CAN'T BEAT THIS SAUCE FOR TASTE OR LOW FAT! IT'S
COURTESY OF ONE OF NASHVILLE'S MOST POPULAR
GOURMET RESTAURANTS, SUNSET GRILLE.

2 teaspoons olive oil
4 large garlic cloves, minced
2 medium onions, minced
1 stalk celery, minced
1 medium carrot, minced
2 (28-ounce) cans whole
    tomatoes

1 cup dry white wine
2 teaspoons sugar
2 teaspoons dried basil
2 teaspoons dried oregano
1 teaspoon salt
Red pepper flakes

1. Heat the oil in a 4-quart nonaluminum pot over medium heat. Add the garlic, onions, celery, and carrot. Cook, stirring often, until onion is tender, about 6 minutes.

2. Meanwhile, drain the tomatoes, reserving liquid. Cut the tomatoes in half crosswise and gently press out and discard the seeds. Chop the tomatoes coarsely.

3. Add tomatoes and their liquid to the pot. Stir in the wine, sugar, basil, oregano, salt, and red pepper flakes to taste.

4. Simmer, uncovered, 1 1/2 hours, stirring occasionally. Do not boil.

❖ Makes 8 cups. Per 1/2 cup serving: 0.8 grams fat (16%); 44 calories; 2 grams fiber; 300 mg. sodium

HERB SALT

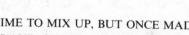

THIS TAKES A LITTLE TIME TO MIX UP, BUT ONCE MADE
IT LASTS FOR MONTHS AND CAN BE USED TO SEASON
ALL KINDS OF FOODS.

1/3 cup salt
1 teaspoon garlic powder
2 teaspoons paprika
2 teaspoons chili powder
1 teaspoon turmeric
1 teaspoon poultry seasoning
1 teaspoon freshly ground
    pepper

1/2 teaspoon ground ginger
1/2 teaspoon dry mustard
1/2 teaspoon celery seed
1/2 teaspoon onion powder
1/2 teaspoon dried dill weed

Combine all ingredients in a small jar; cover and shake to blend. Store in a cupboard at room temperature.

❖ Makes 3/4 cup. Per 1/4 teaspoon: 0 fat; 0 calories; 0 fiber; 235 mg. sodium

LOW-CALORIE EGGNOG

3 cups fresh skim milk
3 tablespoons sugar
3 egg yolks, lightly beaten
3/4 teaspoon vanilla extract
1/4 teaspoon rum flavoring or
   brandy flavoring

1/2 cup evaporated skim milk
1/2 teaspoon unflavored
   gelatin
Grated nutmeg

1. Mix the fresh milk, sugar, egg yolks, vanilla, and rum flavoring in a saucepan. Heat over medium heat for 7 to 8 minutes to just below boiling, or until the mixture starts to coat a spoon. It will thicken slightly. Remove from the heat and let it cool. Place in the refrigerator to chill completely. (This may be prepared a day in advance.)

2. Combine the evaporated milk and gelatin. Let stand 5 minutes. Heat until gelatin is dissolved (about 1 minute in a microwave oven or in a small saucepan on the stove).

3. Using an electric mixer, beat the gelatin mixture on high speed for 5 minutes.

4. Remove the mixture of milk, eggs, and sugar from the refrigerator. Fold the whipped evaporated milk into the egg mixture. Ladle into punch cups, sprinkle with nutmeg, and serve.

❖ Makes 4 cups. Per 1/2 cup serving: 2 grams fat (20%); 85 calories; 0 fiber; 68 mg. sodium

TROPICAL FRUIT SMOOTHIE

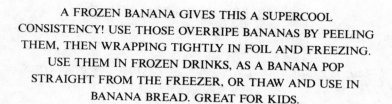

A FROZEN BANANA GIVES THIS A SUPERCOOL
CONSISTENCY! USE THOSE OVERRIPE BANANAS BY PEELING
THEM, THEN WRAPPING TIGHTLY IN FOIL AND FREEZING.
USE THEM IN FROZEN DRINKS, AS A BANANA POP
STRAIGHT FROM THE FREEZER, OR THAW AND USE IN
BANANA BREAD. GREAT FOR KIDS.

*1 large banana, peeled and
frozen
1 cup nonfat yogurt (100-
calorie "tropical" flavored
variety—for example:*

*pineapple, apricot,
strawberry, or banana)
1 cup tropical fruit juice
(orange, strawberry, and
banana blend)*

Break the banana into pieces and combine with the yogurt and fruit
juice in a food processor or blender. Purée until smooth.

❖ Makes 2 servings. Per serving: 0.6 grams fat (3%); 166 calories; 2 grams fiber; 73 mg. sodium

BLUEBERRY YOGURT CUSTARD

3/4 cup egg substitute
3/4 cup sugar
1 cup plain nonfat yogurt

2 cups fresh blueberries, or
   frozen, thawed

1. Spray a 9-inch pie plate with vegetable oil cooking spray.

2. Mix egg substitute, sugar, and yogurt until well blended. Combine with the blueberries, stirring to coat.

3. Pour into the prepared pie plate and bake at 350 degrees for 45 to 55 minutes. Cool and refrigerate until firm.

❖ Makes 8 servings. Per serving: 0.3 grams fat (1%); 165 calories; 1 gram fiber; 89 mg. sodium

PEACH COBBLER

8 cups sliced unsweetened
   peaches, fresh or frozen
1 cup sugar
1 cup all-purpose flour
1 teaspoon baking powder

1 egg, beaten
1/2 cup skim or 1 percent milk
1 tablespoon butter-flavored
   sprinkles
1 teaspoon almond extract

1. Preheat the oven to 350 degrees. Spread the fruit over the bottom of an ungreased 2 1/2-quart casserole.

2. In a bowl, whisk together the sugar, flour, and baking powder. In a separate small bowl, combine the egg, milk, butter flavoring, and almond extract. Add to the flour mixture and stir with a fork to form a stiff dough. Distribute spoonfuls of the dough evenly over the fruit.

3. Bake uncovered until the peaches are tender and the crust is brown (approximately 30 to 40 minutes). Frozen peaches will take longer than fresh. Cool before serving.

❖ Makes 9 servings. Per serving: 0.9 grams fat (3%); 215 calories; 3 grams fiber; 132 mg. sodium

COCOA BROWNIES

THESE ARE EXCELLENT SERVED WARM
WITH FROZEN YOGURT.

4 tablespoons (1/2 stick)	*1 whole egg, lightly beaten*
margarine	*4 egg whites or 1/2 cup egg*
1/3 cup cocoa powder	*substitute*
1/2 cup applesauce	*2 teaspoons vanilla extract*
1 1/2 cups sugar	*1/3 cup all-purpose flour (best*
1/4 teaspoon salt	*if sifted)*

1. Preheat the oven to 350 degrees (325 if you use a glass pan). Coat a 9-inch baking pan with vegetable oil cooking spray.

2. In a medium saucepan, melt the margarine with the cocoa powder over low heat. Stir in the applesauce, sugar, and salt. Add the egg, egg whites, and vanilla; mix well. Stir in the flour just until blended (don't overmix).

3. Pour the mixture into the prepared pan. Bake for 25 minutes. Cool to room temperature in the pan on a wire rack. Cut into squares.

❖ Makes 16 brownies. Per brownie: 3.4 grams fat (24%); 121 calories; 1 gram fiber; 79 mg. sodium

GINGERBREAD

ADAPTED FROM LAURA INGALLS WILDER'S RECIPE.
SERVE THIS MOIST, SWEET CAKE WITH
WARMED APPLESAUCE OR LEMON SAUCE.

1 cup packed brown sugar	*1 teaspoon ground ginger*
3/4 cup applesauce	*1 teaspoon ground cinnamon*
1 cup molasses	*1 teaspoon ground allspice*
2 teaspoons baking soda	*1 teaspoon grated nutmeg*
1 cup boiling water	*1 teaspoon ground cloves*
2 1/4 cups all-purpose flour	*1/2 teaspoon salt*
3/4 cup whole wheat flour	*2 eggs, beaten well*

1. Preheat the oven to 350 degrees. Coat a 9 × 13-inch glass baking pan with vegetable oil cooking spray.

2. Combine the brown sugar, applesauce, and molasses in a large mixing bowl. Stir the baking soda into the cup of boiling water and pour into the sugar mixture. Stir until blended.

3. In another bowl, combine the flours with the spices and salt. Add to the sugar mixture with the eggs and mix well.

4. Pour the batter into the prepared pan and bake for 30 to 40 minutes, until the gingerbread pulls slightly from the sides of the pan and springs back when touched in the center. Cool in the pan on a wire rack.

❖ Makes 16 servings. Per serving: 1.0 grams fat (4%); 186 calories; 2 grams fiber; 189 mg. sodium

MAYONNAISE COCOA CAKE

THIS MOIST CAKE IS GOOD SERVED WARM
WITH LOW-FAT FROZEN YOGURT.

1 cup fat-free mayonnaise   *1 teaspoon vanilla extract*
1 cup sugar   *2 cups all-purpose flour*
2 teaspoons baking soda   *1/4 cup cocoa powder*
1 cup warm water   *1 teaspoon salt*

1. Preheat the oven to 350 degrees. Coat a 9 × 13-inch baking pan with vegetable oil cooking spray.

2. Combine mayonnaise and sugar in a mixing bowl; set aside. In a measuring cup, dissolve the baking soda in the warm water and add vanilla.

3. In a separate bowl, whisk together the flour, cocoa powder, and salt. Beat the liquid into the sugar-mayonnaise mixture alternately with the dry ingredients, beginning and ending with the dry ingredients.

4. Pour the batter into the prepared pan and bake for 35 minutes or until a toothpick inserted in the center comes out clean and the cake shrinks slightly from the sides of the pan. Cool in the pan 5 minutes, then turn out on a rack to cool completely.

❖ Makes 12 servings. Per serving: 0.5 grams fat (2%); 167 calories; 1 gram fiber; 408 mg. sodium

NEW YORK–STYLE CHEESECAKE

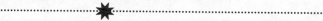

TOP WITH FRESH BERRIES OR OTHER FRUIT FOR A
LIGHT DESSERT EVERYONE WILL ENJOY.

*1 3/4 cups graham cracker
  crumbs
1/3 cup honey
16 ounces yogurt cheese (see
  below) or 16 ounces fat free
  cream cheese and 16 ounces
  "light" ricotta cheese*

*3/4 cup sugar
1 cup fat-free sour cream
2 eggs, lightly beaten
2 teaspoons vanilla extract
2 tablespoons cornstarch*

1. Preheat the oven to 450 degrees.

2. In a bowl, mix graham cracker crumbs and honey. Press mixture onto bottom and sides of a 9-inch springform pan or pie plate sprayed with vegetable oil cooking spray. Chill the crust in the freezer while preparing the filling.

3. In a mixing bowl, beat ricotta cheese and sugar until smooth. Blend in eggs, vanilla, and cornstarch, beating just until blended. If using fat-free cream cheese, blend in along with eggs. If using yogurt cheese, *fold* in with sour cream. Fold in sour cream. Pour the mixture into the prepared crust.

4. Bake for 10 minutes at 450 degrees. Reduce temperature to 200 degrees and bake for 45 minutes. Turn off the oven; allow cake to cool in the oven, with the door opened slightly, for 3 hours. Remove from pan.

❖ Makes 10 servings. Per slice: 4.1 grams fat (12%); 305 calories; 1 gram fiber; 511 mg. sodium

Yogurt Cheese

Invert 32 ounces of plain nonfat yogurt into a strainer lined with coffee filters or cheesecloth. Place over a bowl, cover, and allow to drain in the refrigerator at least 12 hours. Makes 16 ounces yogurt cheese.

Exercise: The Missing Link

It is virtually impossible to be healthy, strong, and lean if you are not physically active. Even if you meticulously follow the nutritional guidelines I have outlined, you cannot sit back and expect good eating to answer all your fitness and weight control prayers. Here are just a few reasons why exercise, too, is essential:

• Exercise promotes both the quality and duration of your life. Put simply, it keeps you feeling good more of the time for more years—and the better you feel, the better you look. According to the Centers for Disease Control, inactivity contributes to 250,000 deaths each year, and some forty-three separate studies have shown that inactive people have twice the risk of coronary heart disease and cancer as those who are physically active. By comparison, regular physical activity directly reduces rates of heart disease, high blood pressure, noninsulin-dependent diabetes, osteoporosis, breast and colon cancer, and depression and other forms of mental illness. Finally, even when people have these conditions and/or a family history of medical problems, if they are fit, they are much less likely to die from these ailments. *Men who burn more than 2,000 calories per week through exercise have been shown to live some two years longer than men who burn only 500 calories per week through exercise.*[1] *Physically fit women are five times less likely to die at any given age than inactive women.* And best of all, it's never too late to gain the benefits of exercise; unfit adults who become physically active have a 36 percent lower death rate than unfit folks who stick to their sedentary ways.

• Exercise builds muscle tissue and bone. In addition to increasing your overall strength and health, this rise in lean body mass helps protect you against some of the problems commonly associated with aging, such as weakening of the bones and muscular wasting. Studies have shown that the elderly reap the same benefits from exercise as younger adults. *There is no age limit to fitness!*

• Exercise keeps you feeling and functioning like a much younger person. Older adults who exercise regularly have the mobility, agility, and physical independence of unfit individuals twenty-five years younger! Exercise is the closest thing we have to a fountain of youth.

• Exercise burns extra calories and fat. The activity itself requires extra energy, and because it maintains and increases lean mass, regular exercise also raises the metabolism of calories and fat between workouts. Studies have found that people who exercise just four hours per week have resting metabolic rates up to 8 percent higher than nonexercisers who eat exactly the same diet.[2] The average weight loss among people who switch from a sedentary to active lifestyle without making any dietary adjustments is about five pounds over the first twelve weeks. **Could this be the answer to *your* Last Five Pounds?**

• Exercise makes you look thinner even if your weight remains unchanged. That's because a pound of lean tissue takes up less space than a pound of fat. So as you build muscle and lose fat, you lose inches. Since the fat that disappears most easily tends to be abdominal fat, you should see the improvement first around your waist.

• Regular exercise is your best protection against regaining weight you've lost in the past. Numerous studies have tracked "graduates" of weight loss programs to determine why some people regain lost weight and others keep it off. The one consistent, critical factor appears to be exercise. People who are physically active on a daily basis reliably keep the weight off. People who give up exercise, on the other hand, triple their likelihood of gaining more than twenty pounds! Exercise needs to be a lifetime habit.

• Regular exercise reduces stress, anxiety, and depression. Not only does this make you feel better about yourself and about life in general, it decreases your susceptibility to binge eating, which is commonly triggered by emotional distress. To keep your stress levels down you do not need to work out intensely or for prolonged sessions, but you do need to exercise at least three to four times a week on a *consistent* basis.

The Mechanics of Exercise

Why does exercise help with weight control? The short answer, of course, is that it burns more calories. But here's what actually happens physiologically when you set off on a brisk morning walk.

As your body goes into motion, your working muscles draw on the glycogen in your bloodstream for instant fuel. This "ignition energy" comes entirely from the carbohydrates your body has stored from recent meals. As you continue your walk and the glycogen in your blood runs low, the next level of glycogen is released from storage within the muscles.

When, you may ask, does this walk start to make a dent in that backside fat you're trying so hard to lose? This depends on how hard you're exercising, but if you maintain a steady, moderate pace, your initial glycogen reserves probably will begin to run low after about twenty minutes, and at that point your body will ignite some of its fat for fuel. While the rate of burn will vary depending on your weight and the exact intensity of activity, most studies suggest that it takes a total of about four to five hours of energetic activity to reduce a pound of fat.

Now, at no point will you burn 100 percent body fat. The caloric expenditure is at best a combination of fat and glycogen. But the longer and more consistent your workout, the more fat you will use. Also, the fitter you are, meaning the more muscle tissue you have, the more fat you will burn to keep those muscles working.

All this helps explain why there's a strong emphasis on aerobic exercise for weight control. Aerobic means oxygen consuming. Your body consumes oxygen in order to burn calories from glycogen and fat. So when you are engaged in aerobic exercise, such as walking, jogging, swimming, or biking, you are burning fat. It's easy to tell aerobic from anaerobic exercise, such as weight lifting. Aerobics force you to breathe steadily in and out, and to keep breathing. Aerobics work your largest muscle groups. Aerobics involve regular, continuous movement. While there is evidence, which we'll get to, that weight training can be an important component of your exercise routine, the mainstay of that routine must be aerobic for you to reap the desired results.

What's the DIF?

Your physical fitness depends on how long you exercise per session, how hard you exercise, and how often you exercise. In other words, it depends on duration, intensity, and frequency: DIF. You need to develop a regular physical activity program that gradually steps up your investment on all three levels in order to build overall fitness.

1. *Duration of activity.* How long do you spend exercising? If you are moderately fit, you will have no difficulty sustaining physical activity for at least thirty minutes at a stretch. If you are very fit, you can work your body for forty minutes to an hour without feeling fatigued. This does not mean that you always exercise for such long stretches or at high intensity. If you spend five minutes scrubbing the kitchen floor or digging in the garden, that qualifies as exercise. The more of these short-duration activities you pack into a day, the more calories you will burn and the fitter you will become, but the longer workouts are also important for building strength and stamina.

2. *Intensity of activity.* How hard do you work when you're working out? If you can comfortably carry on a conversation while exercising, you're probably working at low intensity. If you breathe hard, work up a visible sweat, and really feel your muscles pushing and pulling, you are probably working at moderate to high intensity. The following chart illustrates the calorie-burning benefits when you move up to higher intensity levels. Yes, the harder you work, the more calories you will burn. However, this fundamental truth is deceiving because, unless you are very fit, most of those highest-intensity calories will come from carbohydrate rather than fat. That is, they will come from the glycogen stores in your muscles rather than from your fat stores. If burning up those fat stores is your goal, you will probably see the best results— and possibly enjoy your workout more—if you maintain a steady, moderate pace for a longer period of time. Instead of running hard for fifteen minutes, in other words, you might jog or walk briskly for half an hour.

Exercise Intensity and Calorie Burning

Activity, Intensity	Calories per minute for 130-pound woman
Running, 6-min. mile	15.0
Running, 8-min. mile	12.4
Running, 9-min. mile	11.3
Running, 11.5-min. mile	7.9
Walking, fields and hills	4.8

Exercise Intensity and Calorie Burning   (con't.)

Activity, Intensity	Calories per minute for 130-pound woman
Walking, flat road	4.7
Climbing hills w/ 44-lb. load	8.6
Climbing hills w/ 22-lb. load	8.3
Climbing hills w/ 9-lb. load	7.5
Climbing hills, no load	7.2
Cycling, racing	9.9
Cycling, 9.5 mph	5.6
Cycling, 5.5 mph	3.8
Skiing cross-country, uphill	16.3
Skiing cross-country, lateral	8.5
Skiing cross-country, moderate downhill	7.1
Treading water fast	10.0
Treading water slowly	3.7
Swimming backstroke	9.9
Swimming, fast breaststroke	9.5
Swimming, fast crawl	9.2
Swimming, slow crawl	7.5

3. *Frequency of activity.* How often do you engage in physical activity? If you are moderately fit, you probably exercise about three times a week. If you are very fit, you likely exercise daily. This does not necessarily mean that you take an aerobics class every day, but you might take a class three times a week and on the other days get off the bus or subway a few blocks early to walk the extra distance to work, or spend a half hour walking briskly around the mall at lunchtime. Or maybe you don't take any classes at all, but every morning and evening you take your dog out for a fifteen-minute jog, and every afternoon you play backyard basketball with your son or daughter. Or, going back to my earlier examples, you may devote several hours to vigorous housework or yardwork. The key to fitness is not wearing fancy workout clothes or performing contortions at the gym, it's simply getting your body up and moving as often and as energetically as possible. The more naturally that movement fits into the contours of your daily life, the more likely you are to keep it up. And the fitter you will become.

These three factors work together to make the DIF in your fitness level. The safest and most reliable way to raise your intensity of exercise, for example, is to increase frequency and duration. At Vanderbilt every summer our wellness group sponsors an exercise incentive program. In reviewing the participants' logs, I came across a middle-aged woman who walked five to ten minutes on weekdays, but reported two hours of swimming on Saturday and Sunday. Based on this information alone, I could tell that much of that time at the pool was spent splashing and floating rather than steady swimming. That's because it requires consistent and considerable practice to perform two solid hours of swimming or any other exercise. Duration. Intensity. And frequency.

Exercise and Appetite

Whether it's a legitimate concern or simply an excuse to avoid working out, many people believe that exercise works against weight loss by increasing appetite. The truth is, people who maintain a moderate level of physical activity may eat a little more than those who lead a sedentary lifestyle, but they *lose* a lot more calories in the end.

Research into the precise effect of exercise on appetite has produced conflicting results. Most studies suggest that a strenuous workout will actually *decrease* appetite immediately after exercising, but then a slight increase in hunger will kick in over the following hours. However, while some people eat more than usual when they increase their activity level, others consume less.

My personal observation is that people who are the most calorie conscious—who religiously weigh themselves and calculate calories and fat grams burned and consumed—tend to eat more after exercising. They do this not because the physical activity actually makes them hungrier but because they feel entitled to the extra calories. *I burned up 500 calories running five miles, so why shouldn't I have that hot fudge sundae?* I have done this myself and met dozens of other women who have, too. Surprise, surprise, we found that we gained weight after increasing our exercise level! Of course, it wasn't the exercise that caused the weight gain but the extra treats, which overcompensated for the calories we'd burned off.

The message here, once again, is to forget about counting calories and listen to your body. Ideally, you will choose a form of exercise that you enjoy, and you will work out at a moderate rate that is comfortable at your fitness level. It should not hurt. It should not make you miserable. And it should not be a form of self-punishment after which you yearn to reward yourself with a fattening treat. On the contrary, if you shape the right workout for yourself, it will be fun! And if it is fun, then it's a short step to reconceptualizing the workout itself as your reward. If you feel a little hungrier afterward, then by all means feed your hunger with nourishing low-fat food, but don't let yourself get caught up in calorie computations. And don't use exercise as an excuse to eat every day what should be occasional treats.

When people honestly feel starving after exercising, it's usually because they failed to eat anything beforehand. Believing it's best to exercise on an empty stomach, they may work out early in the morning before breakfast or later in the day only if they've eaten very little. This can lead to a surge in postworkout hunger and it may have a slight negative effect on the caloric benefits of the workout itself.

While it's certainly not advisable to jump in the pool or hit the running track immediately after a four-course meal, researchers at the University of Louisville have shown that exercising one to two hours after a moderate meal (especially one dense in carbohydrates) can increase metabolic rate by about 10 percent more than "exercising on empty."[3] When the subjects of this study walked for twenty minutes before eating, they burned 101.6 calories. But when they walked after eating an 874-calorie meal, they burned 112.2 calories—simply because they ate before instead of after exercising! What was even more surprising, the benefits extended for hours. When the subjects walked without eating beforehand, their resting metabolic rate increased by 5.8 percent, or an extra 12.5 calories, over the following three hours. When they ate the meal without exercising at all, their metabolic rate surged 21 percent to burn an extra 42.3 calories over three hours. But when they took their walk *after* the same meal, their metabolic rate climbed by 29 percent to burn an extra 58.1 calories over three hours. Thus, walking after the meal raised the metabolic rate nearly 4 calories above the predicted rate of 54.8 calories (the sum of increases due to walking alone and the meal alone). These losses may not sound like much, but, combined with the other evidence, they make a strong case for fueling up before working out! Besides, as marathon runners and other athletes have known for years, if you eat a high-carbohydrate meal before exercising, you will have more energy, more stamina, and enjoy your workout more than if you exercise hungry.

Whether you choose to eat before or after working out, whether you eat more or less than you would if not exercising, the important thing is to stay active. You will reap most of the health benefits of exercising even if you do eat a little more. And as long as you don't *try* to make up for the calories you're burning, you should work off more fat than you put back on.

Building an Exercise Habit You Can Live With

Now be honest. Are you physically active enough? If you answer "not really," you have plenty of company. More than half of all Americans— some surveys estimate as many as 70 percent!—lead basically sedentary lives. And the number one reason most give for not exercising more is that they don't have enough time.

I have two responses.

First, every one of us can make the time to exercise if we give our own personal health the priority it deserves. Our health is our most valuable asset. Without it all else loses significance.

Second, while I believe that regular moderate-intensity workouts are important, we can go a long way toward meeting our fitness goals by seizing opportunities to bend, stretch, push, pull, climb, walk, and move through everyday life. The latest scientific research shows that three ten-minute spurts of motion, adding up to thirty minutes per day, will give about the same health benefits as a single thirty-minute workout.

So the time excuse is no excuse. Anybody can find ten minutes for a brisk walk or exercise routine. And anybody can turn those ten minutes into a habit.

As a case in point, one of the nurses I work with at Vanderbilt decided to put the ten-minutes-a-day principle into practice. She dusted off her home treadmill, which she hadn't used since the first month she bought it, and put on her walking shoes. What allowed her to get going was the permission she gave herself to stop after just ten minutes. Not the thirty-five or forty daily minutes that she had long felt she "ought" to do but consistently failed to do. Just ten minutes. She found that once she was actually moving, those ten minutes naturally, painlessly, grew to more.

Once you've established the ten-minute exercise habit, then inch it up to fifteen minutes. After a few weeks at fifteen minutes, push for thirty. You'll find it's easy to do, not because you feel you *should* exercise longer but because it feels good to exercise longer. You'll enjoy it. You'll want to do it. You'll make the time to do it. But the important thing for now is to make those first ten minutes count.

Here are a few suggestions to help you embrace physical activity as a natural and desirable part of your everyday life:

• Have fun! Try out different forms of exercise and select the ones you most enjoy and the ones that fit most easily into your daily life, rather than the ones that are *supposed* to do you the most good. Make those simple, enjoyable activities the mainstay of your exercise routine.

• Get your body moving often and keep it moving as long as possible. The total time spent being active is more important to your health than the intensity of your activity. So if you have to choose between a half-hour walk on your lunch hour every day and a knock-yourself-out aerobics class lasting an hour once a week, take the walk every time. (But recognize that you'll be fitter and leaner if you can manage both.)

• Tailor your activity to your personality, lifestyle, and body. If you have weak ankles or knees, you have no business on the jogging track, but swimming or water workouts would suit you well. If you're a loner, you probably won't last long in a group aerobics class, but you may thrive on daily morning walks or jogs. If you have a family and a full-time job, you may have little time for exercising on your own, but you can get a lot of exercise while playing with your kids—take them swimming or jogging, go sledding with them in the winter, play backyard basketball, or engage the whole family in a game of softball or Frisbee at the park. It's important to be practical and flexible in designing an activity plan that you really can maintain on an ongoing basis.

• Increase your activity level *gradually*. If you're taking an aerobics class for the first time, don't take the advanced step class, and don't force yourself to the point of exhaustion. The benefits of exercise come only over an extended period, so you have to keep it up. If you push yourself too hard, you run a high risk of injuring yourself or burning out— leaving you with zero benefits.

As you juggle your daily schedule to make time for exercise, keep in mind that being fitter will *save* you time in the end by making you better prepared to handle life's everyday physical challenges. I was dramatically reminded of this a few years ago while running through Chicago's O'Hare Airport. I was on a business trip with two colleagues and we had a very tight change of planes. We had to get all the way from one end of the terminal to the other with too many carry-on bags. One of my companions was extremely fit, and he and I started to jog the distance, but my other friend was huffing and puffing after 100 yards. My fit companion and I took this man's luggage to ease his load, but he still couldn't keep up with us, and since we were unwilling to leave without him, we all ended up missing our plane. His lack of fitness cost us four hours as we waited for the next flight. I couldn't help but wonder how many hours this man had wasted over the years because he refused to invest just those few minutes each day on exercise.

Lifestyle Exercises Don't Require a Gym

Not all exercise requires special equipment or scheduling—or even conscious attention. One of the greatest exercise secrets—and an effective weight loss tactic—is fidgeting! Researchers have found that people who fidget burn up to 800 calories more per day than those who tend to sit still. Of course, the tendency to fidget is largely inborn, but so is the tendency to gain fat. One study found that infants who become overweight squirm less than other newborns and have a 21 percent lower energy expenditure.[4]

The message here is not to become a nervous twitcher but simply to recognize and take advantage of the countless opportunities to move your body throughout the day. Even if you work at a desk job, you can periodically stretch your arms and legs. Rearrange your body in your seat. Try pacing when you're thinking through a difficult problem, talking on the phone, or planning your next project. Wiggle your jaw. Twirl your ankle. It may sound ridiculous, but every movement really does count.

Another secret weapon against fat that is available to you twenty-four hours around the clock is *breathing*. Yes, I know, you have to breathe, otherwise you'd die. But how much oxygen do you take in with each breath? Do you really put your energy into that breath or do you let the air slip in and out pretty much on its own? Remember that your body needs oxygen to burn calories and fat, to release the energy you need to think and move. You can feel the results yourself each time you sit up straight and take a deep breath. Try it. Deep breath in. And out. Now slump down in your chair and take a little shallow breath. Feel the difference? The more deeply you breathe, the more energized you will feel. The more energized you feel, the more you will naturally move. The more you move, the more fat you will burn and the leaner your body will be.

Now, here are some other suggestions for spending that extra energy which require no special equipment, no special training, and no special scheduling.

• Become self-sufficient and energy *in*efficient: the less you rely on labor-saving devices, vehicles, machinery, or other people, the more physically active you will, of necessity, become.

• Take the stairs instead of the escalator or elevator. If you're in a hurry, walk up or down the escalator, but don't just stand there!

• At work, make a habit of using the rest room two or three floors up—and take the stairs to get there and back.

• At the airport, theme park, or other major venues, *don't* use the moving walkways or trams between destinations. Use your own muscle power.

• Don't use drive-through windows. Park and get out of your car. Walk in. Walk out. Better yet, don't even drive to the restaurant or bank but walk there.

• Use your bike or your feet instead of your car. Ride your bike or walk to work if at all possible. (Or ride *at* work. As I read over this manuscript I am pedaling away on my exercise bike!)

• Use public transportation, and walk at either end. It may be a short walk from your home to the bus and from the bus stop to your job, but it's bound to be longer than the walk from your front door to your car. Every step counts. As added benefits, by taking public transportation you'll be helping to clean up the air, and you can use your commuting time to read instead of hassling with traffic.

• Park at the far end of the parking lot or mall and walk the extra distance.

• Carry your own bags instead of using shopping carts or letting others help you. Every extra pound you carry burns additional calories.

• Use exercise as entertainment. Instead of attacking the kitchen cabinets, turning on the TV, or going to a movie when you're bored, get out into the fresh air for a walk or bike ride, or head for the gym. Make a date with friends for a swim, tennis, or a game of catch. Go bowling or skating. We often take it for granted that children play physical games for fun, but we forget that adults can have just as much fun at the very same games.

• Stand and move while talking on the phone. If the cord's not long enough, get a cordless phone and walk around the house or yard during your conversation.

• Do something physical while watching TV: pedal your exercise bike, iron, practice your sit-ups, wash the dishes, do floor stretches, dust and straighten up the room—keep moving!

• Go out for a brisk walk at lunchtime or instead of taking a coffee break. Keep a pair of walking shoes in your desk at work so you're always prepared.

• Learn to dance, then head for the dance floor instead of restaurants and movie theaters on your nights out.

• Get a dog. I realize this may not be a practical suggestion for everyone, but if there is room in your home and schedule for this addition, consider that the dog will "force" you to take regular walks, and will give you an excuse to romp in the park. Those obedience classes will occupy time when you might otherwise be snacking, plus dogs are a great conversation-starter if you're trying to meet new people. *And* your new dog will act as a companion as well as a living home security system. (As you can tell, I love my dog!)

• Work in the garden. Weeding, raking, lawn mowing (especially with a hand mower), seeding, pruning, and planting all require hundreds of small and large physical movements that will help bend and stretch you as well as your garden into shape. If you don't have a garden of your own, check around your neighborhood for community garden projects —and if there isn't one, contact your local parks department about starting one!

Caloric Expense of Everyday Activities

Activity	Caloric Cost Per Minute for 130 lbs.
Digging earth	8.5
Climbing a hill	7.2
Lawn mowing by hand	6.6
Scrubbing floors	6.4
Hoeing	5.4
House painting	4.5
Weeding	4.3
Food shopping	4.0
Window washing	3.4
Sitting still	1.2

9

The LFP Workout Guide

While the spontaneous Lifestyle Exercises described in the last chapter can go a long way toward meeting your fitness needs, you will look and feel better—and shed more body fat—if you also work out on a regular, organized basis. The type of exercise you choose should suit your own personal preferences and means, and in a moment I will give the basic information you need to make your selection. But first, it's important for you to envision yourself as a person who *does* exercise.

Why is this so important? Because the second biggest obstacle to physical fitness, after lack of time, is embarrassment. Women especially tend not to think of themselves as athletic or even active. When working with my colleague Dr. Martin Katahn here at Vanderbilt, we would ask weight group members to describe themselves in five adjectives. Words such as "wife" and "mother" came up frequently, as did words describing professions, careers, positions in social organizations and churches. But very rarely did these women use any *active* adjectives to describe themselves. That lack of an active self-concept can be a huge obstacle. Likely, if these women thought of themselves as tennis players, runners, or even golfers, they would find it much more natural to incorporate exercise into their daily life—and to make it a priority.

As an example of how this works, I must tell you about the medical director of the faculty and staff wellness program here at Vanderbilt. She is married with two young children, one of whom is disabled. She is very active in her church and president of the area medical association, *and* a nationally ranked senior tennis player. She walks briskly on her treadmill during the evening news every night without fail. Why? To enhance her tennis game. Because she enjoys being fit. Because the exercise makes her feel better both physically and emotionally, and enhances her sense of independence and self-confidence. Weight control is the natural result, but it is not her primary motivation for exercise.

Some women, unfortunately, have been conditioned to believe it's unfeminine to be strong and active, especially if that activity involves breaking a sweat! Many have been conditioned to feel so ashamed of their bodies that they refuse to wear a swimsuit or leotard in public—and therefore "can't" work out. But the majority simply have never learned *how* to exercise and feel too embarrassed to ask for guidance or to make the inevitable mistakes that we all make when trying a new activity for the first time.

As I say, embarrassment is a powerful obstacle, and it is damaging both to the body and to the soul. But try to remember four things:

1. How, when, and why you exercise is nobody's business but your own. Nobody else has the right to pass judgment on you.

2. You are exercising for yourself, to improve your health, to reduce your stress, and to strengthen and streamline your body. You can achieve all of these goals even if you've never hit a home run in your life. Even if you work out in sweats and an old T-shirt. Even if you don't have an "athletic" or "coordinated" bone in your body.

3. Almost everyone can perform some form of exercise. You don't have to run a marathon or qualify for the Olympics to meet your fitness needs. You just need to get moving, keep moving, and gradually move a little faster.

4. When you get the hang of it, exercise is fun. The only way to claim your share of that fun is to overcome your embarrassment, reconceptualize yourself as a Physically Active Person, and plunge in.

As for myself, I am a jogger and proud of it. I jog three to four miles at least three times a week. I prefer jogging because it burns the most calories in the least amount of time of any exercise that I can do conveniently and consistently. It makes me feel challenged and refreshed. Most of the time, I use a treadmill because it's convenient at work and at home, and I can control my speed and degree of difficulty. When Nashville weather permits (i.e., it's not too hot and humid) I enjoy jogging outside around Vanderbilt's track.

On my "days off" I take walks or do aerobic exercises at home for twenty to thirty minutes in front of the TV using a step or the new side-to-side slide mat (see p. 237). Walking is integrated into the rest of my life. I walk across campus to meetings, or do a few laps around my local mall, or take my dog out around the neighborhood or park.

Now, I do not consider myself to be an exercise fanatic, one of those people who compulsively work out for two or more hours every day (see the end of this chapter), but I can tell you that I feel my best and do my best work after a day's jog. When I go for several days without my routine workout, I tend to feel sluggish and tired. For me, the benefits of physical activity go far beyond the issue of weight control.

Workout Essentials

The following basic rules cover virtually every form of exercise and every personality. They reflect the realities of human physiology and anatomy and will help ensure that you get the greatest possible benefits from your workout without injuring yourself.

• Make a date with yourself to exercise at least every other day, preferably daily, for at least ten minutes, working up to a regular workout of half an hour or more several times a week. I say make a date because you have to *make* time rather than find time. You will never magically find time to exercise, but you will find time for passive activities such as TV watching—so schedule those minutes instead for exercise! Half an hour, your target workout period, is the length of one TV sitcom or the evening news. Instead of sitting still while you watch, ride your exercise bike or step in place. Or split the half hour into two brisk fifteen-minute walks, one in the morning and one after work. The specific timing and type of exercise will depend on your lifestyle and fitness level, but however you set up your workout schedule, make sure you *keep it up.* Just thinking about it will do nothing to increase your physical fitness.

• Don't exercise hungry. Eat a *light* meal or snack that's high in carbohydrates about an hour before your workout. Unless you "prefuel," you won't have the energy you need to ignite the release of calories. The less energized you are, the less you'll feel like exercising. The less you feel like exercising, the more excuses you'll find to avoid working out and the less you'll enjoy the exercise you force on yourself.

• Dress appropriately and use equipment safely and correctly. You needn't spend a lot of money on fancy workout toys, but don't shortchange yourself on necessary equipment. If you take up jogging, wear bona fide running shoes (see p. 228)—and make sure they fit properly. If swimming is your sport, make sure your swimsuit allows a full range of motion, and invest in a pair of goggles so you can see where you're going. If you join a gym that offers circuit training equipment with which you're unfamiliar, have an instructor show you the proper way to use that equipment before you try it yourself. If you buy home or pool exercise equipment, read the instructions thoroughly before your first workout.

• If you are not used to exercising, get your physician's okay before starting a workout program of any kind. This is particularly crucial if you are over fifty or have a preexisting heart condition or history of high blood pressure, chronic illness, chest pain, or injury.

• Establish a sensible goal (length of time or distance you will cover during each workout) based on your current fitness level, and only *gradually* increase intensity and duration over a period of weeks. No one's going to give you a medal for increasing your daily walk or jog from two miles to three. It's something you do for yourself. But if you make that jump too soon, you risk injury and exhaustion. Give yourself at least a couple of weeks to get used to your initial, modest exercise regimen before you add to the demand on your body. Make sure that each new fitness goal you set for yourself is easily attainable. That way you'll be able to progress steadily without suffering unwanted setbacks.

• Breathe! Breathing means taking in oxygen. Just as a flame needs oxygen to burn, your body needs oxygen to burn calories—and fat. Too many people respond to exertion by holding their breath. Don't! As a rule of thumb, try to breathe out as you tighten your muscles, breathe in as the muscles release. When performing a continuous movement, such as walking or jogging, establish a regular rhythm for your breathing and use that rhythm to pace yourself. *If you exercise outdoors in an area with heavy air pollution, time your workout for the least smoggy times of the day: early morning, or evening after rush hour. This will minimize breathing discomfort caused by the smog.*

• Warm up properly. A proper warm-up of five to ten minutes of light movement will prepare you for exercise by gradually increasing your heart rate and blood flow. Also, your muscles, tendons, and ligaments become more flexible and less vulnerable to injury if you warm them up before starting a strenuous workout. Walking, jogging in place, easy cycling, or, in the water, a few laps of slow swimming make the best warm-ups.

• Keep your body in alignment to protect your back. Many Americans suffer from back pain, and when exercise is performed incorrectly it can aggravate that pain. Performed correctly, however, it will help prevent or relieve back pain. The key to protecting your back is to keep your spine as long and straight as possible, tummy tucked in and buttocks tucked down. Whether you're walking, jogging, biking, skiing, swimming, doing aerobics or water aerobics, this rule remains the same. No slumping! No slouching! And no arching your back! If you can't tell whether you're in alignment, imagine someone is holding a plumb line from the top of your head and make sure that your neck, chest, belly, and buttocks all fall into place along that straight line.

• Squeeze and stretch those muscles. Technically, it's called contraction and extension, and it's how you move your body. It's also how you burn calories. Tighten and release. Squeeze and stretch. Pull in, reach out. This is the basic process of exercise.

• Control your movements. You want to aim for steady resistance rather than jerking, flailing, or pounding movements, which can injure muscles. Feel the continuous motion of the bicycle pedal beneath your feet. Push steadily against the water while swimming instead of thrashing about. Consciously press against the ground as you walk or jog, as if it were a treadmill.

• Work as many muscle groups as possible. The more large muscles you use, the more calories you burn now and the more new muscle you build, which will increase your caloric burn in the future. Working muscle groups throughout your body will result in balanced, symmetrical toning. By contrast, exercises such as running, which use only the lower body, tend to build up the thigh and calf muscles but can leave the upper body looking comparatively scrawny. An excellent way to ensure maximum use of muscles throughout the body is to alternate between several different types of exercise, trading off, say, between walking on one day and weight training or swimming on another. Known as cross-training, this strategy is used throughout the athletic world, from Olympians to professional ballplayers.

• Don't lock your joints. Keep elbows and knees, in particular, slightly flexed. When you lock a joint straight you take the strain off the muscles, where it belongs, and grind it instead into vulnerable bones and cartilage. Thus you get less exercise value from your workout and risk doing serious and permanent damage to the joint.

• Check your progress during the workout by monitoring your heart/pulse rate or perceived exertion level. The following charts explain how to take these two basic measurements. In general, the more accurate gauge of intensity is heart rate. However, there is considerable variability in heart rate from one person to the next. Also, for reasons I'll explain later in this chapter, heart rate is most reliable in gauging exertion for exercises performed on land, less accurate in water. Finally, measuring your heart rate requires you to interrupt your activity and take a precise time reading and pulse count. It isn't a practice that many people use outside of a guided workout setting such as an aerobics dance class. Among my many active friends, few ever check their pulse rate—they can feel how hard they are working. This sensation of physical effort is the basis for the perceived exertion scale. Remember, your heart rate will go up with the intensity of your workout whether you check it or not. And it's the intensity of your muscular activity that matters to your figure, not how many heartbeats you can count. Whichever method you use to pace yourself, try to stay within your target range for at least one-third of your total workout. If your fitness level is low to moderate, aim for the lower end of your target range; if you are very fit, aim high. You will know you're exercising at the right pace if you can feel your muscles working and are breathing slightly harder than normal. Do NOT work so hard that you feel dizzy or faint, are gasping for breath or sweating profusely.

Target Heart Rate Chart
No. of Heartbeats Counted for Ten Seconds

Use this chart to target your minimum and maximum *working* heart rates for exercise on land (walking, jogging, cycling, aerobics, etc.) and for water exercise (swimming, water aerobics, etc.)

	Land Exercise		Water Exercise	
Age	Minimum Number Heartbeats	Maximum Number Heartbeats	Minimum Number Heartbeats	Maximum Number Heartbeats
20	17	27	15	25
25	16	26	14	24
30	16	25	14	23
35	15	25	13	23
40	15	24	13	22
45	15	23	13	21
50	14	23	13	21
55	14	22	13	20
60	13	21	12	19
65	13	20	12	18
70	12	20	11	18

Measuring Perceived Exertion

To use perceived exertion as a measure of exercise intensity, simply pay attention to the way your body feels at different levels of activity. You know that if you're walking slowly—strolling—you're not working very hard. That would qualify as a 1 on the Perceived Exertion Scale, or "very easy." Break into a long, regular stride, and you step your exertion level up to "easy." Shorten and quicken your stride and you escalate to "moderate." Now speed up to a jog, and you're up to "somewhat hard." Break into a run, and that's "hard." Move your arms and legs twice as fast: that's "very hard," and it's likely as high as you can or should go on the exertion scale. If, however, you're in excellent shape and can run at racing speed, then when you go flat out in competition, you're working "very, very hard."

As you move up each notch on the scale, your heart rate will climb a little, but what really matters in determining fitness and weight loss is how much oxygen your muscles are burning. The Perceived Exertion Scale relates your exertion level to oxygen use through what's called "VO_2 Max." This is shorthand for the maximum amount of oxygen your body is capable of taking in and delivering to the muscles. If you are working your body to its true max—and burning maximum calories and fat—then you will also be burning 100 percent of your VO_2 Max. Less effort uses less oxygen and burns fewer calories.

Number	Perceived Exertion	% of VO_2 Max
1	Very easy	—
2	Easy	45
3	Moderate	55
4	Somewhat difficult	62
5	Difficult	70
6	Very difficult	85
7	Maximum	100

Perceived exertion can be used for both land and water exercise, and it's certainly easier than counting heartbeats. The more you exercise, the more familiar you will become with your own body's signals and the more reliably you'll be able to tell when you're really making an effort and when you're taking it easy.

- If you are new to exercise, aim to maintain between levels 3 and 4 for the majority of your workout, then gradually ease back down.
- If you are moderately fit, target levels 4 to 5.
- If you are very fit, target levels 5 to 6.

• Drink PLENTY of water before, during, and after your workout, even if you don't feel thirsty. This goes double if you're exercising at high intensity or in hot weather, when your body can lose more than a quart of water in an hour. Fluid loss can cause nausea, lethargy, and contribute to heat exhaustion or heat stroke. Water is the ideal fluid replacement and is generally preferable to so-called sports drinks.

• Cool down and stretch before stopping. Your muscles can seize up if you work them hard, then suddenly quit, so *never stand still immediately after high-intensity exercise.* Use the same easy movements you used for a warm-up to cool down. Then take a few minutes to relax and stretch out the muscles you exercised the hardest.

• Don't ignore or "work through" pain! You should feel the effort of working your muscles, but this should not cause discomfort or pain. If you feel soreness or aching after exercising, it may mean you didn't spend enough time warming up or that you worked yourself too long or too hard. You needn't stop working out, but do slow down until the soreness goes away. DO STOP IF YOU EXPERIENCE MORE ACUTE PAIN. It could signal injury or exhaustion. Know the warning signs: *labored breathing, dizziness, loss of coordination, tightness or pain in your chest, nausea or vomiting, heart rate irregularity, or a stabbing, tearing, or wrenching pain.* If you experience any of these signals, consult a physician as soon as possible, and get a medical okay before resuming exercise.

Optional Workout Guidelines

These suggestions work for many people to make exercising more enjoyable and/or easier. Whether they will work for you, however, depends on your individual personality and lifestyle. Try them. If they prove useful, adopt them.

• Vary your routine. Alternate, for example, between walking one day and swimming the next. You may find this cross-training helps you sustain enthusiasm for exercising. It will also extend the benefits to your body, because each form of exercise uses different muscle groups. The more different activities you perform, the more muscles you will work.

• Try interval training. Alternating three to five minutes of high-intensity movement with up to three minutes of moderate movement may get you in shape faster than maintaining a steady pace for your whole workout. Research suggests this alternating approach produces greater cardiovascular benefits and about the same fat loss results as the steady pace. You may also find it less monotonous.

• Work out with friends. A support system can help relieve the boredom and monotony that sometimes set in with regular exercise. Fitness is more fun if it's also social. And your workout buddy can help boost your momentum when your own motivation starts to flag. Dr. Katahn's wife, a well-known concert pianist and university professor, walks with a group of friends three miles every morning at six A.M. by a scenic lake near her home. They are *accountable* and committed to each other to meet at that lake every day. She's told me that, on many mornings, having her friends there waiting for her is the only thing that keeps her from rolling over and going back to sleep.

• Exercise to music. Regardless of whether it comes at you through headphones or a background stereo, the rhythm in music can help step up the pace of your body and increase the caloric and cardiovascular benefits of your workout. When you hear a strong, steady beat, your arms and legs just naturally start moving in time to it. And, as if you were dancing, you'll hardly notice the extra effort.

Exercise Footwear Guidelines

Wearing the proper shoes is crucial for injury prevention. There is now specialized footwear for virtually every form of exercise. The two basic types of athletic shoes, however, are running and tennis shoes.

Running shoes are designed primarily for forward movement. They are lightweight, with a durable outer sole and a thick heel wedge to tilt the body forward. Running shoes should bend at the ball of the foot, not in the middle. *Running shoes lose about 30 percent of their shock absorption after 500 miles of use, regardless of brand, price, or construction, so they must be replaced regularly.* Walking shoes are a variation on running shoes but generally have a more rigid shank for support.

Tennis shoes are designed for side-to-side movement. They are heavier and stiffer than running shoes, and have reinforcement under the toes. You can use tennis shoes in aerobics classes, which are multidirectional, but not running shoes.

Whatever type of shoe you're looking for, inspect construction carefully when shopping. Make sure the upper is attached correctly—vertically—to the sole. If the heel appears to slant outward or inward, don't buy it.

Cold Weather Workout Guide

It's easy to make excuses when the weather is cold, but you *can* still exercise outside even when the mercury drops below freezing. The key is to dress warmly. Here are some pointers.

- **Don't overdress.** Because exercise lifts your body temperature, dress for weather that's about 30 degrees higher than the actual temperature. If it's 20 degrees out, dress as if it were 50 degrees.
- **Dress in layers.** This creates layers of trapped heat for insulation. Remove the top layer—your outer garment—as soon as you begin to sweat, and carry it or tie it around your waist.

    Layer one, long underwear, should be made of a fabric that draws sweat *away* from your skin. Cpilene, Thermax, or polypropylene will do the trick. Cotton is not advisable, as it holds moisture to your body.

    Layer two should consist of warm clothing—a wool sweater, synthetic turtleneck, or pile jacket on top, and sweat pants or Lycra (not cotton) tights on your legs.

    Layer three, your jacket, should be waterproof and wind resistant, and it should breathe so that moisture won't be trapped inside. The synthetic fabric Gore-Tex is ideal for this purpose.
- **Wear mittens or gloves.** Mittens are warmer because they keep fingers together and have less surface area from which heat can escape.
- **Keep your head covered.** Heat rises and leaves your body through your head. A hat or hood keeps that heat in and will actually help keep your *feet* warm!
- **Wear shoes with good traction and shock absorption.** The ground is harder, more uneven, and often slippery in freezing weather, so you need footwear that grips and cushions well. Cold-weather shoes should be roomy enough so that you can comfortably wear an extra pair of socks.
- **Warm up and cool down *indoors*.** This will minimize discomfort when your body temperature is low.
- **Drink as much water as in hot weather.** You lose extra water in the cold because your body must moisten and warm the cold air you inhale. If you dehydrate, it can impair your body's ability to regulate its internal temperature.
- **Keep moving.** It's your best defense against the cold. If you have to slow down or stop, remember to put back on any clothing you've removed.

Night Workout Safety Tips

You may choose to do your jogging, walking, or cycling after dark, especially during the winter months when days are short. If you share the roadway with car traffic, it's imperative that you take safety precautions so that motorists can see you. Here are a few basic tips.

- Avoid high-traffic thoroughfares if at all possible, and do not use roads with traffic moving faster than 30 miles per hour.
- Wear glow-in-the-dark patches or reflectors on your clothing, headgear, and shoes, back and front, as well as on your bike if you are a cyclist.
- Use direction as a safeguard. Run or walk against the traffic so you can see what's coming. If cycling, ride with the traffic, because drivers will expect you to follow the same rules they do and will predict your movements accordingly.
- Use a light. If on foot, carry a flashlight or clip a flashing light onto your belt or headband. If cycling, equip your bike with a headlight *and* taillight.
- Do not wear headphones. You need to be able to hear as well as see approaching traffic.

Weight Training for Added Benefits

If you're conscientious in your eating habits and perform aerobic activities on a regular basis and *still* have trouble maintaining your figure, strength training could be the secret weapon you've been looking for. Lifting weights, or using Nautilus or resistance equipment that mimics the effect of weight lifting, helps to tone and build muscle, which in turn boosts your metabolism and makes it more difficult for you to gain unwanted fat.

In and of itself, strength training is not a particularly effective way to burn fat because it is anaerobic (does not burn oxygen) and is usually accomplished through quick explosive movements with a lot of stopping and starting. To illustrate, imagine what happens if you repeatedly turn the key on and off in your car; you use plenty of ignition fluid but never really burn gas. Likewise, weight training burns a lot of glycogen (carbohydrates), but not fat. And yet, these exercises offer some real fitness advantages if done *in combination* with a regular aerobic workout.

• Circuit training (using a variety of different weights or machines to work different muscle groups throughout the body) increases muscle tissue. While this might slightly raise your weight, it will decrease fat (remember that muscle, inch for inch, weighs more than fat). It will also increase the total number of calories your body burns each day. Over time, assuming your calorie intake remains stable, this metabolic lift will cause you to burn even more body fat.

• Weight training tones muscles and increases visible definition of muscles, which has a positive effect on body dimensions and on the distribution of fat. While it was once considered unfeminine for women to show their muscles or any evidence of physical strength, that tide has turned. Now the world's most fashionable men and women show off their biceps, triceps, and deltoids with pride. This does not mean that we all should or even could look like Arnold Schwarzenegger—women physiologically cannot build massive muscle bulk! But every one of us *can* increase our muscular strength and improve definition.

• Weight training strengthens muscles and bones. It's not just a matter of fashion but of function. You will be able to do more, lift more, carry more if you have muscular strength. You will be more physically capable and independent. You will stand taller, have better posture, *and* your bones will be less vulnerable to osteoporosis as you get older.

If your chosen exercise is walking or running, one way to combine weight training with aerobics is to carry or wear extra weights as you go. Such weights are available in the form of small dumbbells or wraparound weights for your wrists or ankles. These added weights can enhance the cardiovascular effect of your workout and build muscle strength in the arms, upper back, and legs. You should be aware, however, that they will increase the impact of every step you take and, therefore, add stress on your lower back and joints. In other words, they may also increase your risk of injury. So if you feel yourself straining, cut back on the amount of weight you're carrying.

If you have access to a gym with weight training equipment, my advice is to use that equipment in addition to your regular aerobic workout. Make sure to have a professional at the gym guide you through the instructions and show you the correct setting of equipment for your body *before* you attempt to use it. If used properly, these devices may help protect you against injury by strengthening critical muscles, but every one of them can also hurt you if used incorrectly.

LFP Activity Selection Guide

There is not room in this book to go into exacting instructional detail for all the different forms of exercise that can help keep your body lean. For this I suggest you turn to books dealing exclusively with exercise or, better yet, join a Y, recreation center, or fitness club and get personalized instruction. But before you take that step, you will need to decide which sports to explore. To that end, I've put together an overview of the most popular athletic activities so that you can select those best suited to your lifestyle and fitness goals.

Land Exercise versus Water Exercise

I divide activities into land and water categories in part because I've found that there are "water people," who prefer spending time in a pool, lake, river, or ocean whenever they can, while others tend to be "land people," who can't stand getting wet. There are also practical differences, since not everyone has access to a pool or beach, especially year-round. But the main reason I separate the two categories is that the body behaves very differently in and out of water.

Gravity versus buoyancy. When we exercise on land our bodies work against the force of gravity. Our muscles work to hold us erect, to push us up off the ground with each step, to lift our arms and keep our back vertical. This requires constant, unconscious effort. When we immerse ourselves in water, we become buoyant, effectively eliminating the pull of gravity. The water supports approximately 90 percent of our weight, relieving almost all the stress on joints and permitting a much wider range of motion than we have on land. But this also means that water exercise requires more *conscious* effort than does land exercise to produce noticeable fitness results.

Resistance. The resistance of water is twelve times that of air, greatly increasing the effort required to perform certain movements and multiplying the resulting strength benefits. The resistance is equal in every direction in the water, so that many more muscle groups are exercised than would be if you performed the same movements on land. This represents a trade-off, however, because in the water we do not expend the automatic effort necessary on land to resist gravity.

Temperature control. During land exercise we sweat, in effect creating a layer of water on the skin, to reduce body heat. But when we swim or perform aquatic exercises, the surrounding water is already there, reducing heat buildup and enabling the circulatory system to concentrate on delivering blood to the muscles. When you work out in warm water (83 degrees F or warmer), this enhances the body's fat-burning capacity. Beware, however, if you work out in colder water, especially if you are very lean, because your body may actually retain surface fat just below the skin for insulation. My recommendation? If you like the water, by all means jump in, but remember, if the water is between 80 and 84 degrees it will make it easier to melt away unwanted fat.

Heart rate. When you exercise on land, your heart does most of the work in circulating oxygen-rich blood throughout your body. That is why your pulse is a good way to measure the intensity of land exercise: the higher your heart rate, the harder your body is working. In the pool, however, the pressure of the water against your body acts as an auxiliary pump, relieving the heart of some of its burden and lowering heart rate. When suspended in water your body requires approximately 10 percent fewer heartbeats per minute than it does on land for exactly the same exertion. This does not reduce the number of calories you burn, nor does it diminish the effect of exercise in building muscle tissue, but it does reduce the strain on your heart. It also makes it difficult to gauge your effort through heart rate. You can use the heart rate chart on p. 225, but your water heart rate is affected by a number of additional factors, such as body composition and proportion, which are difficult to calculate. Researchers who study the effects of water exercise now agree that perceived exertion is the better measure of intensity when working out in water.

Fat loss. Studies consistently have shown that water exercise produces about the same fat loss as cycling, but less than walking or jogging. No one is quite sure why this is so. It may have something to do with the lack of gravity. It may be related to the temperature of the water in which swimmers were studied. And it is possible that certain new forms of deep-water resistance exercise (see p. 241–43) will be shown to produce more favorable results for fat loss. But, while you can expect excellent strength training and cardiovascular benefits, don't expect to get the same ultralean results from swimming that you do from jogging.

Land Exercise Balance Sheet

Here, for quick review, is a rundown of the basic pros and cons of the most popular aerobic exercises performed on land, to be followed by a similar balance sheet for aerobic water exercises.

Walking

Fitness benefits: Excellent cardiovascular workout. Tones lower body muscles. Low stress on joints.

Fitness drawbacks: Does not significantly work the upper body or abdominal muscles. Requires brisk pace for noticeable results in fat loss. Lower caloric burn rate than more vigorous exercise.

Practical requirements: Requires no special equipment or training. Can be done virtually anywhere, in all climates. Can be done in street clothes. Can be done in numerous small blocks of time throughout the day. Can be combined with errands and chores. Can also be done on a treadmill at home or at a gym.

Practical drawbacks: Requires a greater time investment than other more intensive exercise before fat loss is achieved.

Jogging/Running

Fitness benefits: Excellent cardiovascular workout. High caloric burn rate. Tones lower body muscles. Requires the least amount of time for the greatest caloric expenditure.

Fitness drawbacks: Does not build or significantly tone upper body or abdominal muscles. Places extreme stress on ankles, knees, hips, and spine, which can lead to injury. May place too much stress on the cardiovascular system if you have preexisting heart condition. May aggravate symptoms of arthritis.

Practical requirements: Wear properly fitted shoes that are designed for running—not regular sneakers or tennis or aerobic shoes. Requires no other special equipment or training. Can be done virtually anywhere, in all climates. Can also be done indoors on a treadmill at home or at a gym. Fat loss can be achieved from relatively short workouts.

Practical drawbacks: Not advisable for anyone who has weak or previously injured ankles, knees, hips, or back. Open-air jogging is not advisable in areas with severe air pollution (nor is any other open-air exercise; the increased oxygen consumption during exercise multiplies the toxic chemicals your body absorbs from the air).

Aerobics

Fitness benefits: Excellent cardiovascular workout. High caloric burn rate. Most workouts exercise muscles throughout the body. Workouts can be performed as high-impact or low-impact workouts, depending on your level of fitness and condition of your back and joints. Use of music and dance movements makes it easier and more fun to increase the pace of activity without noticing the extra exertion.

Fitness drawbacks: Because only about half the class is devoted to strenuous exercise, many aerobics classes may be less effective fat burners than a continuous workout of jogging or running. Significant weight loss requires 30 to 60 minutes of continuous movement at least four times per week. Even low-impact aerobics may place too much stress on the joints if you suffer from arthritis or have weak ankles, knees, hips, or lower back.

Practical requirements: You need music and an instructor, either in person through a class at a fitness center or via video or TV instruction. Wear shoes designed specifically for aerobic exercise.

Practical drawbacks: Many people find it more enjoyable to attend aerobics classes, which offer company, encouragement, and individualized instruction, than to exercise to video instruction, but this means tailoring your daily schedule around a class schedule.

Aerobic Machines: Stairmaster, Stepmaster, Climbers, Rowing and Skiing Machines, Etc.

Fitness benefits: Excellent cardiovascular workout. High caloric and fat burn rate. Most machines tone primarily lower body muscles. Many monitor caloric expenditure, speed, duration, and intensity.

Fitness drawbacks: Machines may cause injury if used improperly. Beware of setting the machine at too high a level; it may drive you to overtrain, causing symptoms such as dizziness, irregular heartbeat, or fatigue. Most machines do not work the abdominal muscles.

Practical requirements: You need access to these machines, either by purchasing them or joining a fitness club.

Practical drawbacks: These machines are costly to buy, and the health clubs that offer them may be costly to join. In many clubs, there are not enough of these machines for all those who use them, so you may have to wait for your turn.

Cycling

Fitness benefits: Excellent cardiovascular workout. Moderate caloric burn rate at most speeds. Tones lower body muscles. Can be used as an alternative form of transportation, allowing you to meet your fitness goals while also traveling to the store or work. Places little stress on vulnerable joints but may intensify lower back pain.

Fitness drawbacks: Does not significantly work upper body or abdominal muscles.

Practical requirements: You need either a stationary bicycle or a functioning bicycle (you can get top-quality exercise benefits from an inexpensive three-speeder as well as from a high-priced racing bike). You will need a reliable bicycle and safety helmet. Special shoes, gloves are optional. You need access to wide and/or low-traffic roads where you can ride without risk of being hit by car traffic.

Practical drawbacks: Not advisable in areas with severe air pollution (see jogging, above). Racing bicycles can be very expensive, though you can achieve the same fitness benefits with an old-fashioned three-speed cycle. Dangerous to ride bikes in crowded city streets.

Tennis/Racquetball/Handball

Fitness benefits: A good cardiovascular workout and calorie burner *if* you keep moving. Tones muscles in both upper and lower body. Uses competitive instinct to increase your exertion level.

Fitness drawbacks: A more intermittent workout, with a lot of stopping and starting, which can cut the cardiovascular and caloric benefits unless you make an effort to stay in motion. Does not work the abdominal muscles. Places stress on ankles, knees, hips, and spine, which can lead to injury. May place too much stress on the cardiovascular system if you have preexisting heart condition. May aggravate symptoms of arthritis.

Practical requirements: You need proper tennis shoes, racquet, balls, and access to a level court. You need at least one partner.

Practical drawbacks: Tennis equipment can be moderately expensive, and must be maintained. Although municipal courts are often free of charge and open to all, tennis clubs are costly to join and may require "tennis white" attire. Scheduling can be an obstacle, since you need to coordinate with your partner and you may have to sign up ahead of time for a public court.

Skiing: Cross-country and Downhill

Fitness benefits: Cross-country uphill skiing has the highest rate of caloric and fat burn of any popular exercise. Works muscles throughout the body.

Fitness drawbacks: Places stress on ankles, knees, hips, and spine, which sometimes leads to injury. May place too much stress on the cardiovascular system if you have preexisting heart condition. May aggravate symptoms of arthritis. High risk of serious injury, especially in downhill skiing, due to falling and collision (with trees, rocks, other skiiers!).

Practical requirements: You need snow, skis, ski boots, gloves, ski poles, warm clothing. You need wide-open space.

Practical drawbacks: Not an available exercise during summer or in warm climates or urban areas. Equipment and lift tickets are expensive.

Team Sports: Basketball, Soccer, Softball

Fitness benefits: Good cardiovascular training if you keep moving. Builds strength and endurance. Burns fat. Develops coordination and team skills.

Fitness drawbacks: A more intermittent workout, with a lot of stopping and starting, which can cut the cardiovascular and caloric benefits unless you make an effort to stay in motion. Does not build or significantly tone abdominal muscles. Places stress on ankles, knees, hips, and spine, which can lead to injury. May place too much stress on the cardiovascular system if you have preexisting heart condition. May aggravate symptoms of arthritis.

Practical requirements: You need to gather a group of players together for at least an hour on a regular basis. You need to understand the rules of the game. You need proper shoes, protective gear, ball, etc.

Practical drawbacks: It may be difficult to gather enough people together unless you participate in a regular game. If you do have a regular game, you must organize your daily schedule to incorporate it.

Golf

Fitness benefits: Cardiovascular and fat loss benefits due primarily to walking the course. Slight benefit in toning upper arm and back muscles. Appropriate for a broad range of fitness levels.

Fitness drawbacks: Provides few benefits if you use caddies and golf carts instead of walking the course.

Practical requirements: You need golf shoes, a set of clubs, supply of golf balls. You must have access to a golf course.

Practical drawbacks: Equipment is expensive to buy, may be expensive to rent. Although many towns have municipal golf courses, golf club memberships are typically very expensive. This is a fair-weather, warm-climate sport.

New Land Exercise Trends

Slide Aerobics

This is one of the hottest new trends, in part because it's fun, in part because it's inexpensive and easy to do at home, in part because it provides excellent conditioning and burns calories. The slide board itself may be between five and eight feet wide. It's a strip of plastic with solid bumpers at each end. The slide comes with soft socks or booties, which you wear over tennis shoes. Then, *following the instructions that come with the slide,* you step on and glide from side to side, as if speed skating, or straight forward and back, as if cross-country skiing. Slide aerobics are designed as low-impact, with no jumping movements, because increased impact would raise the risk of falling on the slippery surface.

Fitness benefits: Excellent cardiovascular workout. High caloric burn rate. Tones lower body muscles and strengthens ankles without high impact. Requires relatively small time investment for high caloric expenditure.

Fitness drawbacks: Does not build or significantly tone upper body or arm muscles. May aggravate any existing arthritis or knee, hip, or ankle problems.

Practical requirements: An aerobic slide and special socks. Wear properly fitted shoes that are designed for tennis—not running shoes. Can be performed at home or in special slide aerobics fitness classes. Slide is portable, requires little storage space. May be combined with handheld weights to add upper body workout.

Practical drawbacks: Not advisable for anyone who has orthopedic problems. Slide equipment costs from $40 to $80, depending on manufacturer.

Step Aerobics

In the past few years, the step has become a familiar component of many aerobics programs. Before that, it was a routine training element for athletes, whose coaches would have them "run the stadium steps" to increase heart rate, endurance, and strength. The new aerobic steps are simple devices made of lightweight plastic and come with adjustable support blocks for changing the height. By continuously stepping up and down for the duration of your workout, you achieve high-intensity exercise with the relatively low impact of walking. You can use handheld or wraparound wrist weights to add upper body conditioning as you step. When steps are used in organized aerobics classes, the movements may be a little more complicated in order to work a wider variety of muscle groups than you would reach by simply stepping forward and back. In general, the higher your fitness level, the more support blocks you will use to increase the height of your step. This is because the higher the step, the more exertion is required from your body. So if you're a beginner, you should exercise with the step at its lowest height, or from four to six inches. At the intermediate level, you can raise the step to between eight and ten inches. If you've used the step for some time and have achieved a high fitness level, you might work out with a step between ten and twelve inches high, but, for safety reasons, no higher and with no more than four support blocks at each end.

Fitness benefits: Excellent cardiovascular workout. High caloric burn rate. Tones legs, hips, buttocks. Requires relatively small time investment for high caloric expenditure.

Fitness drawbacks: Does not build or significantly tone upper body or arm muscles. May place too much stress on the ankles, knees, hips, or back, especially if you have arthritis or preexisting orthopedic problems.

Practical requirements: The step should be placed on a flat, nonskid surface. Wear properly fitted shoes that are designed for running. Can be done at home or in an organized step class.

Practical drawbacks: Not advisable for anyone who has weak or previously injured ankles, knees, hips, or back. Step prices begin at around $30.

NordicTrack

The NordicTrack is the equivalent of a treadmill for skiing. You fit your feet into "skis" and pull on handles or ropes using the same motion you would to pole yourself forward while cross-country skiing. Some versions of the NordicTrack offer additional cross-training features, such as a treadmill and stair-stepper. The NordicTrack is being aggressively marketed as home exercise equipment but is also available in some fitness centers.

Fitness benefits: Overall body conditioning, excellent cardiovascular workout with low impact on joints or back. High caloric expenditure in short periods of time.

Fitness drawbacks: Requires considerable coordination and may be difficult for beginners to learn the proper movements without instruction. Easy to injure yourself (or give up in frustration) if you use the equipment improperly.

Practical requirements: Wear proper running shoes. Options allow you to increase tension to tone arms and legs. Requires about the same floor space as an exercise bike but works more areas of the body. Can be done while watching TV.

Practical drawbacks: Requires greater degree of concentration than many other aerobic workouts. Not available in a wide variety of fitness centers. Expensive for home purchase.

Recumbent Bicycle

This stationary bicycle allows you to work out while lying down! The equipment is low to the ground, the seat tilted so that there is minimum stress on the lower back. Your upper legs do more of the work than they would with an upright bike. Health clubs that specialize in rehabilitative exercise are most likely to offer this equipment.

Fitness benefits: Good leg conditioning, especially for the muscles in the thigh and buttocks. Less stress on the lower back. Good cardiovascular workout.

Fitness drawbacks: Burns fewer calories than an upright bike, and your heart rate will be lower. Does not work the upper body.

Practical requirements: Easy to do. You can read or watch TV while working out.

Practical drawbacks: Some models will be more expensive than upright bikes. Not available in all fitness centers.

Water Exercise Balance Sheet

The one practical requirement common to all the following exercises is, of course, water. However, the amount and depth of water you need will vary widely with the particular form of exercise. And you can engage in several of these activities even if you do not know how to swim.

Swimming

Fitness benefits: Builds muscle strength. Works the widest variety of muscle groups of any exercise. Increases cardiovascular endurance. Burns fat. Recommended if you are recovering from leg or back injury or are pregnant.

Fitness drawbacks: Reduces fat less rapidly than running or cross-country skiing; if you are very thin and swim in a cold pool, swimming may actually cause an increase in surface body fat as insulation.

Practical requirements: You need a swimsuit and a pool or body of water large enough to swim laps, the larger the better. Goggles are not essential, but they will help you to swim more comfortably and therefore more fluidly and longer. Swim fins are beneficial but optional. You should take lessons if you have never learned to do the different strokes properly.

Practical drawbacks: You cannot really swim without getting your head wet, which means that you may need to use special shampoo to get the chlorine or salt out of your hair. The water tends to dry out skin, so you may need to use extra moisturizer. Water can also get into ears, causing discomfort, so you may want to use earplugs during or ear drops after swimming.

Water Aerobics

Fitness benefits: Excellent cardiovascular training. Builds strength and endurance. Burns fat. Water aerobics can be done in deep water with the aid of a flotation belt; this will increase the cardiovascular and muscle toning benefits. Water aerobics classes give you an opportunity to meet and exercise with other people.

Fitness drawbacks: None, assuming your instructor is adequately trained.

Practical requirements: At least initially, you will need to join a class at your local Y or health club in order to learn the basic movements. As water aerobics are typically performed in shallow water, you do not need to know how to swim and you need not get your head wet. Other than a swimsuit, no special equipment is required.

Practical drawbacks: You need to have access to a fitness club that offers water aerobics classes. Once you know the basic workout, you can do it on your own, but most people find it more enjoyable and more challenging to work out to music with a group.

New Water Exercise Trend

Deep-water Resistance Training

One of the latest developments in weight/resistance exercise is the deep-water resistance workout. Olympic athletes have used deep-water resistance as part of their training for years, but it's been only in the last decade that the gear devised for Olympians has been marketed to the general public. Now that equipment is being used for purposes of physical therapy and rehabilitation as well as to reduce fat and increase fitness.

Deep-water exercise uses the natural properties of water to produce similar results as traditional weight training. The difference is that you perform these exercises while suspended in water, which means there is zero impact on your joints and back, and the resistance is constant, so you do not have the stop-start pattern that you have with land weight training. In other words, you simultaneously get strength training and aerobic benefit.

It is important when performing deep-water exercise that you work up to your maximum exertion level. Because you are suspended in water, the sensation is very relaxing and it's tempting just to wave your arms and legs around aimlessly. If you don't use broad, continuous movements so that you really *feel* the water's resistance against your body at all times, then you will not achieve the results you're looking for.

The variety of deep-water gear is multiplying so fast that I can't predict what will be available a year from now, but at the moment, the most popular types of water resistance equipment are:

• Flotation belts (e.g., AquaJogger by Excel Sports of Eugene, OR; Aquatic Exercise Belt by Speedo; Aqua Sprinter Flotation Belt by C & L Aquatics). These suspend you upright in deep water, so you can perform the same motions that you would while walking, jogging, cycling, or cross-country skiing, but without any impact or stress on the joints. The constant lateral resistance of water acts as an opposing weight on your legs, building overall muscle strength more than would the same exercises on land.

• Dumbbells (e.g., DeltaBells by Excel Sports; Hand Buoys by Hydro Fit; Sprint Bells by C & L Aquatics). These are used just like regular dumbbells, except that most movements are reversed to push downward against the resistance of water instead of upward against the resistance of gravity (the basic motion used with weights on land). By using dumbbells in conjunction with a flotation belt, you can get a full workout for your arms, upper back, and chest muscles at the same time you are working your lower body with running, skiing, or cycling movements.

• Swim mitts (e.g., Swim Mitt XT by Speedo; Wave Webs by Hydro Fit; Sprint Aqua Gloves by C & L Aquatics). These are an alternative to the dumbbells and they can also be used to add upper body strengthening while swimming. The webbing between the fingers broadens the surface of the hand so that the sensation as you pull your arm through the water is like pushing against a stubborn door. Some of the mitts come with weighted inserts to add resistance when you lift your arm out of the water as well.

• Water footgear (e.g., AquaRunners by Excel Sports; Speedo Aquatic Exercise Shoe; Buoyancy and Resistance Cuffs by Hydro Fit; Sprint Buoyancy Cuffs by C & L Aquatics). Again, the idea is to widen the surface area of the foot, which in turn increases resistance. The normal running, cycling, or skiing movements require significantly more energy when you wear footgear, thus burning extra fat and building more muscle. Footgear can be used simultaneously with the flotation belt and gloves or dumbbells.

Because these "water toys" are still novelties in most areas, you may feel a little conspicuous being the first in your pool to try them. After just a few weeks of regular use, however, the change in your body will be so dramatic that others will be demanding to know your secret workout. Have the courage to be a pioneer!

Fitness benefits: Burns fat. Produces toning and strengthening of muscles equivalent to moderate weight training. Increases cardiovascular capacity; improves circulation. Works a wide variety of muscle groups. Can be combined with continuous aerobic movement to produce simultaneous cardiovascular, strengthening, and endurance benefits. Deep-water aerobics can produce the same fitness benefits as running, cycling, or cross-country skiing but without straining joints.

Fitness drawbacks: None if the exercises are performed correctly and equipment is used properly.

Practical requirements: You will need flotation equipment, but the combination is up to you: flotation belt, mitts, dumbbells, footgear. These devices are buoyant and, when adjusted properly, they will keep you afloat, but they are not designed for use as lifesaving equipment. You will probably feel more comfortable performing deep-water exercise if you know how to swim. In any case, it is essential that you read all accompanying directions that come with this equipment to ensure that you use it safely. The good news is, you don't have to get your head or hair wet, and you don't need to worry about chlorine in your eyes or water in your ears.

Practical drawbacks: You need access to a body of water at least chin deep and at least ten feet square. Flotation equipment costs about $30–$50 per device.

Exercising with Physical Limitations

I meet people all the time who tell me they "can't" exercise because they have a bad back or bum knees or some other medical ailment. Now, as I've said before, if you have a medical condition of any kind you should consult a physician before starting an exercise program. However, in nine cases out of ten, health problems actually *increase* the need for exercise. Often, exercise decreases symptoms, improves the medical condition, and slows disease progression—or prevents it altogether!

Let me illustrate this point with the story of a friend of mine named Bill, who suffered a stroke at a young age and was almost completely paralyzed from the waist down. Doctors told Bill he would probably never walk again, but as soon as he was released from the hospital he got himself up and moving. Equipped with crutches and braces, he went out for a walk every day. At first it took him three hours to walk to and from the newsstand a block and a half from his home. He put in those three hours every day. After a couple of months he increased his distance. Gradually his pace quickened and his strength and coordination improved. Today, four years after the stroke, Bill walks unaided, a limp the only obvious sign of his handicap. He attributes his recovery entirely to exercise—and persistence.

Another friend, Ann, jogged miles every day for years until she suffered serious damage to one ankle. Surgery failed to mend the damage. Ann was put on prescription medication and alerted that she would probably have to have the ankle fused, which would permanently shorten one leg and prevent her from ever walking normally again. Ann took to the water, swimming and doing deep-water resistance exercises, and began riding an exercise bike on days when she couldn't get to the pool. This daily regimen has stopped the progression of damage and reduced Ann's pain so that she no longer takes prescription pills and is comfortable with just one aspirin per day. Her doctors are amazed that she can even walk.

Am I saying that exercise accomplishes miracles? Well, I might not go quite that far, but I'd come pretty close. If you can move any part of your body, you can exercise. And if you exercise regularly and safely, your body inevitably will grow stronger, healthier, and more flexible. The challenge, of course, is to choose the form of exercise that is best for your particular needs.

If you have arthritis or are recovering from injury to the bones or joints, exercise will help increase your range of motion and encourage the joints to release a special lubricant that reduces inflammation and pain. The object is to move the joints, strengthen the surrounding muscles and connective tissue, and reduce total body weight, but all this must be accomplished without sudden pressure on the joints. The activities most frequently prescribed are water workouts, which effectively cause zero impact. Cycling and walking are also low-impact exercises, and moderate weight training may also be recommended. On the other hand, running, jogging, skiing, high-impact aerobics, tennis, and team sports are exactly the *wrong* exercises if you have any weakening of the bones or joints.

Water workouts are also commonly prescribed for the elderly, people recovering from heart surgery, and people with poor circulation. The water's effect as a "second heart" helps to pump blood throughout the body, allowing a much higher intensity of exercise with less strain on the heart than most land exercises.

The bottom line when it comes to exercise is to be realistic about your body's limitations and flexible in your workout regimen. Time and again I have seen people with chronic joint pain return stubbornly to running and high-impact aerobics because they think those are the only exercises that will help them lose weight, and time and again I have watched those same people reinjure themselves or burn out quickly and stop exercising altogether. *You must listen to your body.* If an activity is causing or aggravating pain, then lower the impact or switch to a different exercise. It's movement itself—not a particular kind of movement—that increases fitness and burns fat, so allow yourself to try a wide variety of activities rather than make a rigid habit of just one.

When Exercise Becomes Unhealthy

There is a tendency in this country to take almost everything to extremes. If a little is good, a lot must be better, or so the thinking goes. When this notion is applied to dieting it can lead to anorexia nervosa— and sometimes death. When turned to exercise, it can lead to anorexia, injury, and addiction. Workout-aholism, I call it.

The first thing you need to understand here is that most of the health and fitness benefits from exercise occur when you step up from a sedentary to a moderately active lifestyle. By moderate, I mean that you work out vigorously for thirty minutes each day, or forty-five minutes to an hour three to five times per week. If you want to boost your activity level above this level, then your best bet is to look for opportunities to get up and stretch and move within your daily routine.

By formally exercising longer or more frequently you will burn more calories and perhaps build more muscle tissue, but you will not gain more significant health benefits. On the downside, you may cut into the time and energy you have for the other important business of living. And you may undermine the positive effect exercise normally has on mood and self-esteem.

A study conducted at the University of South Carolina examined the connection between exercise and body image and came up with some surprising results.[1] Although all the women in the study were within the same average range for body weight and body fat, the women who compulsively exercised every day tended to be more critical of their own body shape than the moderate exercisers. The frequent exercisers also tended to be so obsessive about their workouts that they exercised even when ill.

Other studies suggest that there might actually be a chemical connection between overexercising and compulsive eating. One theory holds that exercisers become addicted to hormones called endorphins,

natural painkillers that are released into the bloodstream during strenuous exertion. Endorphins are responsible for the so-called "runner's
high" experienced by long-distance runners. Strenuous exertion over an
extended period also increases the brain's production of a hormone
called prolactin. And people with high levels of prolactin frequently
display an obsessive preoccupation with diet and/or exercise.

The message in all this is that it is possible to carry a good thing to
unhealthy extremes: sensible, moderate, and consistent exercise should
be your goal, not obsessive, obligatory workouts!

Signs of Workout-aholism

- You use exercise as a purgative—to "get rid of" calories you wish
  you hadn't eaten.
- You use exercise to distract yourself from bad feelings such as
  anxiety or depression, or to avoid problems you don't want to
  deal with.
- You get very upset or anxious if you miss a workout.
- If you're forced to stop exercising you experience withdrawal
  symptoms: confusion, irritability, anxiety, fatigue, depression,
  plummeting self-esteem, and a lack of focus.
- You insist on exercising even if you're sick or injured.
- You organize your life around your workout schedule rather than
  the other way around.
- You base important decisions on how well they can accommodate
  your exercise schedule (e.g., moving to a warm climate so you can
  run through the winter, or refusing a new job because the hours
  conflict with your aerobics class).
- You think it's more important to stick to your workout schedule
  than to see friends or family, or get to work on time.
- Exercise gives you a strong sense of control that evaporates when
  you stop working out for more than a day or two.
- You exercise because you believe you have to, not because you
  want to.

If three or more of these statements apply to you, you may have an
exercise obsession. Try cutting your workouts back to no more than half an
hour five times a week. If you cannot do this without feeling anxious or
depressed, I advise you to get professional counseling. As beneficial as
exercise can be, if done to excess it can be damaging.

10

Family Food and Family Weight

If you have a family, you know how difficult it is to separate your own eating habits from your children's or spouse's. If your husband's favorite food is steak, that makes it tough to run a vegetarian kitchen. If your child will eat only grilled cheese or peanut butter sandwiches, then you probably eat more grilled cheese and peanut butter than you otherwise might. But by the same token, you can have a powerful and positive influence on your family's eating habits. Everything you read in this book applies equally to every member of your family. The LFP plan can make you and your spouse leaner and fitter and at the same time prevent your children from ever becoming overweight!

Women are the gatekeepers for their families' eating habits. Of course, there are some enlightened households where the man does most of the cooking, but in most homes the men and children eat primarily what we women stock and prepare. That means that if we keep a low-fat kitchen for ourselves, then the rest of the family eats low-fat, too. Outside the home, of course, everyone may fend for himself, but we do have considerable veto power over the menu selections of our young children, and we can still exert considerable influence as role models by consistently ordering low-fat selections for ourselves.

Kids and Fat

Gaining fat is a normal and necessary part of childhood growth. During the first six months of life, the number of fat cells in a baby's body increases rapidly. The rate of increase continues, gradually slowing

247

throughout childhood until puberty, when the body again starts mass producing new fat. This is the point at which girls acquire the natural padding that makes them fatter than men for the rest of their lives.

The precise number of fat cells a child will acquire at any given point is determined largely by genetics. But if genetics were the whole story, then children of the current generation should be no fatter or thinner than past generations. This is not the case.

One-third of today's American children are overweight. That's a higher percentage of fat children than of fat adults, and it represents a 50 percent increase since the 1960s. The percentage of superobese kids has increased by *98 percent* during the same period. This is particularly alarming news since 40 percent of children who are obese at age seven will become obese grown-ups, and about 80 percent of overweight adolescents will remain so for life.

Why are so many more kids overweight? Although not definitive, most research has shown that neither obese children nor obese adults eat more calories than their slimmer peers. And while they do tend to be less active overall, overweight kids require more energy to move around and thus end up burning about the same number of calories as their thinner counterparts. But children's eating habits, even more than the rest of ours, have veered dramatically over recent decades toward high-fat foods. Study after study has shown that the only significant dietary factor separating fat kids from thin ones is the proportion of fat they consume. For example, while thinner children typically choose high-carbohydrate treats such as Popsicles and soft drinks as snack foods, obese children reliably prefer high-fat choices such as chips and packaged cakes. Thus, although both groups may eat the same number of calories, overweight children tend to eat more fat.

So one culprit is dietary fat. Another is television. TV has become America's favorite baby-sitter. Kids spend more hours in front of the tube over the course of a year than they spend in school and certainly more than they spend exercising. Each of those hours adds to their risk of developing lifelong obesity.

Television puts children into a veritable trance, reducing their metabolic rate by some 16 percent more than other sedentary activities. At the same time, commercial sponsors prompt young viewers to hunger for packaged treats that are high in fat and low in nutrition. And it seems that the parents who let their kids watch the most TV also tend to honor more of their children's shopping requests than other parents. This contributes directly to the fattening of their children. Which brings us to the family's overall role in childhood weight gain.

Fattening Families

The connection goes well beyond the type of milk Mom buys or how many hot dogs Dad throws on the barbecue. It goes beyond any genetic predisposition to weight gain that may run in the family. When a child gains excess weight, it often means he or she is not getting enough attention—or is getting too much of the wrong kind of attention. And that means that the whole family dynamic needs to change for the child to regain emotional health while losing unwanted pounds.

Psychologists who study weight gain in children have found that rates of obesity tend to be lowest in families where the lines of communication are open and honest between parents and kids. In fact, family cohesiveness seems to be a more reliable criterion than diet or exercise in predicting childhood weight! Since the unity of the family is so important in keeping kids at a healthy weight, it's not surprising that young people frequently gain weight in the face of parental divorce or death in the family. Or that children from abusive families often comfort themselves with food and end up overweight.

There appear to be two typical family patterns that may cause children to overeat. In one pattern, the child is overindulged. This often happens if the parents are estranged and one parent relies on the child for intimacy and companionship that would otherwise come from the marriage. It gives the child far too much power within the family, which is both confusing and threatening. A child who is expected to fill the role of an adult does not feel safe or secure, and may turn to food to soothe this distress.

The second pattern that causes overeating involves emotional neglect. The parents may ignore the child or simply fail to notice when he's feeling troubled or unhappy. They set few limits, so the child may watch TV for hours on end or eat mostly snack foods. His appetite for love and communication could show up as an appetite for cookies and potato chips. (As you may have figured out by now, similar emotional patterns can cause overeating in adults.)

A child can be caught in both patterns. This often happens in divorced families, when one parent becomes overly dependent on the child for emotional support while the other parent emotionally disowns him.

The solution for such a child is not to put him on a diet! NO CHILD SHOULD BE PUT ON A DIET. Even teaching him to eat low-fat foods, turn off the TV, and take up a sport, while important, are all secondary to his need for security and nurturing. The child's weight problem will improve when he's returned to his appropriate role and receives the love and trust and communication he so desperately craves. The first critical step, however, may be to seek family-based therapy.

As I've said before, this is not a psychology book and, even if it were, I cannot tell you how the relationships within your particular family are affecting your children. I can tell you, though, that if your child suddenly gains—or loses—a large, inexplicable amount of weight, you should take it as a warning sign. There might be a medical explanation, so it would be wise first to consult your pediatrician or family physician. But a likely cause could be emotional. *Do not hesitate to get professional help.*

Childhood Fat/Childhood Shame

Whether you are trying to help your overweight child slim down or keep your child at a healthy weight, it's critical that you appreciate the stigma children attach to fatness. From a very young age kids learn that fat is a source of tremendous shame. Elementary school students in several studies ranked obesity as a worse fate than being handicapped or disabled![1] And when asked to name the "worst thing about being fat," sixth grade girls answered that they would be unattractive and unpopular, feel bad about themselves, and that others would tease them.[2] Just as kids are using drugs and alcohol, smoking, and having sex at earlier ages, so, too, are younger and younger children obsessing about their weight.

Of course, the problem is most serious with girls because they pattern their behavior after their mothers and big sisters. They see attractive and *thin* women on TV bemoaning their bodies. They see glamorous celebrities touting weight loss products. They come to a logical conclusion: it's a sign of sophistication to hate their bodies and want to lose weight.

Some 60 percent of girls between grades 1 and 6 fear they are fatter than they really are.[3] A study of public school students in a middle-class area of Boston found that more than half had already dieted by age twelve and still wanted to lose more weight—even though most described their current weight as "about right."[4]

These sixth-grade girls had already absorbed the societal message that would pursue them into adulthood: women should never eat normally or be satisfied with their bodies as they are. They had also adopted a thoroughly "female" dieting mentality: even among those who were not concerned about their weight, most restricted their eating in front of other people; more than half felt "guilty" about overeating; almost all were familiar with calorie counts, tried to avoid high-calorie foods, worried about eating, and thought of exercise as a way to lose weight. As for the self-punishing consequences of dieting—the fatigue, poor concentration, listlessness, and declining grades caused by chronic hunger, the distraction and anxiety caused by the obsession with weight, and the low self-esteem caused by constant self-criticism—these girls, like older, seasoned dieters, accepted it all as part and parcel of being a woman.

The tragedy is that, even if we accept these girls' desire for thinness, their tortured relationship with food is the least efficient way possible to achieve that desire! The root of all this self-abuse is the myth that eating makes us fat. *Eating does not make anyone fat.* Eating fat makes us fat! There is absolutely no reason for young girls or anyone else to starve themselves in order to be thin. But it is our job as informed adults to spread the message of healthy, lean eating to these youngsters before they succumb to the unhealthy cycle of dieting, weight gain, and eating disorders.

Teaching Children About Fat

The need to educate kids about the true causes and remedies for weight gain was brought home to me during a recent "Day on Campus" when groups of sixth-grade students from around Nashville came to visit Vanderbilt. I spoke with these young people about my work at the wellness center and talked a little about the general principles of nutrition. They were surprised to learn that the United States is the fattest country on earth, and even more surprised that Tennessee ranks among the fattest states. Still, they could name lots of solutions to the problem.

People should go on a diet, they said. Or stop eating. Use Ultra SlimFast. Or go to Weight Watchers.

When I asked if these remedies would really work, they shouted back, "No!" Why? "Everybody gains it back." The kids all had parents, neighbors, and relatives who had lost lots of weight only to regain more. What these students didn't know was how much fat they themselves were consuming on a daily basis. So we tallied up a typical school lunch, either brought from home or bought in the school cafeteria. It turned out these kids ate more than 65 grams of fat at lunch—just that one meal!—*every day*. By making a few obvious substitutions, we were able to cut this figure in half. A few more subtle ones could cut it down to 10 to 15 grams of fat, which, in conjunction with other healthful meals and snacks, would bring them into a healthy range for fat intake for the day.

These Nashville kids were extremely receptive to the information I gave them—but few of them had heard much about it before. As adults, we need to do more to wise our children up to proper nutrition *before* they start gaining unhealthy fat.

Changing Children's Eating Habits

Children tend to eat a very limited variety of foods. Many youngsters subsist almost exclusively on bread, cereal, hamburger, cheese, milk, and soda. Very little fruit, few vegetables, and not much in the way of lean protein. Studies have shown that the most popular "kid foods" tend to contain at least 50 percent more fat, saturated fatty acids, and sodium than is recommended. And because children tend to eat such a limited range of foods, consuming the same ones over and over, certain vital nutrients may be missing from the diet entirely.

Your challenge as a parent, then, is to guide your child to eat from a wider, more varied menu and to develop a liking for leaner foods. Note that I did not say "nonfat" foods. Babies and young children especially need some fat. So while you might encourage your teenager to drink skim milk, your two-year-old should drink "low-fat," or 2 percent, milk. For a child under two years of age, your pediatrician would likely encourage whole milk.

The way to encourage low-fat foods is not through lecturing or ultimatums. It is, quite simply, to limit the high-fat foods you keep around the house. Stock up on high-carbohydrate, fat-free snacks such as fruit, Popsicles, frozen yogurt, pretzels, and cereal. Buy lean cuts of luncheon meats and reduced-fat cheeses. Look for reduced- or no-fat baked goods. Pack nutritious, low-fat lunches for school or camp. Modify favorite family recipes to be lower in fat or experiment with new leaner recipes at suppertime. Between meals, encourage your kids to eat whatever's on hand whenever they're hungry. If no high-fat snacks are available, there's no need to restrict them or worry about between-meal pantry raids.

Favorite Kid Foods and Their Better Choices

Typical Kid Food	Better Choice
Pastries and buns	Low-fat, high-fiber breads
Milk	Skim or 1% milk
Ice cream	Nonfat frozen yogurt
Cheese	Partially skim milk and reduced-fat cheese
Hamburger	Extra lean ground beef
	Ground turkey or chicken
Hot dogs	Reduced-fat hot dogs
Chicken	Skinless, light meat chicken
French fries	Oven "fried" potatoes
	Carrot and celery sticks
Cookies	Reduced-fat cookies
	Fresh or dried fruit
Doughnuts	Low-fat muffins
	Bagels w/ low-fat cream cheese
Potato and corn chips	Pretzels
	Air-popped or "light" microwave popcorn
	Low-fat baked chips
Chocolate candy bars	Chocolate syrup on frozen yogurt
	Hard and gummy candies
Soft drinks	Water
	Fruit juice

Make the transition gradually and try the many new lower-fat versions of basic kid staples, such as cookies and chips. These alternatives help make the changes relatively painless. Of course, if your kids show an interest (and the elementary schoolers might) you can explain how and why leaner foods also will make everyone healthier and leaner.

Even if the family embraces nutritional redirection, do not expect to see a big difference in what your children order at restaurants or what they eat at their friends' houses. But do try to shift the emphasis, when the family goes out together, toward restaurants that offer more lower-fat options. Take your kids to menus they haven't seen a thousand times before, and suggest low-fat choices. Introduce them to "lean cuisine" from other countries.

But unless your children do the majority of their eating elsewhere, there's no real need to worry about what they eat when they're away. It's their home eating habits that will make the most difference to their weight, present and future. As they grow more accustomed to the lighter foods, many children will gradually lose some of their affection for high-fat items and will naturally begin making leaner selections most of the time. And even if yours don't make this adjustment, remember that everyone is entitled to splurge every now and then. An occasional cheeseburger or piece of pie won't harm you or your children.

Exercise Is a Family Affair

The time to create a lifetime exercise habit is childhood. Kids have a number of fitness advantages over grown-ups. They tend to be more flexible. Their bodies are smaller, more compact, and more resilient. Children seem to learn new skills and adapt to new and different body movements more easily than adults can. Finally, because kids are naturally learning and trying new experiences all the time, they are less embarrassed to try a new form of exercise—even if they don't do it well—than most grown-ups are.

There is also evidence that people are more likely to continue sports in later life if they start playing them as children. This is particularly true of organized team sports, which have complicated rules of play and expected conduct. It also seems to be true of sports such as swimming, which involve subtleties of form. People who learned to swim as children, particularly those who swam on teams, tend as adults to be much faster, more efficient, and more comfortable in the water than people who begin swimming later in life.

The most compelling reason to get your children into the habit of exercising is simply that fitness is good for everyone at every age. Regular physical activity will make them stronger; leaner, faster, and better coordinated. It will help them think clearly and sleep well. It will boost their self-esteem and reduce feelings of stress. And if you join in their activities, you'll reap the same benefits yourself!

LFP Family Fitness Guide

- Establish a regular mealtime, and include the children in dinner-table conversation.
- Teach your children to appreciate and enjoy good food by including them in meal preparation and exposing them to a wide variety of dishes, but don't insist that they eat everything you put before them.
- Don't establish a Clean Plate Club: let your kids eat until satisfied, even if that requires only a few bites (remember that young children have small stomachs and may need to eat many snack-sized meals throughout the day rather than three large ones).
- Don't use food as a reward, pacifier, or baby-sitter.
- Try to be conscientious rather than controlling in your switch to low-fat nutrition: don't "police" the kitchen.
- Remember that your children's growing bodies may require more food than you do: feed them without overfeeding yourself.
- Set a good example for your family by selecting healthy foods and moderate portions for yourself.
- Get the kids out of the house. From the time they are infants, take them out for walks. Acquaint them with your neighborhood, especially other children in the neighborhood. Walk to nearby playgrounds or parks. Stroll with them around your local mall.
- Play together. Start with friendly roughhousing when your kids are small. Play ball with them as they get older. Take family bicycle rides.
- Don't use TV as the family baby-sitter. *Do limit television viewing and video game time, and keep plenty of safe, active alternatives readily available.* Your children may complain, but in reality they'll be happier playing with you or their friends than staring at the tube. Many parents prohibit TV altogether on weekdays and allow up to four hours on weekends. Others set a daily limit of one to two hours. If you can't seem to get it under control, try unplugging the TV during strategic hours. Or put it in your bedroom so you have more control over it. If all else fails, put the set into storage for a few weeks and see what happens when everyone goes "cold turkey."
- Make play dates for your children. Kids tend to be much more physically active in pairs or groups than they are alone. But children do not often take the initiative in lining up playmates, so you need to help. Get to know your children's friends and encourage dates

LFP Family Fitness Guide   *(con't.)*

with those who enjoy active play (as opposed to watching TV or playing video games).

- Introduce your kids to a wide variety of sports. If you have a regular workout routine, say running or swimming, encourage your child to exercise with you. If you played a sport as a child but have not practiced since, use your child as an excuse to get back in — now as a coach as well as a player. If there's a sport you always wanted to try, learn it now along with your child.
- Sign your child up for team sports. The benefits of team games go well beyond physical fitness. Kids on teams learn to work within a structure of rules and to cooperate toward a common goal. It's also a great way for them to make friends.
- Check the exercise schedule of any camp or after-school program you are considering for your child. Make sure the program offers ample opportunity for kids to play organized athletic games and to develop new physical skills. Look into sports camps and clinics as an alternative to traditional day camps.
- Plan active family vacations. Go hiking or camping or skiing. Vacation at the beach. Bring or rent bicycles so that you can explore the area you're visiting by bike.
- Restrain yourself from pouncing when you feel the urge to criticize your child's habits; instead look for constructive ways to change behavior. (This applies to your own habits and behavior as well!)
- Do set reasonable limits to improve your child's eating habits and encourage exercise. It shows them that you care about them!
- Look for opportunities to praise your child when they are eating well or making the effort to exercise, and never take credit away from your child.
- Pay attention to significant changes in your child's eating or activity level. Help him/her to confront and work through any problems that might be causing these changes, and not to hold feelings inside.

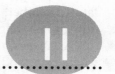

Special Challenges

There are times when you really want to eat light and lean, when you truly *intend* to observe the principles of good nutrition, but somehow your intentions fail you. Other times your intentions remain strong, but you honestly cannot find anything to eat that isn't loaded with fat. Even before you walk into the party or restaurant, before your vacation starts, you can feel your waist inflating. What to do?

The most important thing is, don't despair! Occasional indulgences are what make life fun. They are necessary, and *they will not make you fat* as long as they truly are occasional. Even if you gain a few pounds during a family holiday, the weight will not stick if you quickly return to routine LFP eating habits.

More difficult situations arise when you really don't want to eat high-fat foods but can find little else. This most often occurs at parties and restaurants or when traveling in areas where fat is the mainstay of local cuisine. It's easy to give in because you're *hungry*. But, while it may not be possible to eat as lean as you'd like, there are strategies that allow you to compromise.

Parties

Whether you're host or guest, parties tend to be high-fat situations. Just as most of us equate snack foods with fattening foods, so we associate social gatherings with high-fat "party food." But, in the first place, there is no necessary link between food and social fun. In the

257

second place, the food served at parties doesn't have to be loaded with fat. Remember, most of the people attending any party are trying to hold down their weight.

As always, the rule of thumb is balance. If you're a guest at an event where rich food is served, take a modest helping of high-fat selections if you desire, but try to fill out your plate, according to the 80-20 rule, with leaner choices. If there are no lean choices, wait to go through the buffet line until most others have been served. That way, many of the most tempting choices will be gone, and you'll just be starting when others are already on their second helpings. Take your modest helping of those rich foods and then steer clear of the buffet table. Talk, mingle, dance if that's an option. In short, concentrate on having a good time without stuffing yourself.

Potluck gatherings give you a wonderful opportunity to show off low-fat recipes that you enjoy. Not only does this ensure that you'll have something you want to eat at the party but you'll find that many others also will appreciate the option.

When you're hosting a party, of course, you have maximum control. You can choose not only what is available for your guests to eat but what they'll be doing when they're not eating. You may choose to host a party where there's nothing to eat at all; if the alternatives are entertaining enough, nobody's going to mind.

Here, then, are a few entertainment ideas that deemphasize food:

- Beach or pool parties
- Skating outings
- Group hikes and camping weekends
- Dance parties
- "Social sports" instead of meals: tennis, golf, skiing, racquetball, jogging
- Group excursions: museums, theater, concerts, opera, jazz clubs, lectures

Assuming you do wish to provide your guests with some festive fare, you can start with the basic snack foods you normally eat yourself: pretzels, crackers, low-fat cheeses, sliced fruit and vegetables, baked chips, and low-fat dips. Here are a few more specific suggestions. (Also see Chapter 7 for some great recipes.)

Brunch or midday open house: fresh bagels and low-fat cream cheese and preserves, a medley of fruit, low-fat muffins, cold plate of sliced turkey, chicken breast, and lean ham or Canadian bacon.

Cocktail party: Light cheeses, low-fat crackers, low-fat dips, assorted raw vegetables, cut-up fresh fruit.

Supper party: Pasta, rice, or bean-based dish with low-fat sauce, baked potatoes with a variety of low-fat toppings, fresh baked breads and rolls, vegetable or fruit salads, lean meat or skinless poultry, frozen ices or fruit desserts.

Eating Out

It's difficult to control food choices when you dine out. Restaurant meals are generally larger and higher in fat than meals cooked at home, plus they contain less carbohydrate, fiber, and other vital nutrients. But there is a lot of variability. How well you're able to stick with your routine low-fat eating habits depends on *where* you eat, *what* you order, and *how often* you eat out.

Surprisingly, recent studies have found that women who maintain the best overall nutrition are not those who eat all meals at home but those who eat about 70 percent of meals at home and 30 percent away. That's great news, because most of us fit into this category! The typical American eats out at least four times a week, with at least one of those meals at a fast-food restaurant.

Even ten years ago, such restaurant habits would have virtually guaranteed a jump in average fat intake. Today, however, many restaurants and chains are offering lower-fat, lower-calorie food choices. Thanks to the efforts of health organizations such as the American Heart Association, many moderate and elite restaurants offer "heart-friendly" dishes marked on the menu with a ♥. When I was compiling *The Low-fat Fast Food and Family Restaurant Guide,* I was pleased to discover that lower-fat options are available at almost all of the nation's top fifty restaurant chains. Furthermore, most of the nation's fast-food restaurants now provide consumers with nutrition information about menu items so they can make an informed selection.

Options for lighter, leaner fare extend from main entrees right down to condiments and desserts. Grilled chicken, reduced-fat burgers, and turkey, chicken, and veggie burgers are common alternatives to the traditional fat-heavy cheeseburger. Less saturated vegetable oils seem destined to replace the animal-based shortenings that used to be standard for deep frying (while this does nothing to reduce fat content, it does lower saturated fatty acids and cholesterol). Most establishments have switched from whole to reduced-fat milk. Low-cal, low-fat salad dressings are on the rise, as are lighter desserts, such as mixed fruit and frozen yogurt.

All this means that it's easier to dine lean if you put your mind to it. But as long as the *average American taste preferences* continue to favor more fattening menu items, most restaurants will continue to emphasize those choices. So, when you eat out, you cannot expect the restaurant to protect you from your old fat habits. It's still a jungle out there, and you have to fend for yourself.

Surviving the Fast Food Jungle

Here are some basic tips.

• Try not to be a dining martyr. It is possible to go to a restaurant and have a lean, balanced meal without making a federal case out of it. You know what I mean. You, too, have probably dined with people who deliberate over the menu as if the fate of the universe hangs on their selection. They argue with the serving person to have their selection tailor-made to their particular diet, then send the dish back when it arrives with a tad too much oil. Meanwhile, everyone else at the table gets hungrier and more annoyed—or wants to flee in embarrassment. Don't let your desire to cut fat ruin the pleasure of dining out. Simply try to make the most sensible selections for yourself from the available choices—and remember that it's the *average* content of your overall diet that really matters, not how much fat you do or don't consume in any single dish.

• Select weight-friendly restaurants if and when you have the choice. You're best off with places that offer a varied menu, with at least a few lean options, and that are willing to make reasonable modifications upon request. The typical "greasy spoon" hamburger stand and "meat and three" restaurants, which generally fry, butter, or cream all meats and vegetables, do not meet the basic weight-friendly criteria. But most of the major fast-food chains, most moderate to expensive restaurants, and many diners and coffee shops *are* starting to cater to lower-fat dining preferences. The chart below lists some of the leaner fare now being offered at fast-food restaurants throughout the country.

Top Fast Food Restaurants with Their Leaner Options

Restaurant	Entree	Fat grams per serving
Arby's	Roast chicken salad (light dressing)	8
	Light Menu sandwiches	10
Baskin Robbins	Fat-free dairy desserts	0
Burger King	BK broiler chicken sandwich (no mayo)	8
	Chunky chicken salad (no dressing)	4
Carl's Jr.	Charbroiler BBQ chicken sandwich	6
	Teriyaki chicken sandwich	6
	Chicken Salad-To-Go (reduced-calorie dressing)	10
Chick-Fil-A	Chargrilled chicken garden salad (light dressing)	3
	Chargrilled chicken deluxe sandwich	5
	Grilled 'n' Lites (2 skewers)	2
Dairy Queen	Strawberry Breeze	1
	Frozen yogurt cone or cup	1
	Grilled chicken fillet sandwich	8
Denny's	Beef barley, chicken noodle, or split pea soup	5

Top Fast Food Restaurants with
Their Leaner Options *(con't.)*

Restaurant	Entree	Fat grams per serving
Denny's *(con't.)*	Grilled chicken entree	4
	Pancakes (2, no butter)	4
Domino's Pizza	Cheese pizza (2 slices)	10
	Veggie Feast (2 slices)	13
Dunkin' Donuts	Apple or blueberry muffin	8
	Bran muffin	9
El Pollo Loco	Beans and rice	2
	Chicken salad, flame broiled (salsa as dressing)	4
	Chicken taco	5
Hardee's	Grilled chicken breast sandwich	9
	Grilled chicken salad (fat-free dressing)	4
	Roast beef or turkey sub (no mayo)	7
Jack in the Box	Chicken fajita pita	8
	Side salad (low-cal dressing)	5
Little Caesar's Pizza	Cheese pizza (2 medium round slices)	10
	Cheese pizza (2 medium square slices)	12
Long John Silver	Light Portion baked fish	5
	Ocean chef salad (seafood sauce)	2

Restaurant	Entree	Fat grams per serving
McDonald's	Chunky chicken salad (light dressing)	6
	Fat-free muffin	0
	McLean Deluxe	10
Pizza Hut	Cheese Thin 'n' Crispy (2 medium slices)	17
Red Lobster	Today's Fresh Catch (5 oz., broiled or grilled)	9
Shoney's	Light baked fish, plain baked potato, green salad (low-cal dressing)	2
Taco Bell	Chicken soft taco	10
	Chicken burrito	12
Wendy's	Chili (small)	6
	Grilled chicken sandwich	7

• Learn to decode restaurant menus. Always note how a food is prepared and sauced. If this information is not on the menu, be sure to ask. In one serving of chicken, for example, a "Full Fat-Cat" choice of preparation and saucing could add dozens of fat grams. It's up to you to practice Sauce Control. (See also the LFP Guide to Ethnic Dining under the Travel section of this chapter.)

Low Fat-Cat choices to seek out:

Baked	Steamed	Roasted
Sautéed	Broiled	Poached
Tomato-based	Primavera	Marinara
Wine sauce	Mushroom sauce	Chili

Full Fat-Cat choices to avoid:

Fried	Deep-fried	Smothered
Alfredo	White sauce	Béarnaise
Béchamel	Creamed	Hollandaise
Au gratin	Cheese sauce	Escalloped
Batter-dipped	Tempura	Breaded
Parmigiana	Pesto	Oil and garlic

• Choose pastas with tomato- or vegetable-based sauces, such as marinara and mushroom, rather than meat- or cream-based sauces. If you want extra protein in your sauce, ask for clams or calamari instead of meatballs.

• Try cheeseless, all-vegetable pizza. If you want to add meat, ask for ham or Canadian bacon instead of pepperoni or sausage (2 grams of fat instead of 10 per ounce). If pizza without the cheese just doesn't seem to you like pizza, you *can* ask the kitchen to "go easy on the cheese."

• Order fat-free salad dressing or else take the dressing "on the side" and use it sparingly. Even if you know the restaurant stocks only "regular" dressings, keep asking and the policy might change. If you'll be dining at a place you're sure does not offer lighter dressing, bring your own from home. There are several commercial brands that come in individual serving packets. (See Salad Bar Survival Guide below for more suggestions.)

Salad Bar Survival Guide

We tend to think of salads as "diet food" because the main ingredients, vegetables, are naturally low in fat and calories. But we also tend to dismiss the high-calorie, high-fat "garnishes" we sprinkle on top of those healthy greens. A salad bar meal can and often does contain more fat and more calories than a steak dinner! Below are the typical Low Fat-Cat salad bar choices that are okay in all-you-can-eat quantities, plus the Full Fat-Cat choices that you should use sparingly, if at all.

Low Fat-Cat Choices	Full Fat-Cat Choices
Lettuce, all kinds	Mayo- or oil-based prepared salads
Hard-boiled egg, whites only	Hard-boiled eggs
Raw green vegetables, undressed	
Shredded carrots or beets	Shredded or grated cheese
Garbanzo, navy, or pinto beans	Sunflower or sesame seeds
Raw mushrooms	Marinated mushrooms
Tomatoes	Olives
Raisins	Chow mein noodles
Croutons	Bacon bits or sesame sticks
Ground pepper	Waldorf salad
Fresh fruit	Regular dressings
Low-fat dressing OR	Ranch, Thousand Island, or blue
Vinegar and a little oil	cheese dressing

• Don't be afraid to modify menu items to "hold the fat." Of course, you can't expect the chef to remove oil from preprepared dishes or significantly alter recipes, but the kitchen should be able and willing to make you a sandwich using mustard instead of mayonnaise, refrain from buttering the bun, or simply leave off cheese or sauce. Remember, a single tablespoon of mayo or a single slice of cheese will add 10 grams of fat! So even if the kitchen can't or won't hold the extras, it may be worth it to remove them yourself before eating.

• Watch the "sides." Traditional side orders tend to be high-fat delicacies such as french fries, potato salad, cole slaw, bacon, and sausages. As a low-fat alternative, try ordering a plain baked potato, green salad, soup, chili, baked beans, sliced tomato, or fruit on the side.

• Take full advantage of the bread basket, but leave the butter alone. Each pat of butter contains between 5 and 10 grams of fat—more fat than in ten plain French rolls! Most breads are naturally low in fat and many are high in fiber; the few that are relatively high in fat include croissants (each with 12 fat grams or more), scones, muffins (excluding the new low- and nonfat varieties), corn bread, coffee cakes, and biscuits.

• Choose broth-based or all-vegetable soups instead of cream or cheese-based soups. Hearty soups such as chili, lentil, black bean, and minestrone can all be low-fat meals in themselves.

• Beware of hidden fat in "diet specials." Many so-called diet plates are leftovers from the era of superprotein diets, which minimized carbohydrates while exalting protein foods that are often high in fat. Consider, for instance, the classic "waist watcher's special": a scoop of regular cottage cheese, a ground beef patty, and a hard-boiled egg. That's at least 35 grams of fat! You'd be much better off with a "nondiet" bowl of pasta or a turkey sandwich.

• Balance through portion control as a backup to lean selection. Try not to order items that you know will arrive in gargantuan servings. And, especially if your selection is Regular or Full fat-Cat, do not feel obliged to clean your plate. Stop eating when you're satisfied instead of when you feel stuffed. If you're worried about wasting food, doggie bag the leftovers.

• Split your meal with a dining partner. This is an especially good strategy with entrees if the portions served are large or relatively high in fat. Even with smaller, leaner dishes, the split-a-meal policy can allow you and your partner to sample several different courses instead of just ordering an entree apiece. And it cuts the bill!

• Remember the 80-20 rule, and *do* try to balance out any high-fat choices with lean ones. Don't fall into the trap of thinking, "If I'm going to blow it, I might as well blow it big-time." Perfection is not the goal here, but moderation and common sense are.

• Become an active consumer. Ask the restaurants you frequent to add leaner menu items. Compliment them when they do. Write to the headquarters of national chains to let them know you appreciate their efforts to introduce lighter items.

Holidays

Holidays seem designed to add fat to diets and waistlines. First, there are the rich foods we traditionally eat. Then there are all the social gatherings where we tend to eat more than we otherwise would. And finally, for most of us, there's the stress factor: too much to do in too little time, too many people to meet and greet, too many expectations (mostly other people's) to fulfill. With all the extra food at hand, eating becomes a natural way to "take the edge off" holiday stress. Except, of course, that it ultimately adds stress in the form of unwanted pounds.

The solution is not to restrict but to replace the most fattening holiday foods with leaner substitutes. Again, the 80-20 rule is your guide. Using the basic principles you've learned from earlier chapters of this book, you can:

• Take off all removable fat sources, such as poultry skin, visible meat fat, butter, and cream.
• Look for reduced-fat substitutes, now increasingly available on grocery shelves, for holiday "essentials," such as eggnog, cakes, and cookies.
• Follow reduced-fat recipes for the holiday favorites you create in your own kitchen.
• When there is no substitute for the rich thing, eat a modest portion or skip it and have something entirely different that's equally tasty but lean.

To illustrate how these strategies can lower your holiday fat count, I give you two sample menu plans for a festive Christmas or New Year's day.

Traditional Holiday Feast	*Leaner Holiday Feast*
Breakfast	*Breakfast*
Orange juice	Orange juice
Toast	Toast
Butter	Nonfat cream cheese
Jam	Jam
Eggs scrambled with butter	Oatmeal
Coffee with cream	Coffee with milk
Appetizers	*Appetizers*
Potato chips	Pretzels
Sour cream dip	Dip w/ nonfat sour cream
Crackers	Low-fat crackers
Cheese	Raw vegetable salsa
Eggnog	Reduced fat eggnog
Dinner	*Dinner*
Turkey, light and dark w/ skin	Turkey, white, no skin
Gravy	Reduced fat gravy
Stuffing made w/ butter	Fat-free dressing

Traditional Holiday Feast (con't.)	*Leaner Holiday Feast* (con't.)
Dinner (con't.)	*Dinner* (con't.)
Candied yams	Steamed yams
Creamed onions	Steamed green beans
Rolls	Rolls
Sour cream cranberry sauce	Jellied cranberry sauce
Pecan pie w/ whipped cream	Pumpkin pie (leave the crust)
Champagne	Champagne
Coffee w/ cream	Coffee w/ skim milk
Supper	*Supper*
Cream of mushroom soup	Minestrone
Turkey sandwich w/ mayo	Turkey sandwich w/ mustard
Pecan pie	Fresh fruit
Whole milk	Skim milk

Percent of calories from fat:

45%	11%

Travel

Travel can be either fattening or slimming, depending on how and where you go. If you tend toward low-energy vacations, with eating as a primary form of entertainment, you are likely to come home a few pounds heavier. The gain may be even greater if you holiday in an area known for its high-fat cuisine. On the other hand, if you prefer high-energy vacations, such as hiking tours through wilderness areas or walking tours through the world's great cities, you stand a good chance of losing weight on vacation—or at least breaking even. The amount of exercise you get while traveling really can make a tremendous difference.

If weight control is a serious priority, then consider a vacation that focuses on exercise as the primary recreation. This category includes camping, river rafting trips, cycling tours, and most forms of sight-seeing (cruises only if you really do take advantage of those on-board aerobics classes and fitness centers). Should you opt for a highly athletic trip, however, be forewarned that the muscle you acquire en route may outweigh the fat you burn. I have two friends who decided to circle the globe by bicycle. At the outset my friend Jan was excited by the prospect of all the weight she would lose. But Jan was already slim, her husband a good deal bulkier. They set off, riding up to 100 miles a day, camping most nights, and living on local food along the way. By the end of their journey Jan's husband had lost about thirty pounds, but Jan had *gained* a pound or two—all solid muscle. Their bodies had each found their own Personal Best levels. Having proven it in an extremely grueling, if rewarding, way, Jan finally had to make peace with the fact that her ideal weight did not match the ideal of the fashion magazines.

That, of course, is an extreme example. But whatever you do on holiday, you owe it to your mind and your body to stay physically active. Walk as much as possible. Play tennis or walk the golf course. Rent a bicycle instead of sight-seeing by car. If a pool or beach is available, really swim (don't just float or wade) for at least half an hour a day. Get out on the dance floor at night. Take starlight strolls. With full days at your discretion, you have more time to exercise (and fewer good excuses not to!) while vacationing than you would at home.

Dining when traveling may be a more difficult issue. If you're camping or going by car, of course, you have much more control because you can bring along your own (lean) food and prepare at least some of your meals yourself. When traveling by air, do take advantage of the special meals most airlines offer. For no extra charge, you can either order a low-fat meal or select a particular menu option, such as a fruit or seafood plate. Ask about these options when you make your reservations, either through your travel agent or the airline ticket agent. Ordinarily, special meals must be ordered at least forty-eight hours in advance.

When dining out during an overseas trip, you need to use strategy to maintain the 80-20 rule. The same tips I suggested for American restaurants, of course, apply here as well. But when a cuisine is unfamiliar, it's sometimes hard to tell how a dish is prepared or even what the ingredients are. Eating regional or ethnic cuisine always involves a certain amount of blind faith. That's what makes it exciting. But in order to keep that faith from ending up as fat, remember the following:

• Most cuisines include some form of low-fat carbohydrate as a staple. Steamed rice. Bread. Cooked grains. Potatoes. If in doubt about the rest of the meal, rely on these basic starches in their most naked—least fried—condition.

• In most parts of the world, high-fat meat is considered a delicacy to be served on its own. Leaner meats are generally sliced into dishes with vegetables and starches. So as a rule, you're better off ordering mixed dishes than a straight cut of meat.

• Many cultures rely heavily on beans and legumes as a source of protein. Beans and legumes, you'll recall, are high in carbohydrates as well as protein, but low in fats. Even when these dishes are prepared with oil, they tend to be leaner than dishes with meat.

• Take advantage of local seafood when traveling in coastal regions. Again, try to order it in its freshest and purest (least fried) form.

LFP Guide to Ethnic Dining

Italian

Better Choices (Low or Regular Fat-Cats)
Minestrone, consommé with pastina, cioppino (seafood soup)
Pasta with marinara, pizzaiola, pomodoro, clam, or calamari sauces
Scampi al vino blanco (in wine sauce)
Chicken piccata or cacciatore (remove the skin before eating)
Veal piccata
Italian ices

Occasional Choices (Full Fat-Cats)
Antipasto
Italian sausage
Pasta Alfredo or pesto
Baked and meat pastas: lasagna, manicotti, cannelloni
Eggplant or veal parmigiana
Tira misu, cheesecake

French

Better Choices (Low or Regular Fat-Cats)
Clear soups
Bouillabaise (fish stew); poached quenelles (steamed fish dumplings)
Coq au vin (chicken in wine); pot au feu (stewed chicken)
Chicken or fish en papillote (steamed inside paper)
Ratatouille (mixed vegetables in tomato sauce)
Sorbet; fruit in wine

Occasional Choices (Full Fat-Cats)
Vichyssoise
Rich sauces: hollandaise, béchamel, béarnaise, beurre blanc, velouté,
Mornay, au gratin
Cassoulet (meat and bean casserole)
Poultry or fish en croute (in pastry shell)
Pastries; quiche

Mexican

Better Choices (Low or Regular Fat-Cats)
Salsas
Black bean soup; gazpacho; chili con carne
Ceviche (seafood cocktail)
Tostada (without sour cream or guacamole; leave aside the pastry shell)
Soft tacos; chicken or seafood burritos; enchiladas
Tortillas; black beans; Mexican rice
Arroz con pollo (chicken and rice)
Camarones de hacha (shrimp in tomato sauce); seafood vera cruz
(with vegetables and tomato sauce)
Fruit

Occasional Choices (Full Fat-Cats)
Sour cream; guacamole; tortilla chips
Chile relleno (chile stuffed with cheese)
Chimichangas (deep fried)

Chinese

Better Choices (Low to Regular Fat-Cats)
Won ton, egg drop, hot and sour soups
Steamed or roasted chicken
Steamed dumplings
"Drunken chicken" (Chicken in wine sauce)
Steamed rice
Moo goo gai pan; moo shu chicken; shrimp or chicken with snow peas
or black beans
Lychee; mandarin oranges

Occasional Choices (Full Fat-Cats)
"Crispy" dishes (deep fried)
Sweet and sour dishes

LFP Guide to Ethnic Dining *(con't.)*

Chinese *(con't.)*

Occasional Choices (con't.)
Crispy duck
Spareribs
Pork dishes
Egg foo young
Chow mein
Fried rice

Japanese

Better Choices (Low to Regular Fat-Cats)
Miso soup
Sushi; sashimi
Steamed rice
Teriyaki chicken or beef

Occasional Choices (Full Fat-Cats)
Fried bean curd
Tempura
Agemono and katsu dishes

Thai

Better Choices (Low to Regular Fat-Cats)
Hot and sour soups
Satay (roasted chicken or beef on skewer)
Curries
Pad ka nah (vegetables and noodle in oyster sauce)

Occasional Choices (Full Fat-Cats)
Mee krob (deep fried sweet noodles)
Peanut and coconut sauces
Pad thai (fried noodles)
Fried rice

Indian/Pakistani

Better Choices (Low to Regular Fat-Cats)
Mulligatawny or lentil soup
Chapati (unleavened) and nan (leavened) breads, not fried
Curries
Plain rice

Vegetables masala (with spices)
Tandoori chicken (marinated and baked)

Occasional Choices (Full Fat-Cats)
Fried breads
Coconut soup
Lamb vindaloo (in spicy sauce)

Greek/Middle Eastern
Better Choices (Low to Regular Fat-Cats)
Yogurt and cucumber soup
Pita bread
Shish kebab
Stifado (beef in red wine)
Souvlaki (marinated, roasted chicken or meat)

Occasional Choices (Full Fat-Cats)
Moussaka (baked meat and eggplant with béchamel)
Pastitsio (baked meat and pasta)
Falafel (deep fried chickpea dumplings)
Baklava (puff pastry, nuts, honey)

The LFP Handbook

I'd like this final section to serve as a quick-reference guide recapping key points made in earlier chapters. As I have said all along, you are not likely to achieve your Personal Best body solely by adjusting your eating or solely through exercise. And you probably won't feel satisfied with your body if the rest of your life is a mess. Getting comfortable with your weight is a "whole life" enterprise that encompasses your body, mind, and spirit. So let's take the different phases of this enterprise one by one.

Living Thin

We all confront certain "high-fat-risk" situations in our daily lives. In these situations we eat more than we should or make unwise food choices or exercise less than we should. If these situations crop up only occasionally, this poses no real problem. Remember, it's the amount of fat we eat *on average* and our *overall* activity level that makes the difference, not the eating we do at any single meal or the lack of activity on any single day. It is not necessary to be "perfect" in order to be lean and healthy. However, when it feels as if every day is filled with "high-risk" challenges, then it's important to take preventive measures.

Anticipating these situations and developing strategies to handle them is the first line of defense in thinking thin and staying lean. Here, then, are the forces that most commonly undermine our good intentions.

Negative emotions. When you feel angry, depressed, frustrated, bored, or anxious, or if you're under a great deal of stress, you may eat without paying attention to what or how much you consume and without attempting any control. You are eating not to satisfy hunger but to fill up the empty space around the negative emotion. This is why it is so important to develop coping strategies—problem-solving skills—that a) enable you to externalize your problems and deal with them constructively, and/or b) prompt you to identify the underlying emotions that trigger the urge to eat, and then deal with them through positive, nonfattening activities. Here, for example, are some of the alternatives my weight management groups have found for dealing with problem emotions without eating: a high-energy aerobic workout to vent frustration and anger and reduce stress after a tough day at work; an engrossing novel, a trip through old photo albums, or a leisurely bike ride to satisfy the desire for escape; a hot bubble bath complete with candles or a midday nap under a soft down comforter to satisfy the need for soothing or nurturing. If you have good coping skills you can tell when your problems grow too large for you to handle on your own. You'll acknowledge them and get help to find effective solutions instead of letting your frustration and anxiety fester. You may seek the assistance you need through friends, family, or professional counseling, but you will understand that the answers you need do not lie in ice cream or cookies. This is not to say that you won't still *choose* to eat more when you're distressed—even as you go about the business of confronting your problems. Let's face it, food provides a unique outlet that is immediate, gratifying, sensual, and comforting. So when in need, eat if it helps, but train yourself to reach for lower-fat foods. Even if emotional eating leads to overeating, an excess of low-fat foods will have dramatically less impact on your figure than an excess of high-fat foods!

Social situations. Parties, business meals, family gatherings, and vacation or business travel tend to invite high-fat and irregular eating. You may feel you are expected to eat. You may be overwhelmed by an array of tempting foods. Or you may eat to cover your anxiety in these situations. If you have few of these occasions, then my best advice is to enjoy yourself. Whether you take pleasure in conversation or from the buffet table, the effect on your waistline will be minimal. If, on the other hand, your lifestyle involves a lot of traveling, entertaining, or being entertained, then you will need to develop some strategies for moderation. This means familiarizing yourself with the fat content of foods you typically encounter, and avoiding the highest-fat items. If you are the host, you can build your menu around leaner fare. The key is to work with the situation rather than against it. Total abstinence is not required, and you don't have to make yourself a party martyr!

Tempting fate. Millions of dieters every year act as if, after a diet, they have gone through some magic "cure" and can resume their high-fat, low-exercise lifestyles without putting back their lost pounds. Some do this consciously, "just to see" if they can get away with their former bad habits. Others really believe that weight can be treated like a sickness and, once cured of the extra pounds by a month of stringent dieting and exercise, they can return to life "as usual." They go back to restaurants that serve high-fat dishes. They make excuses to avoid exercising. And they regain the weight. Unfortunately, the surest sign that you need to make permanent changes in your eating and exercise habits is the fact that you've gained unwanted weight in the first place. Once your body has shown that it can gain above a certain level, you have due warning that you won't get away with tempting fate.

Note that these issues are not directly "about" eating or dieting but have to do with the way we feel about ourselves and others and the way we orient our lives. Likewise, the strategies that are most essential in combating "fat risk" have more to do with the way we think and live than what combination of foods we eat.

Physical activity is a vital part of weight loss, weight management, health management, and mental health. In my experience, people who choose not to make time for physical activity on a *consistent* basis rarely if ever succeed in maintaining their desired best weight. If you're serious about losing fat and keeping it off, you must make physical movement a priority. It's like learning a foreign language or an instrument: you have to work at it for a long time before the results are meaningful, and continue working at it regularly to maintain those results. Besides, there is no *good* excuse for not exercising. Most of us can afford half an hour to an hour four times a week for an "official" workout. And "unofficial" but nonetheless effective Lifestyle Exercise can be folded almost invisibly into every single day if you walk whenever possible instead of riding, and avoid labor-saving shortcuts.

Social support from family and friends can help motivate and reinforce your determination to change your eating and exercise habits for the better and sustain those changes. The recommendations in this book are intended not only to help you lose weight but also to improve your health and outlook in general. Your family and friends will be doing themselves a favor if they, too, eat healthier, lower-fat foods and join you in regular physical activity. And their company will help you maintain your new health habits.

Personal motivation is critical to your long-term success. As mentioned in Chapter 1, people give many different reasons for wanting to lose weight, but the only motivation that will ultimately push you to your goal is the belief that you can succeed *for yourself.* Not for your husband, not to prove something to your mother, and not because the dress hanging in your closet is a size too small. If you are to keep these five pounds off for good, you must genuinely believe that you feel better, physically and mentally, at the lower weight. And you must decide that this good feeling is worth more to you than the deep-fried foods and high-fat snacks you have traded for leaner fare. It's encouraging to note that of the more than 80 percent of Americans who regularly use reduced-fat or low-calorie foods, less than a third are dieters; the vast majority use the "light" products with an end goal of improving their health rather than simply losing weight.

A positive attitude means not only believing in your ability to hold your weight down but also recognizing and appreciating the changes that occur as you become leaner. The numbers on the scale are external and ultimately meaningless, but having more energy, lowering your blood pressure, and feeling relaxed in clothes that used to be too tight are *tangible* rewards. If you savor these rewards and take pride in what you have already accomplished, you are far more likely to keep your weight in check than if you constantly berate yourself for the pounds you have yet to lose.

Consistency means making a *permanent* commitment to your health and your goal of leaner living. There is no such thing as a quick fix for weight loss. You cannot stay lean if you slip back into your old habits or if you tilt the 80-20 rule to mean 80 percent fat and 20 percent lean! You need to adopt an active, low-fat lifestyle as your norm and maintain it from now on.

Cooking Thin

The bottom line in cooking thin is to use as little added fat as possible and substitute low-fat products for their high-fat equivalents whenever you can. Beyond that, strive for high-carbohydrate, high-fiber, and diverse menus.

- Use the Fat Master Food Guide at the end of this book to plan menus and fill out your grocery list according to the 80-20 rule (80 percent Low Fat-Cat foods; 20 percent Regular and Full Fat-Cat foods).
- Read nutritional labels and check fat content before selecting packaged food. Emphasize foods with fewer than 3 fat grams per serving.
- Don't put high-fat foods on your weekly shopping list and don't keep them in your house all the time.
- Do stock low-fat foods and fat replacements.
- Cook with nonstick cookware and utensils.
- Bake, broil, steam, or poach instead of frying or sautéing meats and vegetables.
- Remove poultry skin and visible fat from meat before cooking.
- Use nonfat milk and low-fat dairy products instead of the higher-fat versions.
- Use minimal added fats such as butter and oil. If you must use oil, choose an unsaturated vegetable oil such as olive or canola oil.
- Modify favorite recipes to lower the fat content.

Eating Thin

The basic policies for eating thin mirror those for cooking thin: low-fat, high-carbohydrate, high-fiber, and variety of food groups. If in doubt, refer to the Food Guide Pyramid.

- Follow the 80-20 rule every day—even when dining out.
- You don't have to count fat grams, but *do* use the Fat Master Food Guide in this book to familiarize yourself with the general fat content of the foods you encounter most often. Maximize your consumption of Low Fat-Cat choices by experimenting with different types of leaner foods.
- Eat from a variety of food groups according to the U.S.D.A. Food Guide Pyramid (p. 108).
- Emphasize high-fiber foods (grains, fruit, vegetables).
- Eat fruit and cereal or low-fat bread products, such as pretzels or bagels, instead of high-fat snack foods. Surround yourself with these leaner snacks.
- Eat whenever you're hungry.
- Eat slowly. Savor each bite. You'll need fewer bites to feel satisfied.

Moving Thin

Motion is vital for the maintenance of a lean body. You need to *move* throughout the day, not just during isolated workouts. You don't have to be an Olympic athlete. Just think of yourself as an everyday athlete whose "sport" is walking, stretching, reaching, and lifting your own body through space. Your reward, more precious than a medal, will be fitness and improved health.

- Integrate movement into your everyday life by finding ways to *add* physical "labor" to ordinary tasks instead of relying on labor-saving devices.
- Exercise at *least* every other day for at *least* one half hour. Schedule these sessions and hold to your schedule.
- Take advantage of the benefits of cross-training by practicing several different types of activities, such as walking, biking, swimming, or weight training.
- Take up a nonfood hobby such as gardening or jogging to reduce stress and occupy aimless moments.

LFP Fat Loss Laws to Live By

- Lower fat means a leaner body: experiment with low-fat foods to develop leaner taste preferences.
- Pace your progress: losing slowly reduces the chance of regain.
- Stop the gain: stabilizing your weight is the first critical step toward fat loss.
- Gradually increase exercise for long-term results, not short-term goals: pushing yourself too hard will cause you to burn out and give up.
- Perfection is a fool's goal: don't punish yourself for minor slips.
- Redefine your terms of success: it's what you eat, how you feel, and how you look—not what you weigh—that counts.
- Food for fuel, not therapy: personal problems demand solutions, not eating binges.
- Destress: reward and relax yourself by doing things you enjoy instead of eating things you enjoy—and later regret.
- Healthy habits and healthy choices: live right instead of living by the numbers (calories, fat grams, pound counting)!

It's a myth that fitness requires sacrifice. It's a fact that losing weight and keeping it off is your reward for feeling *good*. Fitness is what happens when you take charge of your eating and activity habits. You become responsible for your body. You adopt the practices that make you healthier, happier, more active—and leaner. Once you incorporate these practices into your normal, everyday way of life, you can't help but succeed in losing those last five pounds—and leaving them for good.

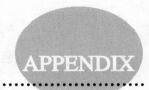

APPENDIX

The Fat Master Food Guide

On the pages that follow you will find a breakdown of over 1,600 foods by Fat-Cat or fat category. I've divided a wide sampling of food items into 1) Low Fat-Cat (3 grams or less of fat per serving); 2) Regular Fat-Cat (between 3 and 7 grams of fat per serving); and 3) Full Fat-Cats (more than 7 grams of fat per serving). Foods that meet the criteria for each section are listed alphabetically within each category according to groups of foods (beverages, breads, cereals, cheeses, etc.). Serving sizes are included followed by total grams of fat, calories, grams of fiber, and milligrams of sodium. I include these numbers for your information and reference, not necessarily for daily counts!

As discussed earlier, at least 80 percent of your daily food choices should come from the Low Fat-Cat, with the remaining 20 percent being made up of selections from the Regular Fat-Cat and occasionally from the Full Fat-Cat. In practical terms, consider that the average woman makes about thirty individual food choices each day—twenty-four (or 80 percent of these choices should come from the Low Fat-Cat, with as many as six (20 percent) from the higher-fat categories. In other words, *most* of your daily food choices should be foods that are low in total fat. And nicely enough, you'll see that most breads, grains, pasta, rice, fruits, vegetables, beans, low-fat dairy products, and lean meats *are* low in fat. In addition, there are literally hundreds (probably thousands!) of low-fat packaged foods on the market today—with no- or reduced-fat alternatives to almost every type of food you can imagine. So, eating by the 80-20 rule certainly doesn't limit your options!

In using the Fat Master Food Guide consider the following:

• This was devised to allow you to achieve a low-fat diet without having to count fat grams. By emphasizing low-fat foods 80 percent of the time, this goal can easily be achieved.

• Make use of food label information to make a quick translation into Fat-Cats. Remember, if it contains less than 3 grams it falls into the Low Fat-Cat and into the Regular Fat-Cat if it's between 3 and 7 grams. Foods that contain more than 7 grams of fat per serving (for an individual food) are classed for LFP purposes as Full Fat-Cat.

• Notice the wide range of fat grams in the Full Fat-Cat. Some foods contain just a few grams over the 7 gram cutoff, while others contain 30, 40, even 50 or more grams of fat. I advise you to look over the list and take note of where some of your typical selections fall.

• The foods are grouped into fat content categories according to the portion sizes listed. If you eat several servings of a Low Fat-Cat food that contains for example, 2 grams of fat, you've easily moved up into the Regular category and possibly up into the Full Fat-Cat for that food. Likewise, if you have a smaller serving of a Regular category item, it might classify as the low-fat category because the fat grams for the portion you chose are less than 3 grams.

• Don't get too wrapped up in "counting" the number of food selections—just familarize yourself with the listings of low fat items and choose these *most* of the time, reserving the higher fat items as "sometimes" choices.

• The listings contain entries that represent traditional recipes or methods of preparation. Your modifications of a favorite recipe from the Combination Foods section could easily drop its fat content and thus change its Fat-Cat. Just use your best judgment! You will achieve your low-fat goals by focusing on a wide variety of the lowest-fat choices.

• Keep balance and nutrition in mind by following the guidelines set forth in the Food Guide Pyramid (p. 108). It represents a healthful, low-fat way of eating.

• Remember that many foods contain very little or no fat but have significant calories. For example, regular soda has no fat, but it contains about 150 calories per 12-ounce serving. Those calories can certainly add up quickly! Also, those 150 calories provide you with nothing in the way of nutrition. Nutritionists call these "empty calorie" foods. So go easy. Just because a food contains no fat doesn't mean you should consume it in unlimited amounts.

LOW FAT-CAT
(0-3 grams of fat per serving)

	SERVING	TOTAL FAT (g.)	CALORIES	FIBER (g.)	SODIUM (mg.)
BEVERAGES					
apple juice	6 oz.	0	90	0	6
beer*					
regular*	12 oz.	0	148	0	19
light*	12 oz.	0	100	0	10
nonalcoholic	12 oz.	0	90	0	5
carbonated drink					
regular	12 oz.	0	152	0	14
sugar free	12 oz.	0	1	0	8
club soda/seltzer	12 oz.	0	0	0	75
coffee, brewed or instant	8 oz.	0	4	0	4
fruit punch	8 oz.	0	120	0	25
grape juice	6 oz.	0	90	0	12
Kool-Aid, from mix, any flavor	8 oz.	0	95	0	8
lemonade, mix or frozen	8 oz.	0	102	0	13
liquor (gin, rum, vodka, whiskey)*	1 oz.	0	70	0	0
orange juice, unsweetened	6 oz.	0	83	0	2
pineapple juice	6 oz.	0	90	0	8
tea, brewed or instant	8 oz.	0	0	0	3
tonic water	8 oz.	0	90	0	10
wine*					
red or rosé	4 oz.	0	85	0	0
white, dry or medium	4 oz.	0	80	0	5
wine cooler	8 oz.	0	83	0	9
BREADS					
bagel, cinnamon raisin	1 medium	1.5	230	2	274
bagel, plain	1 medium	1.4	180	2	300
Boston brown bread, canned	1/2-in. slice	0.6	85	2	100
bread					
French/Vienna	1 slice	1.0	70	1	138
Italian	1 slice	0.5	78	1	151
mixed grain	1 slice	0.9	70	2	103
multigrain, "light"	1 slice	0.5	45	3	117
pita, plain	1 large	0.8	240	2	430
pita, whole wheat	1 large	1.2	236	7	510

*Although alcohol contains no fat, scientific evidence suggests that it may facilitate fat storage and hamper your weight loss efforts. Excessive alcohol intake is detrimental to your health. Use discretion when consuming alcoholic beverages.

(con't.)	SERVING	TOTAL FAT (g.)	CALORIES	FIBER (g.)	SODIUM (mg.)
BREADS					
raisin	1 slice	1.0	70	1	94
rye, pumpernickel	1 slice	0.8	82	2	173
sourdough	1 slice	0.8	68	1	140
wheat	1 slice	1.1	75	1	151
wheat, "light"	1 slice	0.5	45	3	118
white	1 slice	0.9	70	0	136
white, "light"	1 slice	0.5	42	2	91
whole wheat	1 slice	1.2	80	2	180
breadcrumbs	1/2 cup	2.3	196	2	368
breadsticks					
plain	1 small	0.2	23	0	70
crackers					
graham	2 squares	1.3	60	0	66
matzos	1 board	0.9	115	0	75
melba toast	1 piece	0.2	15	0	12
Norwegian flatbread	2 thin	0.3	40	0	32
oyster	33 crackers	0.3	120	0	250
Ryekrisp, plain	2 crackers	0.2	50	0	100
saltines	2 crackers	0.6	26	0	80
soda	5 crackers	1.6	42	0	156
Uneeda	2 crackers	1.0	42	0	67
Wasa crispboard	1 piece	1.0	45	0	50
zwieback	2 crackers	0.7	40	0	20
crêpe	1 medium	1.5	48	0	130
croutons, commercial	1/4 cup	1.9	44	1	115
dumpling, plain	1 medium	1.1	42	0	105
English muffin	1	1.1	135	1	291
flour					
rye, medium	1 cup	1.5	308	13	1
white, all-purpose	1 cup	1.2	418	4	2
white, self-rising	1 cup	1.2	436	4	1,290
whole wheat	1 cup	2.4	399	11	4
French toast made w/ egg substitute	1 slice	3.0	85	1	200
muffins, reduced-fat varieties	1 medium	3.0	110	1	180
pancakes					
"light" from mix	3 medium	2.0	130	5	570
whole wheat, from mix	3 medium	3.0	180	6	410
phyllo dough	2 oz.	3.0	165	1	270

	SERVING	TOTAL FAT (g.)	CALORIES	FIBER (g.)	SODIUM (mg.)
rolls					
brown and serve	1	2.2	100	0	200
French	1	0.4	137	1	287
hamburger	1	3.0	180	1	304
hard	1	1.2	115	1	231
hot dog	1	2.1	116	1	241
kaiser/hoagie	1 medium	1.6	156	1	312
pan type	1 small	1.0	80	0	140
Parker House	1	2.1	59	0	100
raisin	1 large	1.7	165	1	235
rye	1	1.0	79	2	235
sandwich	1	3.0	162	1	312
sourdough	1	1.0	100	1	235
submarine	1 medium	3.0	290	2	580
wheat	1	1.7	52	1	130
white	1	3.0	110	0	175
whole wheat	1	1.1	85	3	184
soft pretzel	1 medium	1.7	190	1	770
tortilla					
corn (unfried)	1 medium	0.8	48	1	38
flour	1 medium	2.5	59	1	63
waffle, frozen	1 medium	2.6	95	1	235
CANDY					
candied fruit					
apricot	1 oz.	0.1	94	1	5
cherry	1 oz.	0.1	96	1	5
citrus peel	1 oz.	0.1	90	1	5
figs	1 oz.	0.1	84	2	5
fondant	1 piece	0.2	116	0	52
Good & Plenty	1 oz.	0.1	106	0	10
gumdrops	28 pieces	0.2	97	0	15
gummy bears	1 oz.	0.1	110	0	13
hard candy	6 pieces	0.3	108	0	9
jelly beans	1 oz.	0	104	0	3
licorice	1 oz.	0.1	35	0	10
Life Savers	5 pieces	0.1	39	0	1
marshmallow	1 large	0	25	0	0
mints	14 pieces	0.6	104	0	10
sour balls	1 oz.	0	110	0	15
Sugar Daddy caramel	1.4 oz.	1.0	150	0	85

(con't.)	SERVING	TOTAL FAT (g.)	CALORIES	FIBER (g.)	SODIUM (mg.)
CANDY					
taffy	1 oz.	1.5	99	0	131
Tootsie Roll pop	1 oz.	0.6	110	0	1
Tootsie Roll	1 oz.	3.0	112	1	56
CEREALS					
All Bran	3/4 cup	1.1	159	19	719
Alpha-Bits	1 cup	0.6	111	1	170
Apple Jacks	1 cup	0.1	110	1	200
Bran, 100%	1/2 cup	1.9	84	9	189
bran, unprocessed, dry	1/4 cup	0.6	29	6	1
Bran Buds	1/3 cup	0.7	72	10	172
Bran Chex	1 cup	1.2	136	9	448
Bran Flakes, 40%	1 cup	0.7	127	6	303
Cheerios	1 cup	1.6	90	2	233
Cocoa Krispies	1 cup	0.5	140	0	275
Corn Chex	1 cup	0.1	111	1	271
cornflakes	1 cup	0.1	108	1	279
corn grits w/o added fat	1/2 cup	0.5	71	1	0
Cream of Wheat w/o added fat	1/2 cup	0.3	67	0	3
Crispix	1 cup	0	110	1	220
Fiber One	1 cup	2.2	128	21	463
Frosted Bran, Kellogg's	2/3 cup	0	100	3	190
Frosted Mini-Wheats	4 biscuits	0.3	102	1	8
Fruit Loops	1 cup	0	111	1	200
fruit squares, Kellogg's	1/2 cup	0	90	2	5
Golden Grahams	3/4 cup	1.1	109	1	178
Grapenut Flakes	1 cup	0.4	116	2	158
Grapenuts	1/4 cup	0.2	104	2	188
Honeynut Cheerios	3/4 cup	0.7	107	1	250
Kix	1 1/2 cup	0.7	110	0	290
Life, plain or cinnamon	1 cup	2.6	162	4	241
Mueslix, Kellogg's	1/2 cup	1.0	140	4	94
Nutri-Grain, Kellogg's					
almond raisin	2/3 cup	2.0	140	3	220
raisin bran	1 cup	1.0	130	5	200
wheat	2/3 cup	0.3	90	3	170
oat bran, cooked cereal w/o added fat	1/2 cup	1.2	55	2	256
oat bran, dry	1/4 cup	1.6	82	3	1

	SERVING	TOTAL FAT (g.)	CALORIES	FIBER (g.)	SODIUM (mg.)
oats					
instant	1 packet	1.7	108	1	105
w/o added fat	1/2 cup	1.2	72	1	1
Product 19	1 cup	0.2	108	1	325
puffed rice	1 cup	0	56	0	0
puffed wheat	1 cup	0.1	44	1	1
Raisin Bran	1 cup	0.8	156	5	296
Rice Chex	1 cup	0.1	111	1	271
Rice Krispies	1 cup	0.2	110	0	291
shredded wheat	1 cup	0.5	85	2	3
Special K	1 cup	0.1	111	0	265
Sugar Frosted Flakes	1 cup	0	147	1	267
Sugar Smacks	3/4 cup	0.5	106	1	70
Team	1 cup	0.5	111	1	175
Total	1 cup	0.7	100	2	280
Wheat Chex	1 cup	1.2	169	6	308
Wheaties	1 cup	0.5	99	2	270
whole wheat, natural, w/o added fat	1/2 cup	0.7	71	2	10
CHEESES					
Alpine Lace, Free 'n' Lean	1 oz.	0	35	0	290
American					
fat free	1 oz.	<0.5	40	0	400
reduced calorie	1 oz.	2.2	50	0	400
Borden's Fat Free	1 oz.	<0.5	40	0	380
Borden's Lite Line	1 oz.	2.0	50	0	420
cottage cheese					
1 % fat	1/2 cup	1.2	82	0	459
2 % fat	1/2 cup	2.2	101	0	459
cream cheese, fat-free varieties	1 oz. (2 T)	0	25	0	390
Healthy Choice fat-free	1 oz.	0	30	0	390
Kraft Free Singles	1 oz.	0	45	0	430
Parmesan, Weight Watchers Fat Free	1 T	1.5	14	0	60
ricotta, "light" reduced-fat	1/4 cup	2.0	55	0	65
Weight Watchers, slices	1 oz.	2.0	50	0	400
COMBINATION FOODS					
baked beans w/ pork	1/2 cup	1.5	100	4	425
baked beans, vegetarian style	1/2 cup	0.5	85	4	390
burrito, bean w/o cheese	1 large	2.8	142	4	510

(con't.) COMBINATION FOODS	SERVING	TOTAL FAT (g.)	CALORIES	FIBER (g.)	SODIUM (mg.)
chicken salad, white meat w/ fat-free mayo	1/2 cup	3.0	100	0	270
chow mein, canned	1 cup	2.3	70	2	850
spaghetti w/tomato sauce	1 cup	1.5	179	2	910
sushi w/fish and vegetables	5 oz.	1.0	210	1	250
tuna salad w/fat-free mayo	1/2 cup	2.0	80	0	120
DESSERTS AND TOPPINGS					
brownie, choc., "light," from mix	1/24 pkg.	2.0	100	0	80
cake					
angel food	1/12 cake	0.2	161	0	161
gingerbread	2 1/2" slice	2.9	267	0	225
pound, Entenmann fat-free	1-oz. slice	0	70	0	100
cookie					
arrowroot	1	0.9	24	0	28
Entenmann's fat-free	2	0	75	0	115
fat-free Newtons	1	0	70	0	95
fig bar	1	0.9	56	1	40
Health Valley fat-free	3	0	75	2	40
frosting/icing, seven-minute	3 T	0	135	0	25
fruit ice, Italian	1/2 cup	0	123	0	0
Fudgesicle	1 bar	0.4	196	1	248
gelatin					
low-calorie	1/2 cup	0	8	0	4
regular, sweetened	1/2	0	70	0	50
Hostess					
cupcake lights	1	2.0	130	0	190
light apple spice	1	1.0	130	0	150
light crumb cake	1	1.0	80	0	95
Twinkie lights	1	2.0	110	0	160
ice cream, Weight Watchers	1/2 cup	0.8	81	0	57
ice cream cone (cone only)	1 medium	0.3	45	0	26
ice milk					
soft serve, all flavors	1/2 cup	2.3	112	0	82
strawberry	1/2 cup	2.5	106	0	60
vanilla	1/2 cup	2.8	92	0	60
ladyfinger	1	2.0	79	0	15
Popsicle	1 bar	0	96	0	0

	SERVING	TOTAL FAT (g.)	CALORIES	FIBER (g.)	SODIUM (mg.)
pudding					
from mix w/ skim milk	1/2 cup	0	124	0	125
Pudding Pop, frozen	1	2.0	75	0	80
sherbet	1/2 cup	1.8	135	0	44
Tasty Kake					
butterscotch Krimpet	1	2.1	118	0	94
jelly Krimpet	1	1.3	96	0	88
light creme-filled cupcakes	1	1.4	100	0	115
toppings					
butterscotch/caramel	3 T	0.1	156	0	109
cherry	3 T	0.1	147	0	10
chocolate syrup, Hershey	3 T	0.6	110	1	54
marshmallow creme	3 T	0	158	0	17
pineapple	3 T	0.2	146	0	20
strawberry	3 T	0.1	139	0	10
yogurt, frozen					
nonfat	1/2 cup	0.2	81	0	39
low-fat	1/2 cup	3.0	115	0	55
EGGS					
substitute, frozen	1/4 cup	0	30	0	80
white	1 large	0	16	0	50
FAST FOODS/RESTAURANTS					
Burger King					
side salad w/diet dressing	1	0	42	NA	750
Chick-Fil-A					
Grilled 'n' Lites	2 skewers	1.8	97	NA	NA
Dairy Queen					
Breeze, strawberry	1 regular	1.0	420	NA	170
ice cream cone, regular yogurt	1	<1.0	180	NA	80
yogurt strawberry sundae	1 regular	<1.0	200	NA	80
Hardees					
bagel, plain	1	2.9	200	NA	350
pancakes	1 order	2.0	490	NA	890
side salad	1	<1.0	19	NA	14
Kentucky Fried Chicken					
corn on the cob	1 ear	2.0	90	1	11
mashed potatoes and gravy	1 order	2.0	71	0	339
Ocean chef salad	1	1.0	110	NA	730
McDonald's					
apple bran muffin	1	0	180	NA	200

(con't.)	SERVING	TOTAL FAT (g.)	CALORIES	FIBER (g.)	SODIUM (mg.)
FAST FOODS/RESTAURANTS					
frozen yogurt cone	1	0.8	105	0	80
garden salad					
w/o dressing	1	2.0	50	1	70
shake					
chocolate	1	1.7	320	0	240
strawberry	1	1.3	320	0	170
vanilla	1	1.3	290	0	170
side salad w/o dressing	1	1.0	30	1	35
sundae					
strawberry	1	1.1	210	0	95
Wendy's					
baked potato, plain	1	0	300	4	20
FATS					
Butter Buds, liquid	2 T	0	12	0	170
butter sprinkles	1/2 t	0	4	0	75
cream substitute					
powdered	2 T	1.4	22	0	8
mayonnaise					
fat-free	1 T	0	12	0	150
no-stick spray (Pam, etc.)	2-sec. spray	0.8	8	0	0
sour cream					
fat-free	2 T	0	16	0	20
reduced-fat	2 T	2.6	30	0	30
FISH					
abalone, canned	3 1/2 oz.	0.3	80	0	298
bass					
freshwater	3 1/2 oz.	2.6	104	0	60
saltwater, black	3 1/2 oz.	1.2	93	0	68
saltwater, striped	3 1/2 oz.	2.7	105	0	60
butterfish					
gulf	3 1/2 oz.	2.9	95	0	80
clams					
canned, solids only	3 oz.	2.5	126	0	95
meat only	5 large	0.9	80	0	70
soft, raw	4 large	1.9	63	0	47
cod	3 1/2 oz.	0.3	78	0	60
crab, canned	1/2 cup	2.1	86	0	283
crab, Alaska king	3 1/2 oz.	1.5	96	0	1,062
crappie, white	3 1/2 oz.	0.8	79	0	225

	SERVING	TOTAL FAT (g.)	CALORIES	FIBER (g.)	SODIUM (mg.)
crayfish, freshwater	3 1/2 oz.	0.5	72	0	42
croaker					
Atlantic	3 1/2 oz.	3.0	60	0	50
white	3 1/2 oz.	0.8	84	0	104
cusk, steamed	3 1/2 oz.	0.7	106	0	110
dolphinfish	3 1/2 oz.	0.7	85	0	86
flatfish	3 1/2 oz.	0.8	79	0	69
flounder/sole	3 1/2 oz.	0.5	68	0	56
gefilte fish	3 1/2 oz.	2.2	82	1	155
grouper	3 1/2 oz.	1.3	87	0	53
haddock	3 1/2 oz.	0.6	79	0	58
halibut	3 1/2 oz.	0.6	79	0	50
lobster, northern	3 1/2 oz.	1.9	91	0	325
muskekunge ("muskie," "skie")	3 1/2 oz.	2.5	109	0	75
mussels, meat only	3 1/2 oz.	2.2	95	0	250
ocean perch	3 1/2 oz.	1.2	88	0	70
octopus	3 1/2 oz.	0.8	73	0	NA
oysters					
canned	3 1/2 oz.	2.2	76	0	100
raw	5-8 medium	1.8	66	0	110
perch, freshwater, yellow	3 1/2 oz.	0.9	91	0	58
pickerel	3 1/2 oz.	0.5	84	0	NA
pike					
blue	3 1/2 oz.	0.9	90	0	45
northern	3 1/2 oz.	1.1	88	0	40
walleye	3 1/2 oz.	1.2	93	0	50
pollock, Atlantic	3 1/2 oz.	1.0	91	0	85
red snapper	3 1/2 oz.	1.0	93	0	60
rockfish, oven steamed	3 1/2 oz.	2.5	107	0	70
scallops	3 1/2 oz.	1.2	81	0	140
sea bass, white	3 1/2 oz.	1.5	96	0	65
shrimp					
canned, dry pack	3 1/2 oz.	1.6	116	0	150
canned, wet pack	1/2 cup	0.8	87	0	1,956
raw or boiled	3 1/2 oz.	1.8	91	0	130
sole, fillet	3 1/2 oz.	0.5	68	0	160
squid	3 oz.	1.2	110	0	49
surimi	3 1/2 oz.	0.9	98	0	142
trout, brook	3 1/2 oz.	2.1	101	0	25
tuna					
canned, light in water	3 1/2 oz.	0.8	115	0	336
canned, white in water	3 1/2 oz.	2.4	135	0	389

FRUIT	SERVING	TOTAL FAT (g.)	CALORIES	FIBER (g.)	SODIUM (mg.)
apple					
dried	1/2 cup	0.1	155	5	56
whole w/ peel	1 medium	0.4	81	4	1
applesauce, unsweetened	1/2 cup	0.1	53	2	0
apricots					
dried	5 halves	0.3	83	6	3
fresh	3 medium	0.4	51	2	1
banana	1 medium	0.6	105	2	1
blackberries					
fresh	1 cup	0.5	74	7	0
frozen, unsweetened	1 cup	0.7	97	7	0
blueberries					
fresh	1 cup	0.6	82	5	9
frozen, unsweetened	1 cup	0.7	80	4	1
boysenberries, frozen, unsweetened	1 cup	0.3	66	6	2
breadfruit, fresh	1/4 small	0.2	99	3	2
cantaloupe	1 cup	0.4	57	3	14
cherries					
maraschino	1/4 cup	0.1	56	1	2
sour, canned in heavy syrup	1/2 cup	0.4	116	1	9
sweet	1/2 cup	0.7	49	2	0
cranberry sauce	1/2 cup	0.2	209	1	40
cranberry-orange relish	1/2 cup	0.9	246	3	44
dates, whole, dried	1/2 cup	0.4	228	8	2
figs					
canned	3 figs	0.1	75	9	1
dried, uncooked	10 figs	1.0	477	16	20
fresh	1 medium	0.2	37	2	1
fruit cocktail, canned	1 cup	0.3	112	5	8
fruit roll-up	1	0	50	0	7
grapefruit	1/2 medium	0.1	39	1	0
grapes, Thompson seedless	1/2 cup	0.3	94	1	7
guava, fresh	1 medium	0.5	45	7	2
honeydew melon, fresh	1/4 small	0.3	33	1	12
kiwi, fresh	1 medium	0.3	46	2	4
kumquat, fresh	1 medium	0	12	1	1
lemon, fresh	1 medium	0.2	17	1	1
lime, fresh	1 medium	0.1	20	1	1
mandarin oranges, canned	1/2 cup	0.1	46	4	7
mango, fresh	1 medium	0.6	135	4	4
melon balls, frozen	1 cup	0.4	55	2	53

	SERVING	TOTAL FAT (g.)	CALORIES	FIBER (g.)	SODIUM (mg.)
mixed fruit					
dried	1/2 cup	0.5	243	6	18
frozen, sweetened	1 cup	0.5	245	2	14
nectarine, fresh	1 medium	0.6	67	2	0
orange					
navel, fresh	1 medium	0.2	65	4	1
Valencia, fresh	1 medium	0.4	59	4	0
papaya, fresh	1 medium	0.4	117	3	8
passionfruit, purple, fresh	1 medium	0.1	18	3	5
peach					
canned in heavy syrup	1 cup	0.3	190	4	16
canned in light syrup	1 cup	0.2	136	4	13
fresh	1 medium	0.1	37	1	0
frozen, sweetened	1 cup	0.3	235	4	16
pear					
canned in heavy syrup	1 cup	0.3	188	6	13
canned in light syrup	1 cup	0.1	144	6	13
fresh	1 medium	0.7	98	5	1
persimmon, fresh	1 medium	0.1	32	3	0
pineapple pieces					
canned, unsweetened	1 cup	0.2	150	2	4
fresh	1 cup	0.7	77	3	1
plantain, cooked, sliced	1 cup	0.3	179	1	8
plum					
canned in heavy syrup	1/2 cup	0.1	119	4	26
fresh	1 medium	0.6	36	3	0
pomegranate, fresh	1 medium	0.5	104	2	5
prickly pear, fresh	1 medium	0.5	42	3	6
prunes, dried, cooked	1/2 cup	0.2	113	10	2
raisins					
dark seedless	1/4 cup	0.2	112	3	8
golden seedless	1/4 cup	0.2	113	3	4
raspberries					
fresh	1 cup	0.2	61	6	0
frozen, sweetened	1 cup	0.4	103	12	1
rhubarb, stewed, unsweetened	1 cup	0	12	6	5
star fruit/carambola	1 medium	0.4	42	2	3
strawberries					
fresh	1 cup	0.2	45	3	2
frozen, sweetened	1 cup	0.3	245	3	3
frozen, unsweetened	1 cup	0.2	52	3	8
sugar apples, fresh	1 medium	0.5	146	4	15

(con't.)	SERVING	TOTAL FAT (g.)	CALORIES	FIBER (g.)	SODIUM (mg.)
FRUIT					
tangelo, fresh	1 medium	0.1	39	3	1
tangerine, fresh	1 medium	0.2	37	3	1
watermelon, fresh	1 cup	0.2	50	1	3
FRUIT JUICE AND NECTARS					
apple juice	1 cup	0.3	116	1	7
apricot nectar	1 cup	0.2	141	1	9
carrot juice	1 cup	0.2	96	1	65
cranberry juice cocktail					
low cal	1 cup	0	45	0	0
regular	1 cup	0.1	147	0	3
cranberry-apple juice	1 cup	0.2	129	1	5
grape juice	1 cup	0.2	155	1	7
grapefruit juice	1 cup	0.3	96	0	2
lemon juice	2 T	0	8	0	0
lime juice	2 T	0	8	0	0
orange juice	1 cup	0.5	111	1	2
orange-grapefruit juice	1 cup	0.2	107	1	8
peach juice or nectar	1 cup	0.1	134	1	17
pear juice or nectar	1 cup	0	149	1	9
pineapple juice	1 cup	0.2	139	1	2
pineapple-orange juice	1 cup	0.1	125	1	26
prune juice	1 cup	0.1	181	1	11
tomato juice	1 cup	0.2	41	2	675
V8 juice	1 cup	0.1	53	2	600
GRAVIES, SAUCES, AND DIPS					
au jus, mix	1/2 cup	0.3	24	0	289
barbecue sauce	1 T	0.3	12	0	127
brown gravy					
from mix	1/2 cup	0.1	4	0	66
homemade	1/4 cup	0.1	16	0	156
chicken gravy					
from mix	1/2 cup	0.9	41	0	566
giblet from can	1/4 cup	2.0	35	0	320
chili sauce	1 T	0	16	0	191
home-style gravy					
from mix	1/4 cup	0.5	25	0	374
jalapeño dip	1 oz.	1.1	33	0	120

	SERVING	TOTAL FAT (g.)	CALORIES	FIBER (g.)	SODIUM (mg.)
mushroom gravy, from mix	1/2 cup	0.4	35	0	701
mustard					
brown	1 T	0.9	14	0	200
yellow	1 T	0.7	11	0	194
onion gravy, from mix	1/2 cup	0.3	40	0	518
picante sauce	6 T	0.6	48	1	480
pork gravy, from mix	1/2 cup	0.9	38	0	617
soy sauce	1 T	0	11	0	1,029
soy sauce, reduced sodium	1 T	0	11	0	600
spaghetti sauce					
"healthy"/"light" varieties	1/2 cup	1.0	50	1	350
meatless, jar	1/2 cup	1.0	70	NA	600
mushroom, jar	1/2 cup	2.0	70	NA	500
steak sauce					
A-1	1 T	0	12	0	400
others	1 T	0	18	0	405
sweet and sour sauce	1/4 cup	0.2	131	0	40
Tabasco sauce	1 t	0	1	0	NA
taco sauce	1 T	0	1	0	52
teriyaki sauce	1 T	0	15	0	690
turkey gravy, from mix	1/2 cup	0.9	43	0	749
Worcestershire sauce	1 T	0	12	0	244
MEATS					
miscellaneous meats					
frog legs, cooked w/o fat	4 large	0.3	73	0	82
venison, roasted	3 1/2 oz.	2.5	157	0	54
processed meats					
chicken roll	2 oz.	2.6	60	0	224
hot dogs/franks					
97 percent fat-free varieties	1	1.6	55	0	515
turkey breast	2 oz.	2.8	95	0	174
MILK AND YOGURT					
buttermilk					
1 % fat	1 cup	2.2	99	0	257
dry	1 T	0.4	25	0	103
evaporated skim milk	1/2 cup	0.4	97	0	15
hot cocoa					
low-cal, mix w/ water	1 cup	0.8	50	0	231
w/ skim milk	1 cup	2.0	158	0	135

(con't.)	SERVING	TOTAL FAT (g.)	CALORIES	FIBER (g.)	SODIUM (mg.)
MILK AND YOGURT					
low-fat milk					
1/2 % fat	I cup	1.0	90	0	125
I % fat	I cup	2.6	102	0	123
Ovaltine, w/ I % milk	I cup	2.8	173	0	201
skim milk					
liquid	I cup	0.4	86	0	126
nonfat dry powder	1/4 cup	0.2	109	0	161
yogurt					
coffee/vanilla, low-fat	I cup	2.8	194	0	149
frozen, nonfat	1/2 cup	0.2	81	0	39
fruit-flavored, low-fat	I cup	2.6	225	0	121
plain (nonfat)	I cup	0.4	127	0	174
MISCELLANEOUS					
baking powder	I t	0	3	0	426
baking soda	I t	0	0	0	821
bouillon cube, beef or chicken	I	0.2	8	0	900
chewing gum	I stick	0	10	0	0
gelatin, dry	I pkg.	0	23	0	0
honey	I T	0	64	0	1
horseradish, prepared	I t	0	2	0	7
jam, all varieties	I T	0	54	0	2
jelly, all varieties	I T	0	49	0	3
marmalade, citrus	I T	0	51	0	3
molasses	I T	0	50	0	3
pickle relish					
chow chow	I oz.	0.4	8	0	400
sweet	I T	0.1	21	0	107
pickles					
bread and butter	4 slices	0.1	18	0	202
dill or sour	I large	0.2	11	0	950
Kosher	I oz.	0.1	7	0	350
sweet	I oz.	0.4	146	0	268
salt	I t	0	0	0	2,132
spices/seasonings	I t	0.2	5	0	0
sugar, all varieties	I T	0	46	0	0
sugar substitutes	I packet	0	4	0	0
syrup, all varieties	I T	0	60	0	0
vinegar	I T	0	2	0	0
yeast	I T	0.1	23	0	10

	SERVING	TOTAL FAT (g.)	CALORIES	FIBER (g.)	SODIUM (mg.)
PASTA, NOODLES, AND RICE					
(all measurements after					
cooking unless otherwise noted)					
macaroni					
semolina	1 cup	0.7	159	1	1
whole wheat	1 cup	0.6	183	5	4
noodles					
egg	1 cup	2.4	200	1	3
manicotti	1 cup	0.4	129	1	1
rice	1 cup	0	140	1	0
rice					
brown	1/2 cup	0.6	116	2	0
long grain and wild	1/2 cup	2.1	120	2	530
Spanish style	1/2 cup	2.1	106	1	547
white	1/2 cup	1.2	111	0	0
spaghetti, enriched	1 cup	1.0	159	1	1
POULTRY					
chicken					
breast, w/o skin, roasted	1/2 breast	2.8	142	0	70
gizzard, simmered	2 oz.	2.1	90	0	32
leg, w/o skin, roasted	1 leg	2.5	76	0	42
turkey					
breast					
oven roasted	3 1/2 oz.	2.8	110	0	786
smoked	3 1/2 oz.	2.9	110	0	910
loaf, breast meat	3 1/2 oz.	1.6	110	0	431
SALAD DRESSINGS					
blue cheese					
fat-free	2 T	0	20	0	28
low-cal	2 T	1.6	22	0	34
French					
fat-free	2 T	0	40	0	24
low-cal	2 T	1.8	44	0	25
Italian					
fat-free	2 T	0	12	0	42
low-cal	2 T	3.0	32	0	256
Kraft, free	2 T	0	40	0	240
Kraft, reduced-cal	2 T	2.0	50	0	240
Russian, low-cal	2 T	1.4	46	0	282
sweet and sour	2 T	1.8	58	0	64
Thousand Island, fat free	2 T	0	40	0	270

	SERVING	TOTAL FAT (g.)	CALORIES	FIBER (g.)	SODIUM (mg.)
SNACK FOODS					
Cracker Jack	I oz.	1.0	114	I	85
popcorn					
air-popped	I cup	0.3	23	I	0
microwave, "light"	I cup	1.0	25	I	35
pretzels	I oz.	1.0	110	0	451
rice cakes	I piece	0.3	35	0	10
tortilla chips, no oil, baked	I oz.	1.4	110	0	120
SOUPS					
bean w/o meat	I cup	2.5	130	5	940
beef broth	I cup	0.5	33	0	642
black bean	I cup	1.5	116	2	1,198
broccoli, creamy w/ water	I cup	2.7	69	I	981
Campbell's Healthy Request					
chicken, cream of, w/ water	I cup	2.0	70	0	490
mushroom, cream of, w/ water	I cup	2.0	60	0	460
tomato, w/ water	I cup	2.0	90	0	430
canned vegetable type, w/o meat	I cup	2.0	67	0	500
chicken and stars	I cup	1.8	55	I	875
chicken and wild rice	I cup	2.3	76	I	815
chicken gumbo	I cup	1.4	56	I	955
chicken noodle	I cup	2.5	75	0	1,107
chicken vegetable	I cup	2.8	74	I	944
chicken w/ rice	I cup	1.9	60	I	814
consommé w/ gelatin	I cup	0	29	0	637
crab	I cup	1.5	76	I	1,234
dehydrated					
asparagus, cream of	I cup	1.7	59	0	801
beef broth cube	I cube	0.3	6	0	1,358
beef noodle	I cup	0.8	41	0	1,041
cauliflower	I cup	1.7	68	0	843
chicken broth cube	I cube	0.2	9	0	1,484
chicken noodle	I cup	1.2	53	0	1,284
chicken rice	I cup	1.4	60	0	980
clam chowder					
Manhattan	I cup	1.6	65	0	1,336
minestrone	I cup	1.7	79	0	1,026
onion					
dry mix	I pkg.	2.3	115	I	3,045
prepared	I cup	0.6	28	0	848
tomato	I cup	2.4	102	0	943
vegetable beef	I cup	1.1	53	0	1,000

	SERVING	TOTAL FAT (g.)	CALORIES	FIBER (g.)	SODIUM (mg.)
gazpacho	1 cup	0.5	40	2	1,183
homemade or restaurant					
chicken broth	1 cup	1.4	38	0	776
Manhattan clam chowder	1 cup	2.2	76	2	1,808
lentil	1 cup	1.0	161	3	1,020
minestrone	1 cup	2.5	105	2	900
mushroom barley	1 cup	2.3	76	1	800
onion	1 cup	1.7	57	1	1,053
pea					
green, w/ water	1 cup	2.9	164	2	987
split	1 cup	0.6	58	1	600
tomato, w/ water	1 cup	1.9	100	0.5	872
tomato rice	1 cup	2.7	120	1	815
turkey noodle	1 cup	2.0	69	1	815
vegetable w/ beef broth	1 cup	1.9	81	1	810
vegetarian vegetable	1 cup	1.0	72	1	823
wonton	1 cup	2.0	92	1	878
VEGETABLES					
alfalfa sprouts, raw	1/2 cup	0.1	5	0	0
artichoke, boiled	1 medium	0.2	53	3	42
artichoke hearts, boiled	1/2 cup	0.1	37	3	55
asparagus, cooked	1/2 cup	0.3	22	2	4
bamboo shoots, raw	1/2 cup	0.2	21	2	3
beans					
all types, cooked w/o fat	1/2 cup	0.4	124	9	1
baked, brown sugar & molasses	1/2 cup	1.5	132	4	516
baked, vegetarian	1/2 cup	0.6	135	5	1,008
baked w/pork & tomato sauce	1/2 cup	1.3	123	5	556
homestyle, canned	1/2 cup	1.6	132	5	550
beets, pickled	1/2 cup	0.1	75	4	301
black-eyed peas, cooked	1/2 cup	0.5	99	2	3
broccoli					
cooked	1/2 cup	0.4	46	7	16
frozen, chopped, cooked	1/2 cup	0.3	25	2	18
frozen in butter sauce	1/2 cup	2.3	51	2	296
raw	1/2 cup	0.2	12	1	12
brussel sprouts, cooked	1/2 cup	0.3	30	2	17
cabbage					
Chinese, raw	1 cup	0.2	10	2	23
green, cooked	1/2 cup	0.2	16	2	14
red, raw, shredded	1/2 cup	0.1	10	2	4

(con't.)	SERVING	TOTAL FAT (g.)	CALORIES	FIBER (g.)	SODIUM (mg.)
<u>VEGETABLES</u>					
carrot					
cooked	1/2 cup	0.1	35	2	52
raw	1 large	0.2	32	2	25
cauliflower					
cooked	1 cup	0.2	30	3	4
raw	1 cup	0.2	12	4	7
celery					
cooked	1/2 cup	0.1	11	1	48
raw	1 stalk	0.1	6	1	35
chard, cooked	1/2 cup	0.1	18	2	158
chilies, green	1/4 cup	0	14	0	3
chives, raw, chopped	1 T	0	1	0	0
collard greens, cooked	1/2 cup	0.1	13	2	36
corn					
corn on the cob	1 medium	0.9	83	4	4
cream style, canned	1/2 cup	0.4	93	4	365
frozen, cooked	1/2 cup	0.2	67	4	4
whole kernel, cooked	1/2 cup	1.1	89	5	14
cucumber	1/2 medium	0.1	8	1	1
dandelion greens, cooked	1/2 cup	0.3	17	2	23
eggplant, cooked	1/2 cup	0.1	13	2	1
endive lettuce	1 cup	0.1	8	1	6
garbanzo beans (chick peas), cooked	1/2 cup	2.1	134	5	6
green beans					
french style, cooked	1/2 cup	0.1	18	2	1
snap, cooked	1/2 cup	0.1	22	2	2
hominy, white or yellow, cooked	1 cup	0.7	138	3	708
Italian-style vegetables, frozen	1/2 cup	7.0	130	2	489
kale, cooked	1/2 cup	0.3	21	2	15
kidney beans, red, cooked	1/2 cup	0.5	112	8	2
leeks, chopped, raw	1/4 cup	0.1	16	1	5
lentils, cooked	1/2 cup	0.4	116	8	2
lettuce, leaf	1 cup	0.2	10	1	6
lima beans, cooked	1/2 cup	0.4	108	5	2
mushrooms					
canned	1/2 cup	0.2	19	1	500
raw	1/2 cup	0.2	9	1	0
mustard greens, cooked	1/2 cup	0.4	13	2	11
okra, cooked	1/2 cup	0.1	25	3	4

	SERVING	TOTAL FAT (g.)	CALORIES	FIBER (g.)	SODIUM (mg.)
onions, chopped, raw	1/2 cup	0.2	27	1	2
parsley, chopped, raw	1/4 cup	0	5	0	12
parsnips, cooked	1/2 cup	0.2	63	3	8
peas, green, cooked	1/2 cup	0.2	67	4	2
pepper, bell, chopped, raw	1/2 cup	0.2	12	2	2
pimientos, canned	1 oz.	0	10	0	5
potato					
baked, w/ skin	1 medium	0.2	220	4	16
boiled, w/o skin	1/2 cup	0.1	116	2	7
pumpkin, canned	1/2 cup	0.3	41	4	6
radish, raw	10	0.2	7	1	9
rhubarb, raw	1 cup	0.2	29	2	2
sauerkraut, canned	1/2 cup	0.2	22	4	780
scallions, raw	5 medium	0.2	45	4	1
spinach					
cooked	1/2 cup	0.2	21	3	29
raw	1 cup	0.2	89	3	22
squash					
acorn					
baked	1/2 cup	0.1	57	4	4
mashed w/o fat	1/2 cup	0.2	41	4	4
butternut, cooked	1/2 cup	0.1	41	4	4
summer					
cooked	1/2 cup	0.3	18	2	1
raw, slice	1/2 cup	0.1	13	1	1
succotash, cooked	1/2 cup	0.8	111	3	16
sweet potato					
baked	1 small	0.1	118	7	12
mashed w/o fat	1/2 cup	0.5	172	5	73
tomato					
boiled	1/2 cup	0.3	30	1	13
raw	1 medium	0.3	24	1	10
stewed	1/2 cup	0.2	34	1	325
tomato paste, canned	1/2 cup	1.2	110	4	86
turnip greens, cooked	1/2 cup	0.2	15	2	21
turnips, cooked	1/2 cup	0.1	14	2	21
water chestnuts, canned, sliced	1/2 cup	0	35	1	6
watercress, raw	1/2 cup	0	2	0	7
wax beans, canned	1/2 cup	0.2	25	2	321
yam, boiled/baked	1/2 cup	0.1	79	3	6
zucchini, cooked	1/2 cup	0.1	14	2	1

	SERVING	TOTAL FAT (g.)	CALORIES	FIBER (g.)	SODIUM (mg.)
VEGETABLE SALADS					
salad bar items					
alfalfa sprouts	2 T	0	2	0	0
bacon bits	1 T	1.6	27	0	181
beets, pickled	2 T	0	18	0	74
broccoli, raw	2 T	0	3	0	3
carrots, raw	2 T	0	6	0	5
chickpeas	2 T	0.4	21	1	75
croutons	1/4 cup	1.9	44	1	115
cucumber	2 T	0	2	0	0
lettuce	1/2 cup	0	4	0	1
mushrooms, raw	2 T	0	2	0	0
onion, raw	2 T	0.1	7	0	0
pepper, green, raw	2 T	0	3	0	0
tomato, raw	2 slices	0	12	0	1
three-bean salad, w/o oil	0.3	0.3	90	3	894

REGULAR FAT-CAT
(3.1–7.0 grams of fat per serving)

	SERVING	TOTAL FAT (g.)	CALORIES	FIBER (g.)	SODIUM (mg.)
BREADS					
biscuit					
baking powder	1 medium	6.6	156	1	344
buttermilk	1 medium	4.8	103	1	366
breadsticks, sesame	1 small	3.7	56	0	85
coffee cake	1 piece	7.0	233	1	160
cornbread, from mix	1/8 mix	4.0	160	1	250
crackers					
Ritz	6 crackers	5.8	108	0	180
Sociables	8 crackers	4.0	95	0	172
Triscuit	6 crackers	3.9	106	0	180
Waverly Wafers	6 crackers	4.8	108	0	240
Wheat Thins	12 crackers	4.2	108	1	180
Wheatsworth	6 crackers	3.6	84	0	162
fruit bread w/o nuts	1 slice	5.9	150	1	100
muffins					
blueberry, from mix	1 medium	4.3	126	0	185
bran, homemade	1 medium	5.1	112	2	160
corn	1 medium	4.2	130	1	192

	SERVING	TOTAL FAT (g.)	CALORIES	FIBER (g.)	SODIUM (mg.)
pancakes, buttermilk	3 medium	6.0	200	4	2
popover	1	5.0	170	0	176
rolls					
cloverleaf	1	3.2	89	0	155
crescent	1	5.6	102	1	256
scone	1	5.5	120	1	189
stuffing, cornbread, from mix	1/2 cup	4.8	198	0	500
toaster pastry, any flavor	1	5.0	195	0	229
waffle, frozen, Eggo	1	5.0	120	1	250
CANDY					
butterscotch					
candy	10 pieces	3.8	180	0	30
chips	1 oz.	6.7	234	0	15
candy bar					
Baby Ruth	1 oz.	6.6	141	1	60
Bit-o-Honey	1 oz.	2.2	121	0	80
Butterfinger	1 oz.	5.5	131	1	46
Milky Way	1 oz.	3.9	118	0	49
Three Musketeers	1 oz.	4.0	140	0	67
candy-coated almonds	1 oz.	5.3	129	1	6
caramels	1 oz.	6.0	120	0	10
choc.-covered cherries	1 oz.	4.9	123	1	52
choc.-covered cream centers	1 oz.	4.9	123	1	52
choc.-covered mint patty	1 oz.	3.2	125	0	10
choc.-covered raisins	1 oz.	4.9	120	1	18
Cracker Jack	1 cup	3.3	170	2	125
English toffee	1 oz.	3.1	113	0	8
fudge	1 oz.	4.5	115	0	45
M&M's, chocolate	1 oz.	5.6	132	1	20
praline	1 oz.	6.9	130	0	18
Tootsie Roll	1 oz.	3.2	112	1	56
CEREALS					
Cap'n Crunch	3/4 cup	3.4	121	0	185
Cracklin' Oat Bran	1/2 cup	4.0	110	4	175
granola, commercial brands	1/3 cup	6.9	186	3	58
wheat germ, toasted	1/4 cup	3.1	108	4	1
CHEESES					
cheese spread (Kraft)	1 oz.	6.0	82	0	381
Cheez Whiz	1 oz.	6.0	80	0	370

(con't.)	SERVING	TOTAL FAT (g.)	CALORIES	FIBER (g.)	SODIUM (mg.)
CHEESES					
cottage cheese, creamed	1/2 cup	5.1	117	0	457
cream cheese, "light" (Neufchâtel)	1 oz. (2 T)	6.6	74	0	113
feta	1 oz.	6.0	75	0	316
hot pepper cheese	1 oz.	6.9	92	0	357
Jarlsberg	1 oz.	6.9	100	0	130
Kraft Light Singles	1 oz.	4.0	70	0	410
Light 'n' Lively singles	1 oz.	4.0	70	0	400
mozzarella					
part-skim, low-moisture	1 oz.	4.9	79	0	150
whole-milk, low-moisture	1 oz.	7.0	90	0	118
ricotta, part-skim	1/4 cup	4.7	85	0	77
Sargento Light					
mozzarella	1 oz.	3.0	60	0	150
Swiss	1 oz.	4.0	80	0	75
smoked cheese product	1 oz.	6.7	91	0	220
Velveeta Light	1 oz.	4.0	70	0	470
COMBINATION FOODS					
chicken & veg. stir-fry	1 cup	6.9	142	3	482
chop suey w/o rice					
fish or poultry	1 cup	6.7	124	4	1,564
chow mein, chicken	1 cup	6.8	200	2	718
curry w/o meat	1 cup	6.6	138	2	294
fish creole	1 cup	5.4	172	2	NA
lo mein, Chinese	1 cup	6.9	185	1	368
shrimp creole w/o rice	1 cup	6.1	146	2	962
spaghetti, w/ red clam sauce	1 cup	6.8	250	2	306
tamale w/ sauce	1 piece	6.0	114	1	356
DESSERTS AND TOPPINGS					
brownie					
chocolate, plain	1 small	3.4	64	0	42
chocolate, w/ nuts & icing	1	5.0	64	0	40
Hostess	1 small	6.0	151	0	50
cake					
devil's food, "light," from mix	1/12 cake	3.5	190	0	350
lemon chiffon	1/12 cake	4.0	190	0	15
sponge	1 piece	3.7	194	0	210
white, "light," from mix	1/12 cake	3.0	180	0	320
yellow, "light," from mix	1/12 cake	3.5	190	0	300

	SERVING	TOTAL FAT (g.)	CALORIES	FIBER (g.)	SODIUM (mg.)
cookie					
animal	15 cookies	4.7	152	0	134
anisette toast	1 slice	3.4	95	0	81
chocolate sandwich (Oreo type)	2	4.2	98	0	60
gingersnap	2	3.2	70	0	80
graham cracker, chocolate covered	2	6.2	125	0	106
macaroon, coconut	2	3.2	110	0	58
molasses	2	4.0	140	0	200
oatmeal	2	6.5	160	0	200
oatmeal raisin	2	6.0	166	0	150
peanut butter	2	6.4	145	2	72
Rice Krispies bar	1 medium	3.1	112	0	97
shortbread	2	4.6	85	0	72
sugar	2	7.0	180	0	120
sugar wafers	3 wafers	3.2	80	0	120
vanilla-creme sandwich	2	6.2	140	0	150
vanilla wafers	5	3.1	85	0	50
Creamsicle	1 bar	3.1	103	0	27
cupcake					
chocolate w/ icing	1	5.5	159	1	110
yellow w/ icing	1	6.0	160	1	108
custard, baked	1/2 cup	6.9	148	0	104
date bar	1 bar	3.1	93	1	49
Dreamsicle	1 bar	6.2	207	0	137
frosting/icing					
"light" varieties, ready-to-spread	3 T	3.2	180	0	90
vanilla or lemon	3 T	4.0	140	0	80
fruitcake	1 piece	6.2	154	1	37
granola bar	1 bar	6.8	141	1	79
Ho Ho	1	6.8	133	1	70
Snoball	1	4.0	150	0	170
Twinkie	1	3.8	144	0	181
ice cream, strawberry (10% fat)	1/2 cup	7.0	128	0	55
ice cream cake roll	1 slice	6.9	159	0	88
ice cream sandwich	1	7.0	169	0	53
ice milk, chocolate	1/2 cup	3.1	91	0	52
lemon bars	1 bar	3.2	70	0	49
Little Debbie					
devil square	1 square	5.2	131	0	75
Dutch apple bar	2 oz.	5.3	207	0	70

(con't.)	SERVING	TOTAL FAT (g.)	CALORIES	FIBER (g.)	SODIUM (mg.)
DESSERTS AND TOPPINGS					
napoleon	1 piece	5.3	85	0	35
pudding, made w/ whole milk					
any flavor except chocolate	1/2 cup	5.5	168	0	142
noodle	1/2 cup	5.3	141	0	158
rice	1/2 cup	5.7	181	0	103
tapioca	1/2 cup	4.6	126	0	150
sopaipilla	1 piece	6.0	88	0	68
soufflé, choc.	1/2 cup	3.9	63	0	31
strudel, fruit	1/2 cup	4.2	80	1	30
toppings					
chocolate fudge	2 T	3.8	97	1	36
milk chocolate fudge	2 T	5.0	124	0	33
pecans in syrup	2 T	3.2	168	0	40
whipped topping					
aerosol	1/4 cup	3.9	46	0	3
frozen, tub	1/4 cup	4.8	59	0	4
"light"	1/2 cup	3.1	30	0	10
EGGS					
boiled or poached	1	5.6	79	0	69
yolk	1 large	5.6	63	0	8
FAST FOODS/RESTAURANTS					
Arby's					
light roast chicken deluxe	1	6.9	276	NA	777
light roast turkey deluxe	1	6.0	260	NA	1,262
Burger King					
BK broiler chicken sandwich	1	8.0	267	NA	728
chunky chicken salad	1	4.0	142	NA	443
garden salad w/o dressing	1	5.0	95	NA	125
Chick-Fil-A					
chargrilled chicken garden salad (w/ Lite Italian dressing)	1	3.1	148	NA	NA
chargrilled chicken sandwich	1	4.8	258	NA	NA
Dairy Queen					
chocolate sundae, regular	1	7.0	300	NA	140
DQ Sandwich, frozen treat	1	4.0	140	NA	135
ice cream cone, regular					
chocolate	1	7.0	230	NA	115
vanilla	1	7.0	230	NA	95

	SERVING	TOTAL FAT (g.)	CALORIES	FIBER (g.)	SODIUM (mg.)
Godfather's Pizza					
cheese pizza, large	1/10 pizza	7.0	228	NA	464
Hardee's					
grilled chicken salad	1	4.0	120	NA	520
ham sub	1	7.0	370	NA	1,400
turkey sub	1	7.0	390	NA	1,420
Kentucky Fried Chicken					
coleslaw	1 order	6.0	114	0	177
Rotisserie Gold chicken White Quarter (skin removed)	1	5.9	199	0	667
Long John Silver's					
coleslaw	1/2 cup	6.0	140	NA	260
Light Portion fish	1 dinner	5.0	270	NA	680
McDonald's					
chunky chicken salad w/o dressing	1	4.0	150	1	230
English muffin w/spread	1	4.0	170	1	285
sundae					
caramel	1	3.0	270	0	180
hot fudge	1	3.2	240	0	170
Wendy's					
breadstick	1	3.1	130	NA	250
Caesar side salad	1	6.0	160	NA	700
chili con carne	1 small	6.0	370	NA	880
deluxe garden salad	1	5.0	110	NA	380
FATS					
cream, light	2 T	5.8	58	0	12
cream substitute, liquid/frozen	2 T	3.2	40	0	24
margarine, reduced-calorie, tub	1 T	6.0	60	0	90
mayonnaise, reduced-calorie, "light"	1 T	4.5	44	0	96
sour cream, cultured	2 T	5.0	52	0	12
FISH					
anchovy, canned	8 fillets	3.6	65	0	1,110
anchovy, paste	1 T	3.1	45	0	NA
bluefish	3 1/2 oz.	3.3	117	0	51
buffalofish	3 1/2 oz.	4.2	150	0	34
carp	3 1/2 oz.	5.8	138	0	54
catfish	3 1/2 oz.	3.1	103	0	50
caviar, sturgeon, granular	1 round T	4.5	78	0	450

(con't.)	SERVING	TOTAL FAT (g.)	CALORIES	FIBER (g.)	SODIUM (mg.)
FISH					
eulachon (smelt)	3 1/2 oz.	6.2	118	0	59
Jack mackerel	3 1/2 oz.	5.6	143	0	360
kingfish	3 1/2 oz.	3.0	105	0	83
mussels, canned	3 1/2 oz.	3.3	114	0	NA
roughy, orange	3 1/2 oz.	6.0	124	0	63
salmon					
Atlantic	3 1/2 oz.	6.3	141	0	43
pink, canned	3 1/2 oz.	5.1	118	0	471
sushi or sashimi	3 1/2 oz.	4.9	144	0	38
swordfish	3 1/2 oz.	4.0	118	0	96
tuna, yellowfin, raw	3 1/2 oz.	3.1	133	0	41
white perch	3 1/2 oz.	3.9	114	0	45
yellowtail	3 1/2 oz.	5.4	138	0	46
GRAVIES, SAUCES, AND DIPS					
beef gravy, canned	1/2 can	3.4	77	0	73
mushroom gravy, canned	1/2 can	4.0	75	0	849
mushroom sauce, from mix	1/4 pkg.	3.2	71	0	479
meat flavor, jar	1/2 cup	6.0	100	1	600
stroganoff sauce, mix	1/4 pkg.	3.2	73	0	493
turkey gravy, canned	1/2 can	3.1	76	0	868
white sauce, thin	1/4 cup	5.2	72	0	200
MEATS (all cooked w/o added fat unless otherwise noted)					
beef, extra lean, ≤ 5% fat					
Healthy Choice lean ground beef	3 1/2 oz.	3.5	114	0	210
round, eye of, lean	3 1/2 oz.	4.2	130	0	60
beef, lean, 5–10% fat					
flank steak, fat trimmed	3 1/2 oz.	6.9	180	0	63
round steak, fat trimmed					
rump, lean, pot-roasted	3 1/2 oz.	7.0	179	0	61
top, lean	3 1/2 oz.	6.4	211	0	60
lamb					
blade chop, lean	1 chop	6.4	128	0	46
beefalo	3 1/2 oz.	6.3	188	0	82
organ meats					
heart					
beef, lean, braised	3 1/2 oz.	5.7	106	0	106
hog, braised	3 1/2 oz.	6.9	195	0	46

	SERVING	TOTAL FAT (g.)	CALORIES	FIBER (g.)	SODIUM (mg.)
kidney, beef, braised	3 1/2 oz.	3.4	144	0	134
liver					
beef, braised	3 1/2 oz.	3.8	140	0	70
calf, braised	3 1/2 oz.	4.7	140	0	45
tongue					
beef, etc., pickled	1 oz.	5.7	75	0	NA
beef, etc., potted	1 oz.	6.4	81	0	20
pork					
bacon bits	3 T	3.0	60	0	543
Canadian bacon, broiled	2 oz.	3.6	86	0	720
ham					
cured, butt, lean	3 1/2 oz.	4.5	159	0	1,255
cured, canned	3 oz.	5.0	120	0	1,255
cured, shank, lean	3 1/2 oz.	6.3	176	0	1,100
fresh, lean	3 1/2 oz.	6.4	222	0	65
ham loaf					
smoked, 95% lean	3 1/2 oz.	5.5	144	0	800
picnic					
shoulder, lean	2 slices	5.4	162	0	50
tenderloin, lean, roast	3 1/2 oz.	4.8	155	0	66
processed meats					
beef, chipped	3 slices	5.4	168	0	2,800
corned beef, jellied	2 oz.	5.8	62	0	300
sausage					
90% fat-free varieties	2 oz.	4.6	86	0	500
turkey ham	2 oz.	3.2	72	0	55
turkey loaf	2 oz.	5.4	86	0	55
turkey pastrami	2 oz.	3.6	80	0	54
veal					
arm steak, lean	3 1/2 oz.	4.8	180	0	70
loin chop	3 1/2 oz.	6.9	220	0	90
sirloin					
lean, roasted	3 1/2 oz.	3.4	175	0	80
sirloin steak					
lean	3 1/2 oz.	6.0	204	0	90
MILK AND YOGURT					
chocolate milk, 2% fat	1 cup	5.0	179	0	150
hot cocoa mix w/ water	1 cup	3.0	110	0	149
low-fat milk					
1.5% fat/acidophilus	1 cup	4.7	122	0	122
2% fat	1 cup	4.7	121	0	122

(con't.)	SERVING	TOTAL FAT (g.)	CALORIES	FIBER (g.)	SODIUM (mg.)
MILK AND YOGURT					
malt powder	2 T	3.2	172	0	206
milk shake, soft serve	1 cup	7.0	218	1	240
yogurt, plain, low-fat	1 cup	3.5	144	0	159
MISCELLANEOUS					
Bac o Bits, General Mills	3 T	3.9	99	0	390
cocoa, dry	1/3 cup	3.6	115	2	2
PASTA, NOODLES, AND RICE					
(all measurements after					
cooking unless otherwise noted)					
noodles					
cellophane, fried	1 cup	4.2	141	0	6
ramen, all varieties	1 cup	6.5	188	1	978
rice, pilaf	1/2 cup	6.8	170	1	600
POULTRY					
chicken					
breast w/o skin, fried	1/2 breast	6.1	179	0	81
fryers w/o skin, roasted	3 1/2 oz.	6.9	180	0	70
leg w/o skin, roasted	1 leg	5.8	112	0	99
liver, simmered	3 1/2 oz.	5.5	157	0	51
wing w/skin, roasted	1 wing	6.6	99	0	28
turkey					
breast, barbecued	3 1/2 oz.	4.0	125	0	860
ham, cured	3 1/2 oz.	5.1	128	0	996
light meat w/o skin, roasted	3 1/2 oz.	3.2	157	0	64
sausage, cooked	2 oz.	6.8	100	0	400
wing drumettes, smoked	3 1/2 oz.	7.0	165	0	60
SALAD DRESSINGS					
Green Goddess, low-cal	2 T	4.0	54	0	35
mayonnaise type, low-cal	2 T	3.6	38	0	224
Thousand Island, low-cal	2 T	3.2	48	0	206
SNACK FOODS					
corn nuts, all flavors	1 oz.	4.0	120	3.0	200
Doo-Dads, Nabisco	1/2 cup	6.0	140	1	393
Funyuns	1 oz.	6.4	140	0	250
popcorn					
caramel	1 cup	4.5	150	1	73

	SERVING	TOTAL FAT (g.)	CALORIES	FIBER (g.)	SODIUM (mg.)
microwave, w/ butter	I cup	4.5	61	1	100
popped w/ oil	I cup	3.0	45	1	86
SOUPS					
asparagus, cream of, w/ water	I cup	4.1	87	1	981
bean w/ bacon	I cup	5.9	173	4	952
beef, chunky	I cup	5.1	171	2	867
beef noodle	I cup	3.1	84	1	952
Campbell's Chunky					
w/ meat	I cup	5.1	170	2	887
w/o meat	I cup	3.7	122	3	1,010
chicken, chunky	I cup	6.6	178	2	887
chicken & dumplings	I cup	5.5	97	0	861
chicken/beef noodle or vegetable	I cup	3.1	83	1	952
chicken noodle, chunky	I cup	6.0	116	2	900
chicken w/ noodles, chunky	I cup	5.0	180	2	850
chicken w/ rice, chunky	I cup	3.2	127	2	1,072
clam chowder					
Manhattan chunky	I cup	3.4	133	1	1,000
New England	I cup	6.6	163	1	960
dehydrated					
bean w/ bacon	I cup	3.5	105	2	928
clam chowder	I cup	3.7	95	0	745
mushroom	I cup	4.9	96	0	1,019
homemade or restaurant style					
gazpacho, traditional	I cup	6.0	90	2	1,183
onion, French w/o cheese	I cup	5.8	93	0	1,053
seafood gumbo	I cup	3.9	155	0	980
mushroom w/ beef stock	I cup	4.0	85	1	970
oyster stew, w/ water	I cup	3.8	59	1	980
pea, split w/ ham	I cup	4.4	189	1	1,008
tomato, w/ milk	I cup	6.0	160	1	932
tomato beef w/ noodle	I cup	4.3	140	1	917
tomato bisque w/ milk	I cup	6.6	198	1	1,048
turkey, chunky	I cup	4.4	136	2	923
vegetable, chunky	I cup	3.7	122	2	1,010
vegetable w/ beef, chunky	I cup	3.1	134	2	1,340
VEGETABLES					
broccoli, frozen w/ cheese sauce	1/2 cup	6.2	116	1	417
cauliflower, frozen w/ cheese sauce	1/2 cup	6.1	114	2	446
Chinese-style vegetables, frozen	1/2 cup	4.7	79	3	120

(con't.)	SERVING	TOTAL FAT (g.)	CALORIES	FIBER (g.)	SODIUM (mg.)
VEGETABLES					
potato					
au gratin, from mix	1/2 cup	6.0	140	2	538
french fries, frozen	10 pieces	4.4	111	2	15
knishes	1	3.2	73	1	83
mashed					
from flakes, w/ milk & margarine	1/2 cup	6.0	124	1	365
w/ milk & margarine	1/2 cup	4.4	111	1	309
scalloped					
from mix	1 serving	5.9	127	1	467
homemade	1/2 cup	4.8	105	1	409
spinach, creamed	1/2 cup	5.7	89	3	312
sweet potato, candied	1/2 cup	3.8	192	5	73
tempeh (soybean product)	1/2 cup	6.4	165	1	5
tofu (soybean curd), raw, firm	4 oz.	5.4	86	1	8
VEGETABLE SALADS					
carrot-raisin salad	1/2 cup	3.7	157	4	762
chef salad w/o dressing	1 cup	4.3	71	1	281
coleslaw w/ vinaigrette	1/2 cup	5.5	77	1	14
gelatin salad w/ fruit & cheese	1/2 cup	4.6	74	0	82
pasta primavera salad	1 cup	5.9	149	3	639
potato salad, German style	1/2 cup	3.5	140	1	NA
salad bar items					
cheese, shredded	2 T	4.6	56	0	85
cottage cheese	1/2 cup	5.1	116	0	458
eggs, cooked, chopped	2 T	1.9	27	0	23

FULL FAT-CAT
(greater than 7 grams of fat per serving)

	SERVING	TOTAL FAT (g.)	CALORIES	FIBER (g.)	SODIUM (mg.)
BEVERAGES					
eggnog, nonalcoholic	8 fl. oz.	19.0	342	0	138
BREADS					
bread, fruit w/ nuts	1 slice	10.1	210	1	140
crackers					
cheese w/ peanut butter	2-oz. pkg.	13.5	283	0	600

	SERVING	TOTAL FAT (g.)	CALORIES	FIBER (g.)	SODIUM (mg.)
toasted w/ peanut butter	1.5 oz. pkg.	10.5	212	0	405
wheat w/ cheese	1.5 oz. pkg.	10.9	212	0	490
croissant	1 medium	11.5	167	1	126
Danish pastry	1 medium	19.3	256	1	103
doughnut					
cake	1 2.2 oz.	16.2	250	1	229
yeast	1 2.2 oz.	13.3	235	1	222
French toast, homemade	1 slice	10.7	172	1	250
funnel cake	6 in. diam.	15.3	285	1	236
hushpuppy	1 medium	11.4	146	1	109
matzo ball	1	7.6	121	0	202
muffins, all types, commercial	1 large	10.3	187	1	263
pie crust, plain	1/8 pie	8.0	125	0	130
rolls					
croissant	1 small	6.1	109	0	106
yeast, sweet	1	7.0	198	1	106
stuffing					
bread, from mix	1/2 cup	12.2	198	0	500
Stove Top	1/2 cup	9.0	176	0	560
sweet roll, iced	1 medium	7.9	198	1	100
turnover, fruit filled	1	15.0	280	1	260
waffle, homemade	1 large	12.6	245	1	303
CANDY					
candy bar					
Almond Joy	1 oz.	7.8	136	2	58
Chunky	1 oz.	8.3	140	1	15
Heath	1 oz.	8.9	142	1	109
Kit Kat	1.13 oz.	9.2	162	0	32
Krackle, Hershey	1 oz.	8.4	145	1	35
Mars	1.7 oz.	11.0	230	1	80
milk chocolate	1 oz.	9.2	147	1	27
Milky Way	1 oz.	3.9	118	0	49
Mr. Goodbar	1 oz.	10.8	154	2	19
Nestle's Crunch	1.06 oz.	8.0	160	1	35
Snickers	1 oz.	7.1	135	1	75
Twix	1 oz.	7.1	140	0	60
carob-coated raisins	1/2 cup	13.5	387	5	83
chocolate chips					
milk chocolate	1/4 cup	11.0	218	1	60
semisweet	1/4 cup	12.2	220	1	10
choc.-covered peanuts	1 oz.	11.7	159	2	17

(con't.)	SERVING	TOTAL FAT (g.)	CALORIES	FIBER (g.)	SODIUM (mg.)
CANDY					
choc. kisses	6 pieces	9.0	154	1	25
choc. stars	7 pieces	8.1	160	1	35
M&M's, peanut	1 oz.	5.6	132	1	20
malted milk balls	1 oz.	7.1	137	1	28
peanut brittle	1 oz.	7.7	149	1	44
Peanut Butter Cups, Reese's	1 oz.	9.2	156	1	82
Reese's Pieces	1.7 oz. pkg.	13.0	240	0	108
yogurt-covered peanuts	1/2 cup	26.0	387	4	30
yogurt-covered raisins	1/2 cup	14.0	313	2	36
CEREALS					
granola, homemade	1/3 cup	10.0	184	2	80
CHEESES					
American, processed	1 oz.	8.9	106	0	406
blue	1 oz.	8.2	100	0	396
brick	1 oz.	8.4	105	0	159
brie	1 oz.	7.9	95	0	178
caraway	1 oz.	8.3	107	0	196
cheddar					
grated	1/4 cup	9.4	114	0	176
sliced	1 oz.	9.4	114	0	176
cheese food, cold-pack	2 T	7.8	94	0	274
cheese sauce	1/4 cup	9.8	132	0	576
Colby	1 oz.	9.1	112	0	171
cream cheese, regular	1 oz. (2 T)	9.9	99	0	84
Edam	1 oz.	7.9	101	0	274
Gouda	1 oz.	7.8	101	0	232
Kraft American Singles	1 oz.	7.0	90	0	390
limburger	1 oz.	7.7	93	0	227
Monterey Jack	1 oz.	8.6	106	0	152
Muenster	1 oz.	8.5	104	0	178
Parmesan	1 oz.	7.3	111	0	454
pimento cheese, spread	1 oz.	9.4	106	0	405
port wine, cold-pack	1 oz.	9.0	100	0	151
provolone	1 oz.	7.6	100	0	248
Romano	1 oz.	7.6	110	0	340
Roquefort	1 oz.	8.7	105	0	513
Swiss	1 oz.	7.8	107	0	74
Velveeta	1 oz.	7.1	100	0	410

	SERVING	TOTAL FAT (g.)	CALORIES	FIBER (g.)	SODIUM (mg.)
COMBINATION FOODS					
(traditional recipe, unless					
otherwise noted)					
beans & franks, canned	1 cup	16.0	366	7	1,105
beans					
refried w/ fat	1/2 cup	13.2	271	7	1,071
refried w/ sausage, canned	1/2 cup	13.0	192	8	825
beef & vegetable stew	1 cup	10.5	218	2	292
beef burgundy	1 cup	21.2	336	1	467
beef goulash w/ noodles	1 cup	13.9	335	2	453
beef noodle casserole	1 cup	19.2	329	2	1,205
beef pot pie	1 cup	25.0	450	2	700
beef stew, canned	1 cup	8.0	184	2	977
beef vegetable stew	1 cup	13.8	244	2	649
beef					
chipped, creamed	1/2 cup	11.0	175	0	681
short ribs w/ gravy, frozen	5 3/4 oz.	25.0	350	0	702
burrito					
bean w/ cheese	1 large	9.7	230	4	642
beef	1 large	24.9	424	2	712
cabbage roll w/ beef & rice	1 medium	8.2	420	1	386
cannelloni, meat & cheese	1 piece	29.7	420	1	597
casserole, meat, veg., rice, sauce	1 cup	12.2	276	3	238
cheese souffle	1 cup	11.0	174	0	118
Chicken a la king	1 cup	25.0	450	1	800
chicken & dumplings	1 cup	10.5	298	1	611
chicken & rice casserole	1 cup	18.0	365	1	600
chicken fricassee	1 cup	20.9	328	1	370
chicken-fried steak	3 1/2 oz.	23.4	355	0	365
chicken noodle casserole	1 cup	10.7	269	2	866
chicken parmigiana	7 oz.	14.8	308	2	620
chicken pot pie	1 cup	25.0	460	1	750
chicken salad, regular mayonnaise	1/2 cup	21.2	271	0	316
chicken tetrazzini	1 cup	19.6	348	1	813
chicken w/ cashews, Chinese	1 cup	10.9	203	3	1,228
chili					
w/ beans	1 cup	14.8	302	6	915
w/o beans	1 cup	19.3	302	3	1,030
chitterlings, cooked	3 1/2 oz.	29.4	303	0	39
chop suey w/o rice, beef	1 cup	17.0	300	3	1,053
corned-beef hash	1 cup	24.4	374	2	1,158
creamed chipped beef	1 cup	22.0	332	0	1,608

(con't.)	SERVING	TOTAL FAT (g.)	CALORIES	FIBER (g.)	SODIUM (mg.)
COMBINATION FOODS					
deviled crab	1/2 cup	15.4	231	1	468
egg foo yung w/ sauce	1 piece	11.5	129	1	492
egg salad	1/2 cup	17.4	212	0	354
eggplant Parmesan, traditional	1 cup	24.0	356	3	1,196
egg roll	1 (3 1/2 oz.)	10.5	153	1	469
enchilada, bean, beef, & cheese	1 piece	14.1	243	3	756
fajitas					
chicken	1	13.5	381	4	363
beef	1	18.2	302	3	761
falafel	1	10.0	150	2	76
fettuccine Alfredo	1	29.7	461	1	912
fritter, corn	1 medium	8.5	132	1	167
frozen dinner					
chopped beefsteak	11 oz.	26.5	443	2	NA
chopped steak	18 oz.	41.0	730	3	NA
fried chicken	11 oz.	31.0	590	2	1,831
meat loaf	19 oz.	57.7	916	3	3,050
meat loaf	11 oz.	29.0	530	2	1,525
Salisbury steak	11 oz.	29.0	500	2	1,340
turkey	11 oz.	11.0	360	2	1,416
green pepper stuffed, w/ rice & beef	1 average	13.5	262	2	986
ham salad w/ mayonnaise	1/2 cup	20.2	277	0	1,300
Hamburger Helper, all varieties	1 cup	18.9	375	1	1,037
hamburger rice casserole	1 cup	21.0	376	3	755
lasagne, homemade w/ beef & cheese	1 piece	19.8	400	2	1,316
lobster					
Cantonese	1 cup	19.6	334	0	1,586
Newburg	1/2 cup	24.8	305	0	670
macaroni & cheese	1 cup	15.0	350	0	900
manicotti, cheese & tomato	1 piece	11.8	238	2	610
meatball (reg. ground beef)	2 medium	10.2	154	0	188
meat loaf, w/ reg. ground beef	3 1/2 oz.	20.4	332	0	696
moo goo gai pan	1 cup	17.2	304	1	595
moussaka	1 cup	8.9	210	3	400
onion rings	10 average	17.0	234	1	263
oysters Rockefeller, traditional	6–8 oysters	14.0	230	1	900
pepper steak	1 cup	21.3	329	1	649
pizza					
cheese	1 slice	10.1	183	1	680

	SERVING	TOTAL FAT (g.)	CALORIES	FIBER (g.)	SODIUM (mg.)
combination w/ meat	1 slice	17.5	272	1	1,000
deep dish, cheese	1 slice	13.5	426	4	1,170
pork, sweet & sour, w/ rice	1 cup	7.5	270	· 1	860
quiche					
Lorraine (bacon)	1/8 pie	43.5	540	1	567
plain or vegetable	1/8 pie	17.6	312	1	539
ravioli w/ meat & tomato sauce	1 cup	9.0	250	2	800
Salisbury steak w/ gravy	8 oz.	27.3	364	1	1,261
salmon patty, traditional	3 1/2 oz.	12.4	239	1	783
sandwiches					
BBQ beef on bun	1	16.8	392	5	1,056
BBQ pork on bun	1	12.2	359	5	895
BLT w/ mayo	1	15.6	282	1	935
bologna & cheese	1	22.5	363	1	1,010
chicken w/ mayo & lettuce	1	14.4	303	1	256
club w/ mayo	1	20.8	590	3	1,396
corned beef on rye	1	10.8	296	1	774
cream cheese & jelly	1	16.0	368	1	421
egg salad	1	12.5	279	1	482
french dip, au jus	1	12.2	360	2	610
grilled cheese	1	24.0	426	1	1,177
ham, cheese & mayo	1	9.8	281	1	412
ham salad	1	16.9	321	1	372
peanut butter & jelly	1	15.1	374	3	406
Reuben	1	33.3	531	6	1,535
roast beef & gravy	1	24.5	429	1	785
roast beef & mayo	1	22.6	328	1	800
sloppy joe on bun	1	16.8	392	5	1,056
sub w/ salami & cheese	1	41.3	766	3	1,842
tuna salad	1	14.2	278	1	443
turkey & mayo	1	18.4	402	1	517
shepherd's pie	1 cup	24.0	407	3	1,158
shrimp salad	1/2 cup	9.5	136	1	1,087
spaghetti					
w/ meat sauce	1 cup	16.7	317	2	1,320
w/ white clam sauce	1 cup	19.5	416	1	436
spanakopita	1 piece	24.1	259	2	354
spinach soufflé	1 cup	14.8	212	2	763
stroganoff, beef w/o noodles	1 cup	44.4	568	1	634
taco, beef	1 medium	17.0	272	2	355
tortellini, meat or cheese	1 cup	15.4	363	1	764

(con't.)	SERVING	TOTAL FAT (g.)	CALORIES	FIBER (g.)	SODIUM (mg.)
COMBINATION FOODS					
tostada w/ refried beans	1 medium	16.3	294	6	249
tuna noodle casserole	1 cup	13.3	315	2	1,209
tuna salad					
oil pack, w/ mayo	1/2 cup	16.3	226	0	351
water, w/ mayo	1/2 cup	10.5	170	0	112
veal parmigiana	1 cup	25.5	485	2	1,028
veal scallopini	1 cup	20.4	429	2	160
Welsh rarebit	1 cup	31.6	415	0	770
wonton w/ pork, fried	2 pieces	8.6	160	0	290
DESSERTS AND TOPPINGS					
apple betty, fruit crisps	1/2 cup	13.3	347	3	114
baklava	1 piece	29.2	426	2	228
brownie					
choc., Little Debbie	2 small	7.3	219	0	135
Pepperidge Farm	1	8.7	168	0	70
cake					
black forest	1/12 cake	14.3	279	1	150
carrot w/ frosting	1/12 cake	19.0	420	3	197
choc. w/ frosting	1/12 cake	17.0	388	2	648
coconut w/ frosting	1/12 cake	18.1	395	2	177
German choc. w/ frosting	1/12 cake	18.5	407	2	600
lemon w/ frosting	1/12 cake	16.0	410	1	160
marble w/ frosting	1/12 cake	16.0	408	1	172
pineapple upside-down	2 1/2" slice	9.2	236	2	165
pound	1/12 cake	9.0	200	1	110
shortbread w/ fruit	1 piece	8.9	344	1	165
spice w/ frosting	1/12 cake	10.9	325	1	155
streusel swirl	1/12 cake	11.0	260	1	163
white w/ frosting	1/12 cake	14.6	369	1	420
yellow w/ frosting	1/12 cake	16.4	391	1	108
cobbler	1/2 cup	9.3	236	3	151
cookies, chocolate chip, homemade	2	7.4	136	0	52
dumpling, fruit	1 piece	15.1	324	2	256
éclair					
w/ choc. icing & custard	1 small	15.4	316	0	147
w/ choc. icing & whipped					
cream	1 small	25.7	296	0	139
frosting/icing					
chocolate	3 T	5.3	148	0	50
cream cheese	3 T	6.8	170	0	43

	SERVING	TOTAL FAT (g.)	CALORIES	FIBER (g.)	SODIUM (mg.)
ready-to-spread	1/12 tub	6.9	169	0	30
Hostess					
cupcake	1	7.4	206	1	250
Ding Dong	1	8.7	170	0	130
fruit snack pie	1	20.2	403	2	449
honey bun	1	33.3	572	2	675
ice cream					
choc. (10% fat)	1/2 cup	7.2	134	1	58
choc. (16% fat)	1/2 cup	11.9	174	0	54
French vanilla soft serve	1/2 cup	11.5	189	0	76
vanilla (10% fat)	1/2 cup	7.2	134	0	58
vanilla (16% fat)	1/2 cup	11.9	175	0	54
ice cream bar					
choc. coated	1 bar	11.5	178	0	28
toffee krunch	1 slice	10.2	149	1	52
ice cream drumstick	1	10.0	188	1	58
Little Debbie					
fudge krispie	2 oz.	7.1	256	1	70
oatmeal creams	2 pieces	12.6	332	1	250
peanut butter bar	2 bars	13.5	265	1	200
mousse, choc.	1/2 cup	15.5	189	1	37
pie					
apple	1/8 pie	16.9	347	3	195
banana cream or custard	1/8 pie	14.0	353	1	300
blueberry	1/8 pie	17.3	387	3	350
Boston creme pie	1/8 pie	8.4	260	1	225
cherry	1/8 pie	18.1	418	2	150
choc. cream	1/8 pie	13.0	311	3	427
choc. meringue, traditional	1/8 pie	18.0	378	1	325
coconut cream or custard	1/8 pie	19.0	365	1	300
key lime	1/8 pie	19.0	388	1	290
lemon chiffon	1/8 pie	13.5	335	1	300
lemon meringue, traditional	1/8 pie	13.1	350	1	260
mincemeat	1/8 pie	18.4	434	3	400
peach	1/8 pie	17.7	421	3	425
pecan	1/8 pie	23.0	510	2	250
pumpkin	1/8 pie	16.8	367	5	338
raisin	1/8 pie	12.9	325	1	336
rhubarb	1/8 pie	17.1	405	3	400
strawberry	1/8 pie	9.1	228	1	250
sweet potato	1/8 pie	18.2	342	2	300
pie tart, fruit filled	1	18.7	362	2	NA

(con't.)	SERVING	TOTAL FAT (g.)	CALORIES	FIBER (g.)	SODIUM (mg.)
DESSERTS AND TOPPINGS					
pudding					
bread	1/2 cup	8.1	219	1	286
choc. w/ whole milk	1/2 cup	8.6	247	1	140
Tasty Kake					
chocolate junior	1	12.2	306	1	298
coconut cream	1	31.2	482	1	286
fruit pie	1	14.3	362	2	370
trifle	1/2 cup	19.5	289	1	81
turnover, fruit filled	1	19.3	226	1	141
whipping cream					
heavy, fluid	2 T	11.2	104	0	12
light, fluid	2 T	9.2	88	0	10
EGGS					
fried w/ 1/2 t fat	1 large	7.8	104	0	144
omelet					
2 oz. cheese, 3-egg	1	37.0	510	0	838
plain, 3-egg	1	21.3	271	0	330
Spanish, 2-egg	1	18.0	250	1	225
scrambled w/ milk	1 large	8.0	99	0	155
FAST FOODS/RESTAURANTS					
Arby's					
baked potato deluxe	1	36.4	621	NA	605
beef 'n' cheddar sandwich	1	26.8	508	NA	1,166
chicken breast sandwich	1	22.5	445	NA	958
curly fries	1 order	17.7	337	NA	167
french fries	1 order	13.2	246	NA	114
ham & cheese sandwich	1	14.2	355	NA	1,400
jamocha shake	1	10.5	368	NA	262
junior roast beef sandwich	1	10.8	233	NA	519
light roast beef deluxe	1	10.0	294	NA	826
potato cakes	1 order	12.0	204	NA	397
roast beef sandwich	1 regular	18.2	383	NA	936
roast chicken club	1	27.0	503	NA	1,143
roast chicken salad	1	7.2	204	NA	508
sausage biscuit	1	31.9	460	NA	1,000
super roast beef sandwich	1	28.3	552	NA	1,174
Burger King					
apple pie	1	14.0	552	NA	412
bacon double cheeseburger	1	30.0	507	NA	809

	SERVING	TOTAL FAT (g.)	CALORIES	FIBER (g.)	SODIUM (mg.)
bacon double cheeseburger					
deluxe	1	39.0	592	NA	804
cheeseburger	1	15.0	318	NA	661
cheeseburger, deluxe	1	23.0	390	NA	652
cheeseburger, double	1	27.0	483	NA	851
chef salad	1	9.0	178	NA	568
cherry pie	1	13.0	311	NA	412
chicken sandwich	1	40.0	685	NA	1,417
Chicken Tenders	1 order	13.0	236	NA	541
Croissan'wich w/ bacon, egg, & cheese	1	23.0	353	NA	780
Croissan'wich w/ham, egg, & cheese	1	22.0	351	NA	1,373
Croissan'wich w/sausage, egg, & cheese	1	40.0	534	NA	985
french fries, medium	1 order	20.0	341	NA	241
french toast sticks	1 order	32.0	538	NA	537
hamburger	1	11.0	272	NA	505
hamburger, deluxe	1	19.0	344	NA	496
mini muffins, blueberry	1 order	14.0	292	NA	244
Ocean Catch fish fillet	1	33.0	479	NA	736
onion rings, regular	1 order	19.0	339	NA	628
shakes					
chocolate	1	10.0	326	NA	198
strawberry	1	10.0	394	NA	230
vanilla	1	10.0	334	NA	213
side salad					
w/ regular dressing	1	22.0	332	NA	400
Whopper	1	36.0	614	NA	865
Whopper w/ cheese	1	44.0	706	NA	1,177
Whopper, double beef	1	53.0	844	NA	933
Whopper, double beef w/ cheese	1	61.0	935	NA	1,245
Chick-Fil-A					
chicken nuggets	8	15.0	258	NA	NA
original chicken sandwich	1	8.5	360	NA	NA
Dairy Queen					
banana split	1	11.0	510	NA	250
Blizzard, strawberry	1 regular	16.0	570	NA	230
breaded chicken fillet sandwich	1	20.0	430	NA	760
breaded chicken fillet sandwich w/ cheese	1	25.0	480	NA	980

(con't.)	SERVING	TOTAL FAT (g.)	CALORIES	FIBER (g.)	SODIUM (mg.)
FAST FOODS/RESTAURANTS					
Buster bar	I	29.0	450	NA	220
cheese dog	I	21.0	330	NA	920
cheeseburger	I	18.0	365	NA	800
cheeseburger, double	I	34.0	570	NA	1,070
chili dog	I	19.0	330	NA	720
Dilly bar	I	13.0	210	NA	50
DQ Homestyle Ultimate burger	I	47.0	700	NA	1,100
fish fillet sandwich	I	16.0	400	NA	630
fish fillet sandwich w/ cheese	I	21.0	440	NA	850
french fries, regular	I order	14.0	300	NA	160
garden salad, plain	I	13.0	200	NA	240
grilled chicken fillet sandwich	I	8.0	300	NA	800
hamburger	I	13.0	310	NA	580
hamburger, double	I	25.0	470	NA	630
hot dog	I	16.0	280	NA	700
hot fudge brownie delight	I	29.0	710	NA	340
ice cream cone, regular					
chocolate dipped	I	16.0	330	NA	100
onion rings	I order	12.0	240	NA	135
Peanut Buster parfait	I	32.0	710	NA	410
shake, regular					
chocolate	I	14.0	540	NA	210
vanilla	I	14.0	520	NA	230
Dominos					
cheese pizza 12"	2 slices	10.0	360	NA	1,000
deluxe pizza 12"	2 slices	23.0	540	NA	1,760
extravaganza pizza 12"	2 slices	24.0	510	NA	1,680
pepperoni pizza 12"	2 slices	15.0	410	NA	1,190
pepperoni/sausage/mushroom pizza 12"	2 slices	20.0	460	NA	1,410
sausage pizza 12"	2 slices	16.5	430	NA	1,270
Vegi Feast pizza 12"	2 slices	13.0	390	NA	1,090
Godfather's Pizza					
combo pizza, large	1/10 pizza	19.0	437	NA	464
Hardee's					
apple turnover	I	12.0	268	NA	245
bacon biscuit	I	21.0	360	NA	950
bacon cheeseburger	I	39.0	610	NA	1,030
bacon/egg/cheese bagel	I	16.0	375	NA	865
Big Cookie Treat	I	13.0	250	NA	239

	SERVING	TOTAL FAT (g.)	CALORIES	FIBER (g.)	SODIUM (mg.)
Big Country Breakfast					
w/ bacon	1	40.0	660	NA	1,540
w/ ham	1	33.0	620	NA	1,780
w/ sausage	1	57.0	850	NA	1,980
Big Deluxe burger	1	30.0	500	NA	760
biscuit 'n' gravy	1	24.0	440	NA	1,250
blueberry muffin	1	17.0	400	NA	310
cheeseburger	1	14.0	300	NA	740
cheeseburger, 1/4 lb.	1	29.0	510	NA	1,060
chef salad	1	13.0	214	NA	910
chicken fillet	1	13.0	370	NA	1,060
chicken stix	6 pieces	9.0	210	NA	678
cinnamon 'n' raisin biscuit	1	17.0	315	NA	515
fisherman's fillet	1	21.0	470	NA	1,140
french fries, regular	1	11.0	230	NA	85
fried chicken breast	1	19.0	340	NA	659
Frisco breakfast sandwich	1	20.0	430	NA	1,110
Frisco burger	1	47.0	730	NA	1,110
Frisco chicken	1	41.0	680	NA	1,680
Frisco club	1	42.0	670	NA	1,870
garden salad	1	12.0	184	NA	250
grilled chicken breast sandwich	1	9.0	310	NA	890
hamburger	1	10.0	260	NA	510
Hash Rounds	1 order	14.0	230	NA	560
hot dog	1	16.0	290	NA	760
mushroom 'n' Swiss burger	1	28.0	490	NA	940
rise 'n' shine biscuit	1	18.0	320	NA	740
roast-beef sandwich	1	11.0	280	NA	870
sausage biscuit	1	28.0	440	NA	1,100
steak biscuit	1	29.0	500	NA	1,320
turkey club sandwich	1	16.0	390	NA	1,280
Kentucky Fried Chicken (KFC)					
breast, extra crispy	1	23.0	365	0	640
breast, hot & spicy	1	26.0	382	0	905
breast, original recipe	1	14.0	260	0	609
Chicken Little sandwich	1	10.0	169	1	331
chicken nuggets	6 nuggets	18.0	284	0	865
Colonel's chicken sandwich	1	27.0	482	1	1,060
crispy fries	1 order	17.0	294	1	761
drumstick, extra crispy	1	14.0	205	0	292
drumstick, hot & spicy	1	14.0	207	0	406

(con't.)	SERVING	TOTAL FAT (g.)	CALORIES	FIBER (g.)	SODIUM (mg.)
FAST FOODS/RESTAURANTS					
drumstick, original recipe	1	9.0	152	0	269
french fries	1 order	12.0	244	1	139
Hot Wings	6	33.0	471	0	1,230
Rotisserie Gold Chicken					
Dark Quarter (as served)	1	23.7	333	0	980
Dark Quarter (skin removed)	1	12.2	217	0	772
White Quarter (as served)	1	18.7	335	0	1,104
White Quarter (skin removed)	1	5.9	199	0	667
thigh, extra crispy	1	31.0	414	0	580
thigh, original recipe	1	21.0	287	0	591
wing, extra crispy	1	17.0	231	0	319
wing, original recipe	1	11.0	172	0	383
Long John Silver's					
baked chicken dinner	1	15.0	550	NA	1,670
batter-dipped fish	1 piece	11.0	180	NA	490
batter-dipped shrimp	4 pieces	8.0	120	NA	320
Chicken Plank	2 pieces	12.0	240	NA	800
Chicken Planks (dinner)	3 pieces	44.0	890	NA	2,000
chicken sandwich	1	8.0	280	NA	790
clam dinner	1	52.0	990	NA	1,830
corn cobbette	1	8.0	140	NA	10
fish and fries	2-piece	37.0	610	NA	1,480
Fish & More dinner	2-piece	48.0	890	NA	1,790
fish sandwich (w/out sauce)	1	13.0	340	NA	890
fish w/ lemon crumb	1 dinner	12.0	570	NA	1,470
french fries	1 order	15.0	250	NA	500
hush puppies	3	9.0	210	NA	75
seafood gumbo	7 oz.	8.0	120	NA	740
seafood salad	1	31.0	380	NA	980
shrimp dinner	1	47.0	840	NA	1,630
McDonald's					
Big Mac	1	26.0	500	1	890
biscuit w/ bacon, egg, & cheese	1	26.4	440	1	1,215
biscuit w/ sausage	1	28.0	420	1	1,040
biscuit w/ sausage & egg	1	33.0	505	1	1,210
biscuit w/ spread	1	12.7	260	1	730
breakfast burrito	1	17.0	280	1	580

	SERVING	TOTAL FAT (g.)	CALORIES	FIBER (g.)	SODIUM (mg.)
cheeseburger	I	13.8	305	0	725
chef salad w/o dressing	I	9.0	170	I	400
chicken fajitas	I	8.0	185	I	310
Chicken McNuggets	6 pieces	15.0	270	0	580
cookies					
chocolate chip	I box	15.0	330	0	280
McDonaldland	I box	9.2	290	0	300
Danish, all varieties	I	18.0	420	0	400
Egg McMuffin	I	11.2	290	0	710
Filet-O-Fish	I	18.0	370	0	730
french fries					
small	I order	12.0	220	I	110
medium	I order	17.1	320	I	150
large	I order	21.6	400	I	200
hamburger	I	9.0	255	0	490
hash browns	I order	7.3	130	0	130
hotcakes w/ margarine and syrup	I	12.0	440	0	685
McChicken sandwich	I	20.0	415	0	830
McLean Deluxe	I	10.0	320	NA	670
McLean w/ cheese	I	14.0	370	NA	890
pie, apple	I	14.8	260	0	240
Quarter Pounder	I	20.7	410	I	645
Quarter Pounder w/ cheese	I	28.0	520	I	1,110
sausage, pork	I	15.0	160	0	310
Sausage McMuffin	I	20.0	345	I	770
Sausage McMuffin w/ egg	I	25.0	430	I	920
scrambled eggs (2)	I order	9.8	140	0	290
Pizza Hut					
Hand-Tossed pizza					
cheese, medium	2 slices	20.0	518	NA	1,276
pepperoni, medium	2 slices	23.0	500	NA	1,267
supreme, medium	2 slices	26.0	540	NA	1,470
Pan pizza					
cheese, medium	2 slices	18.0	492	NA	940
pepperoni, medium	2 slices	22.0	540	NA	1,127
supreme, medium	2 slices	30.0	589	NA	1,363
Thin 'n' Crispy pizza					
cheese, medium	2 slices	17.0	398	NA	867
pepperoni, medium	2 slices	20.0	413	NA	986
supreme, medium	2 slices	22.0	459	NA	1,328

(con't.)	SERVING	TOTAL FAT (g.)	CALORIES	FIBER (g.)	SODIUM (mg.)
FAST FOODS/RESTAURANTS					
Taco Bell					
burrito, bean	1	14.0	381	1	1,148
burrito, beef	1	21.0	431	NA	1,311
burrito, chicken	1	12.0	334	NA	880
burrito, combo	1	16.0	407	NA	1,136
burrito, Supreme	1	22.0	440	NA	1,181
chilito	1	18.0	383	NA	893
cinnamon twists	1 order	8.0	171	NA	234
Mexican pizza	1	37.0	575	NA	1,031
MexiMelt, beef	1	15.0	266	NA	689
MexiMelt, chicken	1	15.0	257	NA	779
nachos	1 order	18.0	346	NA	399
nachos, Supreme	1 order	27.0	367	NA	471
pintos 'n' cheese	1 order	9.0	190	NA	642
soft taco	1	12.0	225	NA	554
soft taco, Chicken	1	10.0	213	NA	615
soft taco, Supreme	1	16.0	272	NA	554
taco	1	11.0	183	1	274
taco salad	1	61.0	905	NA	910
tostada	1	11.0	243	NA	596
Wendy's					
baked potato, w/ cheese	1	24.0	550	4	640
Big Classic	1	23.0	480	NA	850
breaded chicken sandwich	1	20.0	450	1	740
cheeseburger, single	1	21.0	420	1	770
cheeseburger, junior	1	13.0	320	NA	760
chicken club sandwich	1	25.0	520	NA	980
country fried steak sandwich	1	26.0	460	NA	880
crispy chicken nuggets (6)	1	20.0	280	NA	600
fish fillet sandwich	1	25.0	460	NA	780
french fries (small)	1	12.0	240	NA	145
Frostie, choc., small	1	10.0	340	0	200
grilled chicken salad	1	8.0	200	NA	690
hamburger, single	1	15.0	350	1	510
hamburger, double	1	27.0	540	1	730
hamburger, junior	1	9.0	260	NA	590
taco salad	1	30.0	640	NA	960
FATS					
bacon fat	1 T	14.0	126	0	126
beef, separable fat	1 oz.	23.3	216	0	5

	SERVING	TOTAL FAT (g.)	CALORIES	FIBER (g.)	SODIUM (mg.)
butter	1 T	12.3	108	0	78
chicken fat, raw	1 T	12.8	115	0	0
cream, medium (25% fat)	2 T	7.4	74	0	12
half and half	1/4 cup	7.1	80	0	24
margarine, solid (corn), stick	1 T	12.0	105	0	90
mayonnaise, regular (soybean)	1 T	11.0	99	0	78
oil					
canola	1 T	14.0	120	0	0
corn	1 T	14.0	120	0	0
olive	1 T	14.0	119	0	0
safflower	1 T	14.0	120	0	0
soybean	1 T	14.0	120	0	0
pork, backfat, raw	1 oz.	25.4	192	0	7
pork fat (lard)	1 T	12.8	116	0	0
salt pork, raw	1 oz.	23.8	219	0	404
sandwich spread (Miracle Whip type)	1 T	7.1	69	0	84
shortening, vegetable	1 T	12.0	106	0	0
FISH					
butterfish, northern	3 1/2 oz.	10.2	184	0	59
crab					
deviled	3 1/2 oz.	9.9	188	0	450
fried	3 1/2 oz.	18.0	273	0	NA
crab cake	3 1/2 oz.	10.8	178	0	225
eel, American	3 1/2 oz.	18.3	260	0	82
fillets, frozen					
batter dipped	2 pieces	31.0	440	0	552
light and crispy	2 pieces	23.0	311	0	345
herring					
canned or smoked	3 1/2 oz.	13.6	208	0	734
cooked	3 1/2 oz.	11.3	176	0	90
pickled	3 1/2 oz.	15.1	223	0	786
lobster, northern, broiled w/fat	12 oz.	24.0	308	0	NA
mackerel					
Atlantic	3 1/2 oz.	12.2	191	0	80
Pacific	3 1/2 oz.	7.3	159	0	80
oysters, fried	3 1/2 oz.	13.9	239	0	426
pompano	3 1/2 oz.	9.5	166	0	65
salmon					
chinook, canned	3 1/2 oz.	14.0	210	0	800
smoked	3 1/2 oz.	9.3	176	0	471

(con't.)	SERVING	TOTAL FAT (g.)	CALORIES	FIBER (g.)	SODIUM (mg.)
FISH					
sardines					
Atlantic, in soy oil	6 sardines	8.4	150	0	360
Pacific	3 1/2 oz.	8.6	160	0	310
shrimp, fried	3 1/2 oz.	10.8	225	0	186
smelt, canned	4-5 medium	13.5	200	0	NA
trout, rainbow	3 1/2 oz.	11.4	195	0	46
tuna					
albacore, raw	3 1/2 oz.	7.5	177	0	542
canned, light in oil	3 1/2 oz.	8.1	197	0	351
canned, white in oil	3 1/2 oz.	8.0	185	0	393
FRUIT					
avocado					
California	1 (6 oz.)	30.0	306	4	21
Florida	1 (11 oz.)	27.0	339	4	14
GRAVIES, SAUCES AND DIPS					
béarnaise sauce, mix	1/4 pkg.	25.6	263	0	474
brown gravy, homemade	1/4 cup	14.0	164	0	NA
chicken gravy, canned	1/2 can	8.5	118	0	859
dip made w/ sour cream	1/4 cup	9.6	106	0	600
guacamole dip	1 oz.	12.0	108	0	370
hollandaise sauce	1/4 cup	18.5	180	0	332
onion dip	1/4 cup	8.0	120	0	520
pesto sauce, commercial	1 oz.	14.6	155	0	244
sour-cream sauce	1/4 cup	11.9	124	0	126
spaghetti sauce					
homemade, w/ reg. ground beef	1/2 cup	18.7	243	1	505
spinach dip (sour cream-mayo)	1/4 cup	14.2	158	2	276
tartar sauce	1 T	7.9	70	0	75
white sauce, thick	1/4 cup	10.4	130	0	222
MEATS					
beef, lean, 5-10% fat (cooked)					
arm/blade, lean pot roast	3 1/2 oz.	9.4	207	0	60
hindshank, lean	3 1/2 oz.	9.4	207	0	70
porterhouse steak, lean	3 1/2 oz.	10.4	225	0	60
rib steak, lean	3 1/2 oz.	9.4	207	0	70
round					
bottom, lean	3 1/2 oz.	9.4	207	0	51
roasted	3 1/2 oz.	7.4	189	0	64

	SERVING	TOTAL FAT (g.)	CALORIES	FIBER (g.)	SODIUM (mg.)
short plate, sep. lean only	3 1/2 oz.	10.4	225	0	60
sirloin steak, lean	3 1/2 oz.	8.9	201	0	67
sirloin tip, lean, roasted	3 1/2 oz.	9.4	207	0	62
tenderloin, lean, broiled	3 1/2 oz.	11.1	219	0	60
top sirloin, lean, broiled	3 1/2 oz.	7.9	201	0	60
beef, regular, 11-17.4% fat (cooked)					
chuck, separable lean	3 1/2 oz.	15.2	268	0	70
club steak, lean	3 1/2 oz.	12.9	240	0	60
cubed steak	3 1/2 oz.	15.4	264	0	45
hamburger					
extra lean	3 oz.	13.9	253	0	49
lean	3 oz.	15.7	268	0	56
rib roast, lean	3 1/2 oz.	15.2	264	0	75
sirloin tips, roasted	3 1/2 oz.	15.2	264	0	50
stew meat, round, raw	4 oz.	15.3	294	0	50
T-bone, lean only	3 1/2 oz.	10.3	212	0	66
tenderloin, marbled	3 1/2 oz.	15.2	264	0	61
beef, high-fat, ≥ 17.5% fat (cooked)					
arm/blade, pot-roasted	3 1/2 oz.	26.5	354	0	50
chuck, ground	3 1/2 oz.	23.9	327	0	65
hamburger, regular	3 oz.	19.6	286	0	60
rump, pot-roasted	3 1/2 oz.	19.6	286	0	60
short ribs, lean	3 1/2 oz.	19.6	286	0	60
sirloin, ground	3 1/2 oz.	26.5	354	0	50
beef, highest-fat, ≥ 27.5% fat (cooked)					
brisket, lean and marbled	3 1/2 oz.	30.0	367	0	55
chuck, stew meat	3 1/2 oz.	30.0	367	0	55
corned, medium fat	3 1/2 oz.	30.2	372	0	1,726
ribeye steak, marbled	3 1/2 oz.	38.8	440	0	60
steak, chicken-fried	3 1/2 oz.	30.0	389	0	370
lamb					
leg, lean	3 1/2 oz.	8.1	180	0	60
loin chop, lean	3 1/2 oz.	8.1	180	0	68
rib chop, lean	3 1/2 oz.	8.1	180	0	60
shoulder, lean	3 1/2 oz.	9.9	248	0	70
miscellaneous meats					
frog legs					
flour-coated and fried	6 large	28.6	418	0	NA
rabbit, stewed	3 1/2 oz.	10.1	216	0	35

(con't.)	SERVING	TOTAL FAT (g.)	CALORIES	FIBER (g.)	SODIUM (mg.)
MEATS					
organ meats					
brains, all kinds, raw	3 oz.	7.4	106	0	106
heart					
calf, braised	3 1/2 oz.	9.1	208	0	112
liver					
beef, pan fried	3 1/2 oz.	10.6	229	0	106
calf, pan fried	3 1/2 oz.	13.2	261	0	82
pork					
bacon cured, broiled	3 slices	9.3	105	0	303
blade, lean	3 1/2 oz.	9.6	219	0	70
Boston butt, lean	3 1/2 oz.	14.2	304	0	65
ham					
ham loaf, glazed	3 1/2 oz.	14.7	247	0	811
smoked	3 1/2 oz.	11.0	175	0	800
loin chop, lean	1 chop	7.7	170	0	40
picnic, cured, lean	3 1/2 oz.	9.9	211	0	920
pig's feet, pickled	2 oz.	8.2	112	0	522
rib roast, trimmed	3 1/2 oz.	10.0	204	0	65
sausage					
brown and serve	2 oz.	18.8	210	0	732
patty	1	8.4	100	0	349
regular link	2 oz.	14.8	208	0	680
spareribs, roasted	6 medium	35.0	396	0	93
top loin roast, trimmed	3 1/2 oz.	7.5	187	0	65
processed meats					
bacon substitute					
(breakfast strips)	3 strips	7.0	85	0	450
beef breakfast strips	3 strips	10.8	160	0	560
beef jerky	2 oz.	8.0	218	0	560
bologna, beef/beef & pork	2 oz.	16.0	170	0	400
bratwurst					
pork	2-oz. link	22.0	256	0	473
pork & beef	2-oz. link	19.5	226	0	778
braunschweiger	2 oz.	15.6	130	0	948
corn dog	1	20.0	330	0	1,252
hot dog/frank					
beef	1	13.2	145	0	504
chicken	1	8.8	116	0	616
turkey	1	8.1	102	0	454
kielbasa (Polish sausage)	2 oz.	16.6	160	0	610
knockwurst/knackwurst	2-oz. link	18.0	209	0	560

	SERVING	TOTAL FAT (g.)	CALORIES	FIBER (g.)	SODIUM (mg.)
liver pâté, goose	1 oz.	12.4	131	0	192
pepperoni	1 oz.	13.0	148	0	600
salami, dry/hard	2 oz.	20.0	262	0	800
sausage					
Italian	2-oz. link	17.2	216	0	618
smoked	2-oz. link	20.0	229	0	642
Vienna	4 sausages	16.0	180	0	608
Spam	2 oz.	14.8	95	0	864
turkey roll	2 oz.	9.0	144	0	53
turkey salami	2 oz.	7.2	110	0	53
veal					
blade, lean	3 1/2 oz.	8.4	228	0	80
chuck, med. fat, braised	3 1/2 oz.	12.8	235	0	NA
cutlet					
breaded	3 1/2 oz.	15.0	319	0	NA
round, lean	3 1/2 oz.	12.8	194	0	90
flank, med. fat, stewed	3 1/2 oz.	32.0	390	0	80
rib chop, lean	3 1/2 oz.	7.6	225	0	90
rump, marbled, roasted	3 1/2 oz.	11.0	225	0	80

MILK AND YOGURT

	SERVING	TOTAL FAT (g.)	CALORIES	FIBER (g.)	SODIUM (mg.)
chocolate milk, whole-milk	1 cup	8.5	250	0	149
condensed milk, sweetened	1/2 cup	14.0	323	0	49
evaporated milk, whole	1/2 cup	10.0	126	0	99
hot cocoa, w/ whole milk	1 cup	9.1	218	0	123
malted milk	1 cup	9.9	236	0	223
milk shake					
chocolate, thick	1 cup	17.2	341	1	333
vanilla, thick	1 cup	14.7	274	0	299
whole milk					
3.5% fat	1 cup	8.0	150	0	122
dry powder	1/4 cup	8.6	159	0	119
yogurt, plain, whole milk	1 cup	7.4	139	0	105

MISCELLANEOUS

	SERVING	TOTAL FAT (g.)	CALORIES	FIBER (g.)	SODIUM (mg.)
chocolate, baking	1 oz.	15.0	143	1	1
olives					
black	4 large	8.0	74	1	480
Greek	3 medium	7.1	67	1	631
green	5 medium	8.0	75	0	950

	SERVING	TOTAL FAT (g.)	CALORIES	FIBER (g.)	SODIUM (mg.)
NUTS AND SEEDS					
almond paste	2 T	9.0	160	2	4
almonds	12-15	9.3	104	1	0
Brazil nuts	4 medium	11.5	114	1	0
cashews, roasted	6-8	7.8	94	2	2
coconut, dried, shredded	1/3 cup	9.2	135	1	6
hazelnuts (filberts)	10-12	10.6	106	1	0
macadamia nuts, roasted	6 medium	12.3	117	1	0
mixed nuts					
w/ peanuts	8-12	10.0	109	2	2
w/ out peanuts	2 T	10.1	110	2	2
peanut butter, creamy or chunky	2 T	16.0	186	1	150
peanuts					
chopped	2 T	8.9	104	2	3
honey roasted	2 T	8.9	112	2	150
in shell	1 cup	17.7	209	2	156
pecans	2 T	9.1	90	1	0
pine nuts (pignoli)	2 T	9.1	85	2	0
pistachios	2 T	7.7	92	1	1
poppy seeds	2 T	7.4	88	1	6
pumpkin seeds	2 T	7.9	93	1	4
sesame seeds	2 T	8.8	94	1	6
sunflower seeds	2 T	8.9	102	1	1
trail mix w/seeds, nuts, carob	1/4 cup	10.2	174	2	6
walnuts	2 T	7.7	80	1	0
PASTA, NOODLES, AND RICE					
(all measurements after					
cooking unless otherwise noted)					
noodles					
Alfredo	1 cup	29.7	462	3	844
almondine, from mix	1/4 pkg.	12.0	240	1	700
chow mein, canned	1/2 cup	8.0	153	0	210
romanoff	1 cup	23.0	372	3	774
rice, fried	1/2 cup	7.2	181	1	550
POULTRY					
chicken					
breast					
w/ skin, fried	1/2 breast	10.7	236	0	77
w/ skin, roasted	1/2 breast	7.6	193	0	72

	SERVING	TOTAL FAT (g.)	CALORIES	FIBER (g.)	SODIUM (mg.)
fryers					
w/ skin, batter dipped, fried	3 1/2 oz.	17.4	289	0	85
w/o skin, fried	3 1/2 oz.	11.1	237	0	60
w/ skin, roasted	3 1/2 oz.	13.6	239	0	75
giblets, fried	3 1/2 oz.	13.5	277	0	113
heart, simmered	3 1/2 oz.	7.9	185	0	67
leg					
w/ skin, fried	1 leg	8.7	120	0	92
roll, light meat	3 1/2 oz.	7.4	159	0	662
stewers					
w/ skin	3 1/2 oz.	18.9	285	0	73
w/o skin	3 1/2 oz.	11.9	237	0	78
thigh					
w/ skin, fried	1 thigh	11.3	180	0	55
w/ skin, roasted	1 thigh	9.6	153	0	52
wing					
w/ skin fried	1 wing	9.1	121	0	25
duck					
w/ skin, roasted	3 1/2 oz.	28.4	337	0	59
w/o skin, roasted	3 1/2 oz.	11.2	201	0	65
pheasant, w/ or w/o skin, cooked	3 1/2 oz.	9.3	211	0	98
quail, w/o skin, cooked	3 1/2 oz.	9.3	213	0	95
turkey					
dark meat					
w/ skin, roasted	3 1/2 oz.	11.5	221	0	76
w/o skin, roasted	3 1/2 oz.	7.2	187	0	79
ground	3 1/2 oz.	14.0	225	0	105
light meat					
w/ skin, roasted	3 1/2 oz.	8.3	197	0	63
patties, breaded/fried	1 patty	16.9	266	0	500
roll, light meat	3 1/2 oz.	7.2	147	0	489
SALAD DRESSINGS					
blue cheese, regular	2 T	16.0	144	0	30
buttermilk, from mix	2 T	11.6	116	0	27
Caesar	2 T	14.0	140	0	28
French					
creamy	2 T	13.8	140	0	37
regular	2 T	12.8	134	0	39
Green Goddess, regular	2 T	14.0	136	0	34
honey mustard	2 T	13.2	178	0	64

(con't.)	SERVING	TOTAL FAT (g.)	CALORIES	FIBER (g.)	SODIUM (mg.)
SALAD DRESSINGS					
Italian					
creamy	2 T	9.0	104	0	34
regular zesty, from mix	2 T	18.4	170	0	246
mayonnaise type, regular	2 T	9.8	114	0	210
oil and vinegar	2 T	15.0	138	0	0
ranch style, prep. w/ mayo	2 T	11.4	108	0	210
Russian, regular	2 T	15.6	152	0	266
sesame seed	2 T	13.8	136	0	206
Thousand Island, regular	2 T	11.2	118	0	218
SNACK FOODS					
bagel chips or crisps	1 oz.	8.8	149	1	140
Bugles	1 oz.	8.0	150	0	150
Cheese Puffs, Cheetos	1 oz.	10.0	159	0	348
cheese straws	4 pieces	7.2	109	0	433
corn chips, Frito's	1 oz.	9.7	155	0	233
party mix (cereal, pretzels, nuts)	1 cup	23.0	312	3	722
pork rinds, Frito-Lay	1 oz.	9.3	151	0	570
potato chips	1 oz.	11.2	159	1	182
potato sticks	1 oz.	10.2	152	0	71
Tostitos	1 oz.	7.8	145	0	140
SOUPS					
asparagus, cream of, w/milk	1 cup	8.2	161	1	982
bean					
w/ franks	1 cup	7.0	187	3	1,092
w/ ham	1 cup	8.5	231	3	1,800
cheese w/ milk	1 cup	14.6	230	0	1,020
chicken					
cream of, w/ milk	1 cup	11.5	191	0	1,046
cream of, w/ water	1 cup	7.4	116	0	986
chicken mushroom	1 cup	9.2	150	1	900
hmde or restaurant style					
beer cheese	1 cup	23.1	308	1	725
cauliflower, cream of, w/ whole milk	1 cup	9.7	165	1	800
celery, cream of, w/ whole milk	1 cup	10.6	165	1	1,010
clam chowder, New England	1 cup	14.0	271	1	914
corn chowder, traditional	1 cup	12.0	251	3	632
fish chowder, w/ whole milk	1 cup	13.5	285	1	710
hot & sour	1 cup	7.1	134	1	1,209

	SERVING	TOTAL FAT (g.)	CALORIES	FIBER (g.)	SODIUM (mg.)
mock turkey	1 cup	15.5	246	2	939
oyster stew, w/whole milk	1 cup	17.7	268	0	980
mushroom					
condensed	1 can	23.1	313	1	2,000
w/ milk	1 cup	13.6	203	1	1,076
w/ water	1 cup	9.0	129	1	1,031
potato, cream of, w/ milk	1 cup	7.4	157	2	1,000
shrimp, cream of, w/ milk	1 cup	9.3	165	1	976
VEGETABLES					
miso (soybean product)	1/2 cup	8.0	284	4	5,032
mushrooms, fried/sautéd	4 medium	7.4	78	1	0
onions, canned, french-fried	1 oz.	15.0	175	0	334
potato					
french fries					
homemade	1/2 cup	9.3	160	1	528
hash browns	1/2 cup	10.9	163	2	101
pan fried, O'Brien	1/2 cup	12.1	157	3	421
potato pancakes	1 cake	12.6	495	1	388
potato puffs, frozen, prep. w/ oil	1/2 cup	11.6	183	3	462
scalloped, w/ cheese	1/2 cup	9.7	177	1	370
twice-baked potato, w/ cheese	1 medium	9.9	180	1	55
VEGETABLE SALADS					
Caesar salad w/o anchovies	1 cup	7.2	80	1	145
macaroni salad w/ mayo	1/2 cup	12.8	200	1	157
potato salad, w/ mayo dressing	1/2 cup	11.5	189	1	662
tabbouleh salad	1/2 cup	9.5	173	3	542
taco salad w/ meat and taco sauce	1 cup	14.0	202	2	404
three-bean salad	1/2 cup	11.2	145	3	307
Waldorf salad w/ mayo	1/2 cup	12.7	157	2	123

NOTES

Chapter 1
[1]George et al., "Effect of Dietary Fat Content on Total and Regional Adiposity in Men and Women," *Intl Jnl Obesity* 14 (1990):1085–93.
[2]Ibid.
[3]Williamson et al., "Recreational Physical Activity and 10-Year Weight Change in a US National Cohort," *Intl Jnl Obesity* 17 (1993):270–86.
[4]DiPietro et al., "Behavioral Risk Factor Surveillance Survey, 1989," *Intl Jnl Obesity* 17 (1993):69–76.
[5]Gortmaker, Dietz, Cheung, "Inactivity, Diet, and the Fattening of America," *Perspectives in Practice*, vol. 90, no. 9, Sept. 1990.

Chapter 2
[1]Walker et al., "Potentiating Effects of Cigarette Smoking and Moderate Exercise on the Thermic Effect of a Meal," *Intl Jnl Obesity* 16 (1992):341–47.
[2]Perkins, K A, "Metabolic Effects of Cigarette Smoking," *Jnl Applied Physiol* 72 (Feb. 1992):401–9.
[3]Slattery et al., "Associations of Body Fat and Distribution with Dietary Intake, Physical Activity, Alcohol, and Smoking in Blacks and Whites," *Am Jnl Clin Nutr* 55 (May 1992):943–49.
[4]Selby et al., "Genetic and Behavioral Influences on Body Fat Distribution," *Intl Jnl Obesity* 14 (1990):593–602.
[5]McPhillips et al., "Dietary Differences in Smokers and Nonsmokers from Two New England Communities," *Jnl Am Diet Assoc*, vol. 94, no. 3 (1994):287–92.

Chapter 3
[1]Fisher et al., "Eating Attitudes, Health-risk Behaviors, Self-esteem, and Anxiety among Adolescent Females in a Suburban High School," *Jnl Adolescent Health* 12 (Jul 1991):377–84.
[2]Casper and Offer, "Weight and Dieting Concerns in Adolescents, Fashion or Symptom?" *Pediatrics* 86 (Sept. 1990):384–90.
[3]Frank et al., "Weight Loss and Bulimic Eating Behavior," *Southern Med Jnl* 84 (Apr. 1991):457–60.
[4]Dewey et al., "Maternal Weight Loss Patterns During Prolonged Lactation," *Am Jnl Clin Nutr* 58 (1993):162–66.
[5]Kaye et al., "Association of Body Fat Distribution with Lifestyle and Reproductive Factors in a Population study of Postmenopausal Women," *Int Jnl Obesity* 14 (1990):583–91.
[6]Colditz et al., "Patterns of Weight Change and their Relation to Diet in a Cohort of Healthy Women," *Am Jnl Clin Nutr* 51 (1990):1100–5.

[7]Anderson et al., "Influence of Menopause on Dietary Treatment of Obesity," *Jnl Int Med* 227 (March 1990):173–81.

[8]Voorrips et al., "History of Body Weight and Physical Activity of Elderly Women Differing in Current Physical Activity," *Intl Jnl Obesity* 16 (1992):199–205.

[9]Moses et al., "Fear of Obesity Among Adolescent Girls," *Pediatrics* 83 (March 1989):393–98.

[10]Abbott, Shirley. "Healthy Eating: How Do You Rate?" *Glamour*, Nov. 1993:254ff.

Chapter 4
[1]"Biology, Culture, Dietary Changes Conspire to Increase Incidence of Obesity," *Jnl Am Med Assoc* 256 (Oct. 24, 1986):2157–58.

Chapter 5
[1]Colditz et al., "Patterns of Weight Change and their Relation to Diet in a Cohort of Healthy Women," *Am Jnl Clin Nutr* 51 (1990):1100–5.

[2]Katzeff and Danforth, "Decreased Thermic Effect of a Mixed Meal During Overnutrition in Human Obesity," *Am Jnl Clin Nutr* 50 (1989):915–21.

[3]George et al., "Effect of Dietary Fat Content on Total and Regional Adiposity in Men and Women," *Intl Jnl Obesity* 14 (1990):1085–94.

[4]Slattery et al., "Associations of Body Fat and Its Distribution with Dietary Intake, Physical Activity, Alcohol, and Smoking in Blacks and Whites." *Am Jnl Clin Nutr* 55 (1992):943–49.

Chapter 8
[1]Paffenbarger et al., "Physical Activity, All-cause Mortality, and Longevity of College Alumni," *New Eng Jnl Med* 314 (1986):605–13.

[2]Van-Dale et al., "Does Exercise Give an Additional Effect in Weight Reduction Regimens?" *Intl Jnl Obesity* 11 (1987):367–75.

[3]Walker et al., "Potentiating Effects of Cigarette Smoking and Moderate Exercise on the Thermic Effect of a Meal," *Intl Jnl Obesity* 16 (1992): 341–47.

[4]Gortmaker, Dietz, Cheung, "Inactivity, Diet, and the Fattening of America," *Perspectives in Practice*, Sept. 1990, vol. 90, no. 9.

Chapter 9
[1]Imm and Pruitt, "Body Shape Satisfaction in Female Exercisers and Non-exercisers," *Women and Health* vol. 17, no. 4 (1993):87–96.

Chapter 10

[1]Moses et al., "Fear of Obesity among Adolescent Girls," *Pediatrics* 83 (March 1989):393–98.

[2]Koff and Rierdan, "Perceptions of Weight and Attitudes Toward Eating in Early Adolescent Girls," *Jnl Adol Health* 12 (1991):307–12.

[3]St. Jeor, Sachiko, "The Role of Weight Management in the Health of Women," *Jnl Am Diet Assoc*, vol. 93, no. 4 (1993):1007–12.

[4]Koff and Rierdan.

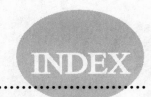

INDEX

Knockwurst, 332
Kool-Aid, 285
Kumquat, 294

Lamb, 310, 331
Lard, 95
Lasagne, 318
  spinach, 191
Laval University, 72, 90
Laxatives, 43
Leeks, 302
Legumes, 101, 270, 301, 302
Lemon, 294
Lemon juice, 296
Lentils, 302
Life cereal, 288
Life problems
  coping skills in, 45, 275
  and weight gain, 13, 63, 64, 79,
    274–75
Lifestyle
  exercise, 26, 75–77, 217–19
  weight gain, 12, 27
Light (lite) products, 122
Lima beans, 302
Limburger, 316
Lime, 294
Lime juice, 296
Little Caesar's Pizza, 262
Little Debbie products, 307, 321
Lobster, 293, 318, 329
Lo mein, 306
Long John Silver's, 262, 309, 326
Low-calorie products, 123
Low-cholesterol products, 123
Low-fat baking
  substitutions in, 130–32
  tips, 128–29
Low-fat cooking
  meats, 127–28
  recipe modification in, 147–48
  substitutions in, 130–32
  tips, 277–78
  vegetables/salads, 129–30
Low-fat foods, 91, 92, 93, 103, 115,
    278
  airline, 269
  brunch, 258
  calories in, 284
  for children, 252–54
  cocktail party, 259
  content labels, 122–23
  entrees, 118

Fat Master food guide to, 285–304
  in holiday feasts, 266–68
  pantry supplies, 118–21
  products, 123
  refrigerator items, 120–21
  replacements, 116–17, 120–21,
    130–32
  seasonings/spices, 121
  shopping for, 121–26
  snack, 134, 139, 146
  staples, basic, 120
  supper party, 259
  See also Restaurants, low-fat dining
Low saturated fat products, 123
Luncheon meats, 126, 311, 333
Lunch menus, 139–45

Macadamia nuts, 334
Macaroni, 299, 318
McDonald's, 263, 291–92, 309,
    326–27
Mackerel, 310, 329
Mademoiselle, 57
Mall food, 134
Manicotti, 318
Mansfield, Jane, 57
Margarine
  low-fat, 128, 129, 131, 309
  solid, 329
Marinated/marinades
  carrots, 195
  fat-free, 128
Marmalade, 298
Marriage, and weight gain, 12, 33
Matzo ball, 315
Mayonnaise, 130, 131, 292, 309, 312,
    329, 336
Meal planning
  benefits of, 110–11
  checklist, 115–16
  and eating patterns, 111–12
  and fat content, 115, 116–18
  menus, 137–45
  and portion control, 112–14, 115
Meat
  full fat-cat, 330–31
  low fat-cat, 126, 127–28, 297
  oven-frying, 128
  processed, 297, 332–33
  protein content, 100, 101
  regular fat-cat, 310–11
  shopping guidelines, 124, 126
  See also Beef; Pork